University of Chester

CHESTER CAMPUS
LIBRARY
01244 392738

This book is to be returned on or before the last date stamped below. Overdue charges will be incurred by the late return of books.

INTENSIVE RESPIRATORY CARE

Second Edition

JOHN M. LUCE, M.D.

Professor of Medicine and Anesthesia
University of California, San Francisco;
Associate Director, Medical-Surgical Intensive
Care Unit, San Francisco General Hospital
San Francisco, California

DAVID J. PIERSON, M.D.

Professor of Medicine, University of Washington;
Medical Director, Respiratory Care Department
Harborview Medical Center
Seattle, Washington

MARTHA L. TYLER, M.N., R.N., R.R.T.

Assistant Professor of Nursing
Adjunct Assistant Professor of Medicine
University of Washington
Seattle, Washington

W.B. SAUNDERS COMPANY
A Division of Harcourt Brace & Company
Philadelphia, London, Toronto, Montreal, Sydney, Tokyo

W.B. SAUNDERS COMPANY
A Division of
Harcourt Brace & Company

The Curtis Center
Independence Square West
Philadelphia, PA 19106

Library of Congress Cataloging-in-Publication Data

Luce, John M.

Intensive respiratory care / John M. Luce, David J. Pierson, Martha L. Tyler.–2nd ed.

p.   cm.

Includes bibliographical references and index.

ISBN 0–7216–4270–5

1. Respiratory intensive care.   I. Tyler, Martha L.   II. Pierson, David J.
    III. Title.   [DNLM: 1. Critical Care—handbooks.   2. Respiratory Care Units—
    handbooks.   3. Respiratory System—physiology—handbooks.   4. Respiratory
    Tract Diseases—therapy—handbooks.   WF 39 L935i]

RC735.R48L83 1993   616.2′00428—dc20

DNLM/DLC   92–48898

INTENSIVE RESPIRATORY CARE   ISBN   0–7216–4270–5

Printed in the United States of America.

Last digit is the print number: 9   8   7   6   5   4   3   2   1

PREFACE

This handbook is written for clinicians—physicians, nurses, and respiratory therapists—at the student and practitioner level. It is intended to furnish them with practical diagnostic and therapeutic information regarding the intensive respiratory care of adult, and to a lesser extent, pediatric patients. Although its chapters stand as separate entities, they are tied together by the common thread of applied respiratory physiology. This approach provides a conceptual framework for our topics and should prompt the administration of respiratory care in a flexible and intellectually satisfying manner. We have found the approach helpful with students from all the health professions. We hope it allows readers to use this handbook not only as a ready resource but also as an introduction to the remarkable biology that underlies respiratory care.

We would like to thank our colleagues in the Division of Pulmonary and Critical Care Medicine and the Department of Respiratory Care at San Francisco General Hospital and Harborview Medical Center for helping to shape and refine our approach to this subject and prepare this second edition of *Intensive Respiratory Care*.

CONTENTS

5

A PHYSIOLOGICAL APPROACH TO RESPIRATORY DISEASE 62

6

METHODS OF DIAGNOSING RESPIRATORY DISEASE 79

1

RESPIRATION AND THE ANATOMY OF THE RESPIRATORY SYSTEM

RESPIRATION

EXTRACELLULAR AND INTRACELLULAR RESPIRATION

In its broadest sense, the word respiration describes the exchange of oxygen (O_2) and carbon dioxide (CO_2) between an animal, such as man, and its environment. This process also is called extracellular respiration, because it includes the entire body. Within individual cells, respiration involves the chemical combustion of O_2 and foodstuffs—carbohydrate, fat, and protein—to form CO_2 and water (H_2O) and to generate energy. Some of this energy is lost as heat; the remainder is used to run the complex machinery of the cells.

OXYGEN CONSUMPTION AND CARBON DIOXIDE PRODUCTION

The volume of O_2 consumed each minute by intracellular respiration is denoted $\dot{V}O_2$, whereas the volume of CO_2 produced is $\dot{V}CO_2$. The ratio $\dot{V}CO_2/\dot{V}O_2$, which is called the respiratory quotient (RQ), varies with the type of foodstuff being metabolized; it equals one when carbohydrate is burned and is less than one when fat and protein are used. For the body as a whole, $\dot{V}CO_2/\dot{V}O_2$ relates the volume of CO_2 expired to the volume of O_2 inspired and is called the respiratory exchange ratio (R). This value reflects intracellular respiration and is equal to RQ in steady state conditions. However, R may vary transiently with factors other than metabolism. For example, it may exceed one during exercise, when an individual continues to excrete CO_2 while contracting an O_2 debt. After exercise, R falls as the debt is repaid. The resting value for $\dot{V}CO_2$ in a normally sized male adult is 200 milliliters per minute (ml/min) compared with a $\dot{V}O_2$ of 250 ml/min. As a result, R normally equals 0.8.

1

RESPIRATORY GASES

PARTIAL PRESSURES

When several gases exist in the same volume, as occurs with the gaseous components of air, each exerts a tension, or partial pressure (P_{GAS}), that is the same as if it had the entire space to itself. These partial pressures depend upon the concentration of the gases and their kinetic energy; they are a reflection of the gases' ability to travel by diffusion and hence a reflection of their availability to participate in chemical reactions. The sum of the partial pressures of the gases in a system makes up the total pressure. When the pressure goes up or down, as occurs if a volume of air is compressed or expanded, the partial pressures of the individual gases increase or decrease proportionately. Since each partial pressure is a set fraction of the total pressure, the partial pressure can be figured by multiplying the total pressure by the fractional concentration of a single gas (F_{GAS}).

ATMOSPHERIC PRESSURE

Atmospheric pressure is the total pressure of all the molecules of all the gases in the atmosphere brought to bear on any one point. The major gases present in the atmosphere are nitrogen (N_2) and O_2; CO_2 exists only in minute quantities. Atmospheric pressure is commonly referred to as barometric pressure (P_B). In a barometer, a sealed tube from which air has been evacuated, it will raise a column of mercury a certain number of millimeters. At sea level, or one atmosphere, P_B averages 760 millimeters of mercury (mmHg). Since O_2 makes up 21 per cent of the atmosphere at any given P_B, the fraction of O_2 in inspired air (F_IO_2) is 0.21. Thus, the PO_2 for inspired air (P_IO_2) at sea level is the F_IO_2 of 0.21 times 760, or approximately 160 mmHg. The P_B will double to 1520 mmHg under 33 feet of water, since this amount adds the equivalent of another atmosphere of pressure. At a pressure of two atmospheres, the P_IO_2 is 320 mm Hg. At higher altitudes, where the air is thinner, P_B falls. It is 640 mmHg in Denver, the "Mile-High City," where the P_IO_2 is 134 mmHg (Fig. 1–1). At 5500 meters in the Peruvian Andes, the highest point of human habitation, P_B is 380 mmHg and the P_IO_2 is 70 mmHg in dry air.

ACCOUNTING FOR WATER VAPOR

The aforementioned description of partial pressures is expressed in terms of dry air. Yet the atmosphere is not dry: It contains

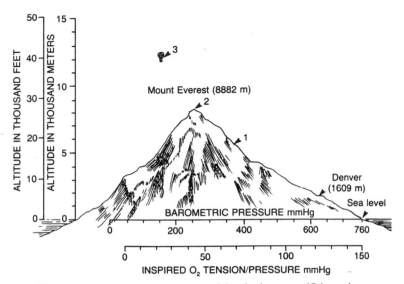

Figure 1–1. Barometric pressure and inspired oxygen (O_2) tension or partial pressure in millimeters of mercury (mmHg) related to altitude in thousands of feet and in meters. Point 1 is the highest point of continuous human habitation; even at elevations well below this, unacclimatized individuals usually feel breathless and may lose consciousness. Supplemental O_2 is usually required at Point 2, although Mount Everest has been climbed without O_2. Point 3 represents the highest ascent with O_2 but without superatmospheric pressure.

water vapor. A vapor is a substance that evaporates at a given temperature and exerts a pressure that is independent of PB. Since vapor molecules occupy a certain space under the right temperature conditions, they limit the total pressure available to the other gases. The pressure of water (PH_2O) in the human respiratory tract, in which the temperature is 37° C and the air is fully saturated with vapor, is 47 mmHg. As a result, the PO_2 of air entering the lungs at sea level is approximately 150 mmHg ($0.21 \times (760-47)$). This PO_2 is similar to the PO_2 immediately above the surface of a pond.

EVOLUTION OF THE RESPIRATORY SYSTEM

Single-celled spherical animals with low metabolic needs living on a pond surface can take in O_2 and give off CO_2 simply by passive diffusion. This is a process by which gas molecules move by random motion from areas of high partial pressure to areas of low partial pressure. However, it is estimated that a larger animal with a radius greater than one centimeter and a higher $\dot{V}O_2$ and $\dot{V}CO_2$ would require a pressure difference of 25 atmospheres, or 19,000 mmHg, to supply O_2 to its center by diffusion alone. Because this pressure gradient is not available, large animals have evolved complex systems to aid respiration. The focal point of the system in air breathers is the lung, which places respiratory gases and circulating blood in approximation and provides a vast surface area for diffusion to occur.

ANATOMY OF THE RESPIRATORY SYSTEM

THORACIC CAGE

The thoracic cage, or skeleton, is composed of the anterior sternum and the posterior thoracic vertebrae, which are linked by C-shaped ribs. All 12 ribs articulate with the thoracic vertebrae, but only the first seven have flexible cartilaginous connections with the sternum. In addition to housing the heart, lungs, and other vital structures, the ribs provide attachments for the respiratory muscles. Since the ribs angle downward from back to front and from the midline to the side, their elevation by the respiratory muscles causes the thorax to increase in both an anterior-posterior and a transverse dimension.

RESPIRATORY MUSCLES

Inspiratory Muscles

Although their actions are complex, the muscles of respiration may be divided simply into those that function primarily in inspiration or in expiration. Inspiration is always an active event involving muscular contraction (Fig. 1–2). The diaphragm generally performs most ventilatory work, and the other muscles improve its efficiency by stabilizing the chest wall. They may be called upon to assume a greater burden during exercise or when diaphragmatic function is impaired.

Diaphragm. This is a thin sheet of muscle that is inserted onto the inferior surface of the lower ribs and is dome-shaped in the resting position. When the diaphragm contracts, its dome moves down, increasing the vertical dimension of the thoracic cavity and generating a negative pleural pressure that inflates the lungs. In its descent the diaphragm also pushes down on the abdominal viscera;

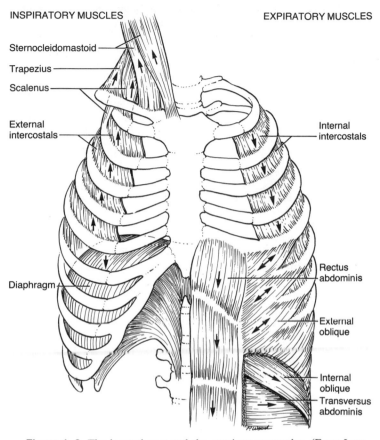

INSPIRATORY MUSCLES   EXPIRATORY MUSCLES

Sternocleidomastoid

Trapezius

Scalenus

External
intercostals   Internal
                                                                intercostals

                                                                Rectus
                                                                abdominis

Diaphragm   External
                                                                oblique

                                                                Internal
                                                                oblique
                                                                Transversus
                                                                abdominis

Figure 1–2. The bony thorax and the respiratory muscles. (From Luce JM, and Culver BH: Respiratory muscle function in health and disease. *Chest,* 81:82–90, 1982.)

this increases the intra-abdominal pressure, displaces the abdominal wall outward, and increases the transverse dimension of the lower ribs.

Although the diaphragm is primarily an inspiratory muscle, it has an expiratory action on the thoracic cage when its dome is flattened, as occurs in patients who breathe at high lung volumes. In such persons, the negative pleural pressure generated by the diaphragm sucks in the lower part of the chest, and the thoracic cage may decrease in its transverse dimension. Because the diaphragm is innervated by the phrenic nerves from cervical roots three through five, it remains functional in patients with spinal injuries below the midcervical level. However, the long course of the phrenic nerves along the mediastinum makes them vulnerable to interruption by disease, injury, or chest surgery.

External and Parasternal Intercostal Muscles. External and parasternal intercostal muscle contraction elevates the anterior ends of the ribs, causing them to move upward and outward and increasing the anterior-posterior dimension of the thorax. The external and parasternal intercostal muscles are supplied by nerves that come off the spinal cord at the same first through twelfth thoracic levels as the muscles; they therefore may cease to function in spinal cord injuries.

Accessory Muscles of Respiration. The accessory muscles include the scalene muscles, which elevate the first two ribs; the sternocleidomastoid muscles, which raise the sternum, and the trapezius muscles, which fix the shoulders. These muscles are recruited at high levels of inspiratory activity and become hypertrophied in some patients with respiratory disease. The muscles are innervated by cranial and high cervical nerves and are therefore preserved in spinal cord injuries.

Expiratory Muscles

In contrast to inspiration, expiration is a passive event in healthy persons during quiet breathing, because muscular contraction is not needed to return the lung and the thoracic cage to their resting positions. However, expiration often becomes an active event requiring muscular effort during airflow obstruction or exercise.

Internal Intercostal Muscle. Internal intercostal muscle contraction pulls the ribs down and in, decreasing their anterior-posterior dimension during forceful expiration.

The Abdominal Respiratory Muscles. The abdominal respiratory muscles include the rectus and the transverse abdominis and the internal and external oblique muscles. Contraction of these muscles depresses the lower ribs, forces the diaphragm up by increasing intra-abdominal pressure, and decreases the vertical dimension of the thoracic cavity. The abdominal muscles also serve an inspiratory function by forcing the diaphragm into a domed position and increasing its efficiency. Because these muscles are supplied by nerves originating from the sixth thoracic through the first lumbar vertebrae, their function is impaired in thoracic cord injury.

PLEURAL SPACE

The pleura is a continuous membrane that lines the outside of the lungs (visceral pleura) and the inside of the thoracic cavity (parietal pleura), creating a potential pleural space that resembles the inside of an empty, flat, sealed envelope. The pleural surfaces of the right and left lungs are distinct entities separated by the mediastinum, which contains the heart and great vessels, the trachea and main bronchi, and the esophagus. The pleura is bounded inferiorly by the diaphragm; its apex reaches above the clavicle. The pleura is moistened by fluid that facilitates movement of the lungs in the thorax, so that air is not normally present in the pleural space. In certain disease states, the pleural space may fill with fluid (pleural effusion) or with air (pneumothorax), which interferes with lung expansion. (These and other pleural abnormalities are discussed in Chapter 19.)

LUNGS

Lobes

The lungs are conical structures whose apices extend above the first rib and whose bases touch the diaphragm. The lungs are divided into five lobes, three of which are on the right and two of which are on the left (Figs. 1–3 and 1–4). Both lungs are divided

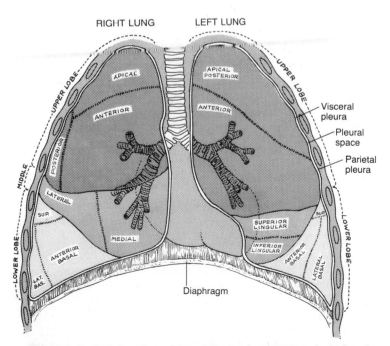

Figure 1–3. Anterior view of lung lobes and segments and of pleural surfaces.

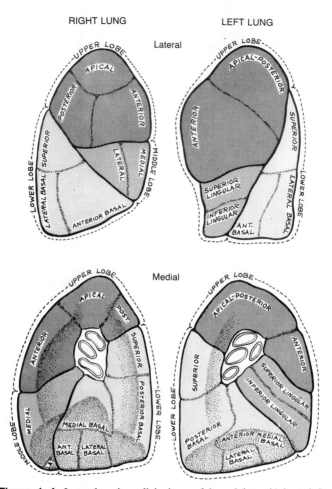

Figure 1–4. Lateral and medial views of lung lobes. (Adapted from Johnson J, et al.: *Surgery of the Chest: A Handbook of Operative Surgery,* 4th ed. Copyright © 1970 by Year Book Medical Publishers, Inc., Chicago.)

by an oblique fissure that runs down from back to front. The right and left lower lobes extend to the level of the fourth rib posteriorly. On the right side only, the horizontal fissure intersects the oblique fissure and separates the right middle lobe from the right upper lobe. The left upper lobe fills all the space above the left oblique fissure. Its inferior portion, the lingula, is the anatomical correlate of the right middle lobe. Each lobe receives gas from a lobar bronchus, is nourished by a lobar branch of the pulmonary artery, and is drained by a lobar branch of the pulmonary vein.

Segments

The basic anatomical units of the lung are the bronchopulmonary segments, each of which is served by a segmental branch of the pulmonary artery. The lower lobes of each lung are divided into superior segments occupying their upper portions and four basal segments in contact with the diaphragm (two of these may be combined on the left). The right middle lobe has two segments, as does its counterpart, the lingula. The right upper lobe and the remaining portion of the left upper lobe have anterior, posterior, and apical segments (the latter two are combined on the left). Because the segments have separate airways and blood supply, they may be resected individually.

UPPER AIRWAYS

Nasal Cavity

Gas is inspired and expired through either the mouth or the nose (Fig. 1–5). In the nasal cavities it passes over an extensive membrane containing ciliated and mucus-secreting cells. Small particles not filtered in the openings of the nose, or nares, are

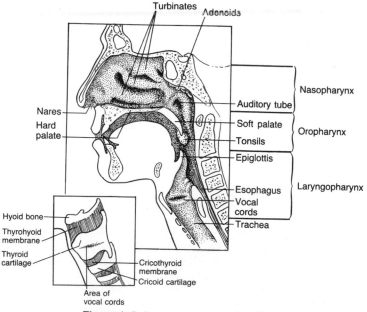

Figure 1–5. Lateral view of upper airways.

trapped in mucus and passed posteriorly by cilia to the oropharynx, where they are swallowed. Inspired air is also humidified by contact with the mucus membrane and is warmed by heat from the vascular network that underlies it. The outpouchings of the nasal mucosa, called turbinates, increase the surface area for filtering and for moisture and heat exchange.

Pharynx

The pharynx is a sac between the mouth and the nares and the esophagus. At the base of the nasal cavity and above the level of the soft palate is the nasopharynx, which contains the adenoids and the auditory or eustachian tube. This tube connects the nasopharynx and the middle ear and opens during swallowing to equalize the pressure across the middle ear. Middle ear pain or infection may develop if the auditory tube is swollen shut by an upper respiratory infection or occluded by an endotracheal tube. The oropharynx lies between the soft palate and the upper edge of the epiglottis. It contains the tonsils and is the center of the swallowing or gag reflex, an important pulmonary defense mechanism that propels food into the esophagus and simultaneously closes the larynx to prevent aspiration of food into the lower airways. The laryngopharynx contains the larynx and the esophagus, a part of the alimentary canal.

Larynx

Situated above the trachea and below the root of the tongue, the larynx serves as the organ of voice and as a defense against aspiration. It is composed of several cartilages: the thyroid cartilage, commonly referred to as the Adam's apple; the cricoid cartilage, which forms a complete ring and is the narrowest portion of the upper airway in infants; the arytenoid cartilage, to which the posterior ends of the vocal cords are attached; and the vocal cords themselves. The cricothyroid membrane, an avascular structure joining the thyroid and cricoid cartilages, is below the level of the vocal cords and may be pierced (cricothyroidotomy) to provide access to the lower airways in an emergency. The combination of the vocal cords and the opening between them, the glottis, is the narrowest portion of the upper airway in adults.

Muscles of the Upper Airway

For completeness, the muscles of the upper airway should be thought of as respiratory muscles. They include the muscles of the mouth (innervated by cranial nerves nine and ten), uvula and palate (cranial nerve eleven), tongue (nine and twelve), and larynx (first cervical nerve). Although these muscles do not have a direct action on the thorax, they are essential in keeping the upper airway open. Also, by affecting airway resistance and airflow, they may affect lung volume.

LOWER AIRWAYS

Trachea

The trachea begins at the lower border of the cricoid cartilage of the larynx, at the level of the sixth cervical vertebra, and ends by dividing into the right and left main bronchi at the carina, which is located at the level of the sternal angle (Fig. 1–6). The trachea is supported by 18 to 20 C-shaped cartilaginous rings, the second of which is usually incised in creating a tracheostomy. The posterior membrane of the tracheal cartilages contains smooth muscle that is shared by the esophagus; the cuff of an endotracheal tube may erode through this membrane, creating a tracheoesophageal fistula.

When intrathoracic pressure exceeds the pressure in the tracheal lumen, the membrane may become invaginated and the lumen may be significantly reduced in size. This is particularly pronounced during cough, a reflex initiated by irritation of nerve receptors in the upper and lower airways. Cough is characterized by a sudden, strong contraction of the abdominal muscles that forces the diaphragm upward. The resulting high intrathoracic pressure compresses the airways and increases the pressure within them. This

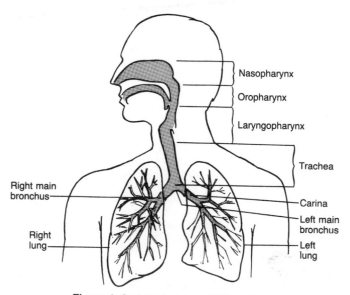

Figure 1–6. Anterior view of lower airways.

and the invagination of the membranous trachea, which reduces the airway diameter, greatly augments the velocity of airflow and propels unwanted substances out of the mouth.

Bronchi

The right and left main bronchi are lined with a mucociliary membrane, similar to that in the nasal cavity, that filters and humidifies gas being conducted to the lungs. The right main bronchus continues more directly from the trachea than the left main bronchus does after the carinal bifurcation; therefore it is more likely to receive material aspirated from the pharynx or to be entered by an endotracheal tube. The main bronchi divide into five lobar bronchi that enter the upper, middle, and lower lobes of the right lung and the upper and lower lobes of the left lung. The lobar bronchi divide in turn into the segmental bronchi, ten on the right and eight on the left, which are named after the lung segments they supply. The cartilage of these lobar bronchi is nearly circumferential and resists collapse. The bronchi are invested with circumferential smooth muscle that contracts under the influence of certain stimuli. They are nourished by the bronchial arteries that branch from the aorta and are not part of the pulmonary circulation. Because they lack alveoli and are not exposed to pulmonary arterial blood, the bronchi cannot participate in gas exchange.

Bronchioles

The next order of airways, the bronchioles, lack cartilage, have limited smooth muscle, and are not held open by structural rigidity but by the elastic recoil of the surrounding lung. They are divided into the terminal bronchioles and the respiratory bronchioles. The walls of the respiratory bronchioles contain alveoli that participate in gas exchange, whereas the walls of the terminal bronchioles do not. Beyond the bronchioles are the alveolar ducts, the alveolar sacs, and the individual alveoli.

The entire respiratory unit served by one terminal bronchiole is called an acinus. This is the smallest lung component that can be visualized roentgenographically and is around 5 mm in diameter. The number of airway generations required to reach an acinus varies with the pathway length, but there may be 24 or more in the periphery of the lung. Although the size of the airways becomes smaller peripherally, their number doubles with each generation so that the total cross-sectional area increases rapidly.

ALVEOLI

Alveoli are irregular polyhedrons, approximately 250 micrometers in diameter, that abut one another like the individual units of a honeycomb (Fig. 1–7). They increase in number until late adolescence and number 300,000,000 in an adult. Lying free in the alveolar spaces are alveolar macrophages, scavenger cells that engulf and carry off invading microorganisms and other foreign particles. The cells lining the alveoli include the Type I epithelial cells, whose pancake-like cytoplasm covers most of the alveolar surface, and the cuboidal Type II epithelial cells, which produce surfactant and differentiate into Type I cells after injury. Surfactant is a substance that lowers surface tension in the alveolus as the alveolus becomes smaller, as occurs when the lungs deflate, and thereby prevents the delicate structure from collapsing.

The alveoli are surrounded by pulmonary capillaries. The capillaries are so interconnected that, when engorged, they cover the alveolar wall in a veritable sheet of blood. Along the thin portion of the wall, the capillary endothelial cells and the alveolar epithelial cells share a common basement membrane with no intervening interstitial space, so the diffusion distance from alveolar gas to red blood cells is less than a single red cell's diameter. In the thick portion of the wall, in which the endothelium and epithelium do not share a basement membrane, the interstitial space contains

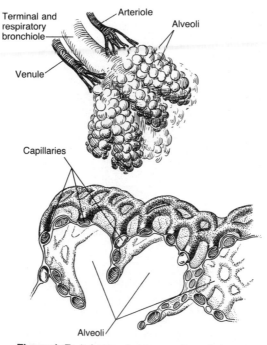

Figure 1–7. Acinus and close-up view of alveoli.

scavenger cells and collagen. Edema fluid may fill this space in certain disorders and also may spill over into the alveoli.

CARDIOVASCULAR SYSTEM

Overview of the Cardiovascular System

The human cardiovascular system contains a single divided heart and two circulations, the systemic circulation and the pulmonary circulation, arranged in series (Fig. 1–8). The muscular heart consists of two atria that both store blood returning from the circulations, two ventricles that pump blood through the circulations, and a pacemaker and a conducting system that stimulate the chambers to contract rhythmically. Each circulation is composed of three parts: arteries and their smaller branches, the arterioles,

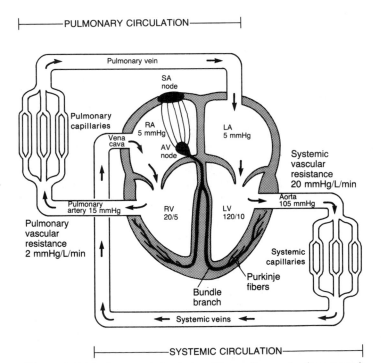

Figure 1–8. The heart and circulation. The cardiac conduction system is shown, including sinoatrial (SA) and atrioventricular (AV) nodes, bundle branches, and Purkinje fibers. RA = right atrium; LA = left atrium; RV = right ventricle; LV = left ventricle. Pressures in the right and left atria and in the pulmonary artery and the aorta are mean pressures.

that carry blood away from the ventricles and whose walls can constrict and dilate and thereby regulate circulatory resistance; capillaries, tiny muscle-less vessels that are the site of gas exchange; and veins and venules, their tributaries, that return blood to the heart and serve as capacitance vessels because they can accept a large volume of blood without an increase in their intraluminal pressure.

Flow Through the System

Like flow in any hydraulic system, blood flow ($\dot{Q}$) across each circulation is directly proportional to the mean pressure drop (P) from one end of the circulation to the other and inversely proportional to the resistance (R) of its vessels. This is symbolized by the formula $\dot{Q} = P/R$. Rewriting this formula reveals that $R = P/\dot{Q}$. Although the heart beats intermittently, continuous flow through the circulation occurs by virtue of distension of the aorta, the pulmonary artery, and their branches during ventricular contraction (systole) and by virtue of elastic recoil of the walls of the arteries, which causes forward propulsion of the blood during ventricular relaxation (diastole).

Systemic Circulation

The systemic circulation begins in the aorta, which receives the output of the left ventricle, and ends in the right atrium. Systolic pressure in the aorta and other major arteries averages 120 mmHg, diastolic pressure averages 80 mmHg, and mean arterial pressure (MAP) is around 105 mmHg. Mean right atrial pressure approximates 5 mmHg. The wide pressure drop of 100 mmHg across the systemic circulation means that systemic vascular resistance (SVR) amounts to 100 mmHg divided by the left ventricular output of 5 L/min, or 20 mmHg/L/min; this usually is multiplied by 80 and expressed as 1600 dynes sec/cm^{-5}. The SVR is relatively high because the systemic circulation must overcome the effects of gravity to maintain blood flow to the head and must regulate flow through numerous capillary beds in response to stress and exercise.

Pulmonary Circulation

The pulmonary circulation starts in the pulmonary artery and ends in the left atrium. The right ventricle pumps blood through the pulmonary circulation at a systolic pressure of 20 mmHg and a diastolic pressure of 5 mmHg in the pulmonary artery. Mean pulmonary artery pressure is approximately 15 mmHg and left atrial pressure is 5 mmHg in the resting state, so pulmonary vascular resistance (PVR) is 10 mmHg divided by the right ventricular output of 5 L/min, or 2 mmHg/L/min; this usually is multiplied by 80 and expressed as 160 dynes sec/cm^{-5}. This is one-tenth the resistance in the systemic circulation, reflecting that the pulmonary circulation has less need—and fewer mechanisms—than the systemic circulation for regulating regional blood flow.

VENTILATORY REGULATION

Ventilatory Control Center

Unlike the pacemaker of the heart, the pacemaker of the respiratory muscles is not found in those organs but is instead located in the medulla of the brainstem (Fig. 1–9). It is composed of several subcenters that interact to produce rhythmical breathing. The output of this center is transmitted down the phrenic nerves to the diaphragm and down the other nerves that innervate the remaining respiratory muscles. Although the respiratory center has inherent neurological activity that normally guarantees involuntary ventilation when people are asleep or unconscious, its output is affected by higher cortical centers and by mechanical and chemical stimuli.

Cortical Centers

The cerebral cortex has input into the ventilatory center. As a result, breathing is partially under voluntary control.

Mechanical Reflexes

Mechanical reflexes emanate from skeletal muscle spindles and from pulmonary vessels and tissue. The pulmonary reflexes are activated by the stretching and altering of tissues, as occur during lung inflation, and pass to the ventilatory center via the vagus nerve. Deformation of these pulmonary stretch receptors may be responsible for the increased ventilation seen in patients with interstitial fibrosis and other forms of restrictive lung disease.

Central Chemoreceptors

Certain cells lying near the ventilatory control center are primarily sensitive to changes in the pH of brain extracellular fluid. These pH changes are influenced by changes in the PCO_2 of arterial blood, because CO_2 may be converted into carbonic acid. As a result, ventilation usually increases in response to increasing amounts of CO_2 in blood and decreases when the CO_2 level falls.

Peripheral Chemoreceptors

The peripheral chemoreceptors are cells located at the bifurcation of the carotid arteries and along the arch of the aorta. The

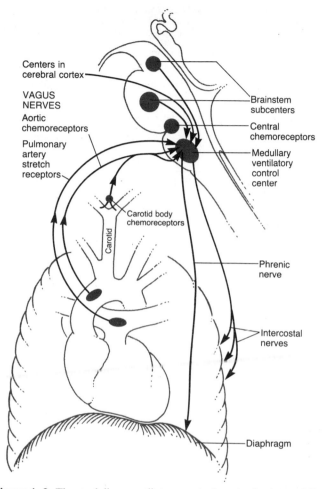

Figure 1–9. The medullary ventilatory control center in the medulla of the brainstem and the output from it.

rate of blood flow in the carotid bodies is extremely high in relationship to their size; this allows for a rapid ventilatory response to changes in the PO_2 of arterial blood and, to a lesser extent, to changes in the PCO_2.

RECOMMENDED READING

1. Comroe JH: *Physiology of Respiration,* 2nd ed. Chicago, Year Book Medical Publishers, 1974.

2. Culver BH (ed.): *The Respiratory System: Syllabus for Human Biology 540.* Seattle, University of Washington, Lecture Notes, 1982.
3. Heath D, and Williams DR: *Man at High Altitude.* Edinburgh, Churchill Livingstone, 1977.
4. Luce JM, and Culver BH: Respiratory muscle function in health and disease. *Chest,* 81:82–90, 1982.
5. Murray JF: *The Normal Lung,* 2nd ed. Philadelphia, W. B. Saunders Co., 1986.
6. Proctor DF: The upper airways and breathing mechanics. *In* Murray JF, and Nadel JA (eds.): *Textbook of Respiratory Medicine.* Philadelphia, W. B. Saunders Co., 1988, pp. 3–11.
7. Reid L: The lung: Its growth and remodeling in health and disease. *Am J Roentgenol,* 129:777–795, 1977.
8. Roussos C, and Macklem PT: The respiratory muscles. *N Engl J Med,* 307:786–797, 1982.
9. Shapiro BA, et al.: *Clinical Application of Respiratory Care,* 2nd ed. Chicago, Year Book Medical Publishers, 1979.
10. Shoene RB, and Hornbein TF: High altitude adaptation. *In* Murrary JF, and Nadel JA (eds.): *Textbook of Respiratory Medicine.* Philadelphia, W. B. Saunders Co., 1988, pp. 196–220.
11. Staub NC, and Albertine KH: The structure of the lungs relative to their principal function. *In* Murray JF, and Nadel JA (eds.): *Textbook of Respiratory Medicine.* Philadelphia, W.B. Saunders Co., 1988, pp. 12–36.
12. West JB: *Respiratory Physiology.* Baltimore, Williams & Wilkins, 1974.

2

PHYSIOLOGY OF THE RESPIRATORY SYSTEM

STEPS OF RESPIRATION

OVERVIEW

Respiration in man may be divided into five separate steps or processes. These are:

1. Ventilation, the exchange of respiratory gases between the atmosphere and the lungs.

2. Pulmonary perfusion, the flow of mixed venous blood through the pulmonary circulation to the alveolar capillaries and the return of arterialized blood from the capillaries to the left atrium.

3. Pulmonary gas exchange, the transfer of oxygen (O_2) and carbon dioxide (CO_2) across the alveolar-capillary membrane in the lungs.

4. Gas transport and uptake, the conveying of arterial blood from the left ventricle to the peripheral tissues, which extract O_2 and release CO_2 for transport back to the right atrium.

5. Regulation of ventilation, the control of blood acidity-alkalinity and respiratory gas tensions by increasing or decreasing ventilation.

VENTILATION

Ventilatory Mechanics

Elastic Recoil Properties. The properties of the lung and the thoracic cage that affect the exchange of respiratory gases with the atmosphere are called the mechanics of ventilation. Of these properties, the most important is elastic recoil, the tendency of the lungs and chest wall to return to a resting position after their form has been altered (Fig. 2–1). Resting positions may differ dramatically: When the lungs are removed from the thoracic cage, their elasticity causes them to collapse to a smaller volume; when the

NORMAL   COLLAPSED LUNG

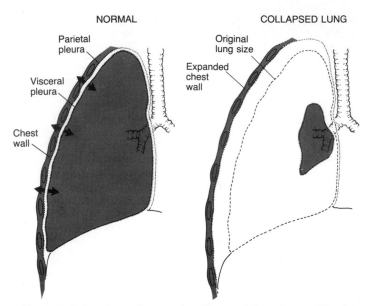

Figure 2–1. Elastic recoil properties of lung and thoracic cage. The chest wall springs outward when the lung collapses; the lung collapses when the chest wall is removed.

thoracic cage no longer houses the lungs, it recoils outward. Normally, these opposing elastic forces balance one another at the pleural space at the end of a quiet expiration. The lung volume at this point is called the functional residual capacity (FRC). Atmospheric pressure, measured at the mouth, is 760 mmHg at FRC, but pressure in the pleural space is subatmospheric, around 755 mmHg (by convention, this pleural pressure is expressed as −5 mmHg compared with atmospheric pressure, which arbitrarily is said to be zero).

Inspiration. During inspiration from FRC, diaphragmatic contraction pushes down on the abdominal viscera and displaces the chest wall outward. The diaphragm also lifts the lower ribs laterally while the external intercostals lift the ribs upward and outward and stabilize the thoracic cage. Expansion of the thorax opposes the elastic recoil of the lungs, creates a more negative pleural pressure, and increases the pressure difference between the pleural space and alveoli; this difference might be called the transpulmonary pressure. Thoracic expansion might pull the pleural surfaces apart if the pleural space did not contain liquid that is incompressible and inexpandable; instead, the expansion enlarges the lungs. Lung enlargement in turn creates a subatmospheric pressure in the alveoli, into which air flows because the pressure in the lungs is lower than that at the mouth. Inflation to total lung capacity (TLC) requires sustained inspiratory muscle activity.

Expiration. After muscle contraction concludes at the end of inspiration, airflow ceases because a pressure gradient no longer exists between the alveoli and the mouth. The elastic recoil of the lungs then causes alveolar pressure to exceed atmospheric pressure, and air flows out of the lungs until the pressure gradient no longer exists at FRC. Although the respiratory muscles are passive during a relaxed exhalation, contraction of the abdominal muscles will force the lungs to their residual volume (RV) (Fig. 2–2).

Tidal Breathing. The difference between TLC and RV, and hence the greatest amount of air that can be inhaled or exhaled, is the vital capacity (VC) (Fig. 2–3). Normal breathing involves a tidal volume (V_T) that is only 10 per cent of the VC, although the V_T may increase to 50 per cent or so of the VC during exercise. The

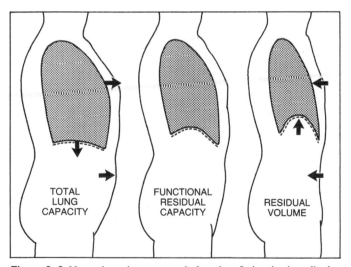

TOTAL LUNG CAPACITY

FUNCTIONAL RESIDUAL CAPACITY

RESIDUAL VOLUME

Figure 2–2. Normal respiratory muscle function. In inspiration, diaphragmatic contraction pushes down on the abdominal viscera and displaces the chest outward. In addition, the diaphragm lifts the ribcage upward and outward and inflates the lung toward its total capacity while intercostal and accessory muscles stabilize the chest wall. In expiration, the diaphragm and other inspiratory muscles relax, and contraction of the abdominal muscles helps the lung deflate to residual volume. In this illustration the arrows represent the direction of movement, not the muscular force applied. (From Luce JM, and Culver BH: Respiratory muscle function in health and disease. *Chest*, 81:82–90, 1982.)

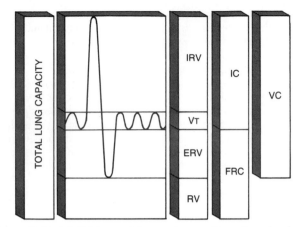

Figure 2–3. Subdivisions of lung volume with unforced spirometric tracing. IRV = inspiratory reserve volume; VT = tidal volume; ERV = expiratory reserve volume; RV = residual volume; IC = inspiratory capacity; FRC = functional residual capacity; VC = vital capacity. (Spirometry is discussed in Chapter 6.)

word tidal is useful, because the VT may be likened to a tide refreshing a tidal pool: It mixes fresh gas with residual gas but never really empties the lungs. As noted above, the volume of gas contained in the lungs at this end-tidal position after a normal exhalation is the FRC. The volume that can be inhaled from the FRC is the inspiratory capacity (IC). Increases in the VT occur by utilizing parts of the inspiratory reserve volume (IRV) and the expiratory reserve volume (ERV).

Minute Ventilation

Minute ventilation ($\dot{V}E$) is the volume of air moved in and out of the mouth (i.e., the volume exchanged) in a given minute; it is the product of VT and the ventilatory frequency (f). Thus, $\dot{V}E$ = VT × f.

Dead Space Ventilation

Although $\dot{V}E$ is convenient to measure, it does not necessarily reflect the gas available for exchange deep in the lungs. As a result, $\dot{V}E$ must be divided into two components: alveolar ventilation ($\dot{V}A$), which participates in gas exchange, and dead space ventilation, which does not. Dead space ventilation ($\dot{V}D$) includes anatomical dead space ventilation, the volume of air that remains in the airways at the end of inspiration and hence is not exposed to pulmonary capillary blood, and alveolar dead space ventilation, the volume of air that reaches the alveoli but is not exposed to pulmonary capillary blood because perfusion in certain alveoli is limited. Together, the anatomical and alveolar dead space are referred to as the physiological dead space. Anatomical dead space totals about 2 milliliters per kilogram (ml/kg) of body weight, or about 150 ml in an average man. Alveolar dead space is insignificant in health but increases in diseases that affect the pulmonary circulation. The per-breath ratio of V_D to V_T is called the dead space fraction (V_D/V_T). It normally averages 0.3.

Alveolar Ventilation

Alveolar ventilation ($\dot{V}_A$) is the volume of air that participates in gas exchange because it is in contact with alveoli perfused by pulmonary capillary blood. Because the body's CO_2 production ($\dot{V}CO_2$) is eliminated only by ventilation and the amount of CO_2 inhaled from the atmosphere is negligible, the partial pressure of CO_2 in the alveoli (P_ACO_2) is approximately equal to $\dot{V}CO_2$ divided by $\dot{V}_A$. Furthermore, because the CO_2 in the alveoli and the pulmonary capillary blood is in equilibrium across the alveolar-capillary membrane, the P_ACO_2 and the partial pressure of CO_2 in arterial blood ($PaCO_2$) leaving the lung are the same. These relationships are symbolized in the alveolar ventilation equation: $P_ACO_2 = PaCO_2 = \dot{V}CO_2/\dot{V}_A$.

Alveolar Hyperventilation and Hypoventilation

In health the body maintains a normal $PaCO_2$ of approximately 40 mmHg by adjusting $\dot{V}_A$ for $\dot{V}CO_2$ through the process of ventilatory regulation discussed below. Alveolar hyperventilation is $\dot{V}_A$ in excess of metabolic needs and is reflected in a $PaCO_2$ of less than approximately 40 mmHg. Conversely, alveolar hypoventilation is $\dot{V}_A$ inadequate for metabolic needs and is reflected in a $PaCO_2$ greater than approximately 40 mmHg. Since $\dot{V}_A = \dot{V}_E - \dot{V}_D$, $\dot{V}_A$ can be altered by changes in $\dot{V}_E$, $\dot{V}_D$, or both variables. It should be noted that the terms "hyperventilation" and "hypo-ventilation" do not describe visible breathing behavior and should be used only if the $PaCO_2$ is known. Furthermore, although the $PaCO_2$ is useful in appraising the adequacy of $\dot{V}_A$, it does not indicate the actual volume of expired CO_2 inasmuch as it reflects only the ratio of $\dot{V}CO_2$ and $\dot{V}_A$.

Under resting conditions, $\dot{V}CO_2$ is relatively constant. People whose $\dot{V}_A$ increases initially will exhale CO_2 faster than it is produced, so their $PaCO_2$ will fall. As it does, however, the CO_2 exhaled per breath gradually decreases until $\dot{V}_A$ again equals $\dot{V}CO_2$ and a new steady state is reached. On the other hand, people whose $\dot{V}_A$ decreases initially exhale CO_2 slower than it is produced. Their $PaCO_2$ then rises until CO_2 excretion again equals $\dot{V}CO_2$ and each liter of gas leaving the alveoli carries more CO_2. In this fashion, some patients with lung diseases that cause a high work of breathing can excrete their $\dot{V}CO_2$ at relatively less energy by increasing their $PaCO_2$.

PULMONARY PERFUSION

Mixed Venous Blood

Blood returning from peripheral tissues to the right atrium contains individual streams from a multitude of capillary beds, each with its own PO_2 and PCO_2 levels. Capillary blood cannot be obtained easily, and samples of the individual venous streams may differ markedly. However, mixed venous blood can be sampled in the pulmonary artery after mixing of the streams has occurred in the right ventricle. The PO_2 of mixed venous blood ($P\bar{v}O_2$) averages 40 mmHg under normal conditions; normal mixed venous PCO_2 ($P\bar{v}CO_2$) is 46 mmHg. These blood gas tensions are an approximation of those generally available for diffusion of O_2 into and of CO_2 out of peripheral tissues. They also are the tensions to which alveolar gas is exposed.

Pulmonary Vascular Resistance

Blood Flow in the Pulmonary Circulation. As discussed in Chapter 1, the pulmonary circulation originates in the pulmonary artery and ends in the left atrium. At its center are the pulmonary capillaries, which function less as individual vessels than they do as a continuous sheet of blood that covers the alveoli. Blood flow or perfusion ($\dot{Q}$) across the pulmonary circulation is equal to the pressure difference across it (P) divided by the pulmonary vascular resistance (PVR). Pulmonary vascular resistance therefore equals mean pulmonary artery pressure (15 mmHg) minus mean left atrial pressure (5 mmHg) divided by the right ventricular output of 5 liters per minute (L/min), or 2 mmHg/L/min. This low resistance reflects the relative simplicity of the pulmonary circulation, as noted in Chapter 1.

Factors Affecting Pulmonary Blood Flow. Despite the simplicity of the pulmonary circulation, PVR can be altered by several factors. One is increased pulmonary arterial or venous pressure, which forces blood through previously empty vessels and thereby lowers PVR by a process called vascular recruitment. Another factor is lung volume: Extra-alveolar vessel walls are tethered open when lung volume increases, thereby lowering resistance, and collapse at low lung volume. However, since the pulmonary capillaries are surrounded by alveolar gas, they also collapse when pressure in the alveoli exceeds that in their lumens. Alveolar pressure normally exceeds intraluminal pressure in the upright position only at the lung apices, where pulmonary arterial pressure is lower than it is at the lung bases because of gravitational forces. As a result, there is comparatively less blood flow to the top of the lung unless pulmonary artery pressure rises.

The final determinant of PVR is the smooth muscle tone of the pulmonary arteries and arterioles. This muscle dilates in response to beta-adrenergic agents, such as isoproterenol, and constricts in response to alpha-adrenergic agents, such as norepinephrine. However, the strongest stimulus causing vessel constriction is a low PO_2 in adjacent alveoli. This phenomenon is called hypoxic pulmonary vasoconstriction and is a basic defense mechanism of the lung.

Hypoxic Pulmonary Vasoconstriction. If the alveoli in only one lung or in a single segment or lobe of a lung have a low PO_2, hypoxic pulmonary vasoconstriction may force blood to another region of the lung or to the other lung, where ventilation is more adequate. This matching of ventilation and perfusion results in exposure of the mixed venous blood being exposed to the highest possible alveolar PO_2. However, if all the alveoli have a low PO_2, as occurs when overall alveolar ventilation is reduced or when the inspired gas has a decreased PO_2, hypoxic pulmonary vasoconstriction may be distributed over the lungs. This increases PVR and pulmonary artery pressure. Although this may be helpful initially because perfusion of the lung apices and recruitment of capillaries for gas exchange take place, sustained severe pulmonary hypertension causes the thin-walled right ventricle to hypertrophy and dilate and, in some circumstances, to fall.

PULMONARY GAS EXCHANGE

Diffusion Across the Alveolar-Capillary Membrane

Respiratory gases that have traveled through the upper and lower airways by the ventilatory process must pass the final distance through the alveoli, across the alveolar-capillary membrane, and into the red blood cells by passive diffusion alone. Normally the distances involved are small, and because red blood cells spend nearly a full second in the capillaries during resting conditions, ample time is available for O_2 and CO_2 molecules to diffuse. Furthermore, the membrane area is the most important factor governing diffusion, because its tremendous surface, which is estimated to be 70 square meters, greatly facilitates gas exchange. As a result, only when the travel time of red blood cells through the lungs is markedly shortened (as occurs with an increased cardiac output during strenuous exercise at altitude), or when the membrane is severely reduced in size (as might happen in pulmonary vascular disease), is diffusion limited across the alveolar-capillary membrane. Although theoretically diffusion limitation would offset the equalization of O_2 and CO_2 tensions across the membrane, other factors generally account for incomplete gas equilibration in the lung.

Equilibration Across the Alveolar-Capillary Membrane

Assuming that diffusion is not limited, the O_2 and CO_2 that reach the lungs from the peripheral tissues in mixed venous blood ($P\bar{v}O_2$ = 40 mmHg, $P\bar{v}CO_2$ = 46 mmHg) should equilibrate completely with the O_2 and CO_2 arriving in the alveolus (inspired PO_2 [PIO_2] = 150 mmHg after correcting for water vapor, inspired PCO_2 [$PICO_2$] = 0 mmHg) until new alveolar and capillary (Pc) values are reached (PAO_2 = PcO_2 = 100 mmHg, $PACO_2$ = $PcCO_2$ = 40 mmHg). The arterialized pulmonary capillary blood then courses through the pulmonary veins to the left atrium.

Complete equilibration of CO_2 between alveolus and capillary does occur in most situations, so that, as noted above, $PACO_2$ and $PaCO_2$ are assumed to be the same. However, before the pulmonary capillary blood leaves the left atrium it meets a small amount of blood, including that from the bronchial veins, that has bypassed the pulmonary circulation and has not been oxygenated. The addition of this shunted blood with a low mixed venous O_2 tension causes the PO_2 in the arterial blood leaving the left ventricle to be less than that in the alveolus. This difference is called the alveolar to arterial O_2 gradient [$P(A-a)O_2$]. It is 10 mmHg in normal young adults, whose PaO_2 is approximately 90 mmHg.

Ventilation-Perfusion Abnormalities

General Principles. Although equilibration is assumed to exist in individual alveolar-capillary units, it may be impaired in the entire lung owing to regional differences in ventilation and perfusion ($\dot{V}A/\dot{Q}$) that cause the $P(A-a)O_2$ to widen. These regional differences encompass a spectrum of physiological abnormalities.

Shunt. At one extreme is shunt, a condition in which capillary blood perfusion is normal but ventilation is totally lacking in certain alveoli. As noted above, a small amount of shunt normally occurs because blood from sources such as the bronchial veins bypasses the pulmonary capillaries. Abnormal shunt is seen when the alveoli are filled with inflammatory cells or edematous fluid. In such circumstances, large amounts of unoxygenated venous blood mix in the left atrium and left ventricle with blood that is fully oxygenated.

It should be emphasized that the PaO_2 resulting from this mixture does not equal the average of its PO_2's. Rather, it reflects the sum of the actual amounts of O_2, the O_2 content, of the oxygenated and unoxygenated blood. As described further on (see Oxygen-

Hemoglobin Interaction), the O_2 content of blood is determined largely by the saturation of its hemoglobin molecules with O_2. The O_2-hemoglobin dissociation curve is S-shaped, so arterial O_2 saturation (SaO_2) falls drastically when PO_2 is low. The addition of desaturated blood yields a low total SaO_2 that causes the final PaO_2 to be lower than if the PaO_2's of the two streams of oxygenated and unoxygenated blood simply were averaged. Furthermore, no amount of supplemental O_2 can improve the PaO_2. This occurs in part because the shunted blood is not exposed to O_2-containing alveoli and its O_2 content cannot increase. At the same time, increasing the PO_2 in well-ventilated alveoli does not improve arterial oxygenation because the hemoglobin exposed to these alveoli already is saturated with O_2 (Fig. 2–4).

Low Ventilation-Perfusion Mismatching. In this condition, ventilation to certain alveoli is reduced in comparison with perfusion but is not abolished entirely. The $\dot{V}A/\dot{Q}$ mismatching increases the $P(A-a)O_2$ and decreases the PaO_2 by a mechanism similar to shunt, but the fall in PaO_2 can be overcome if the PIO_2 is increased

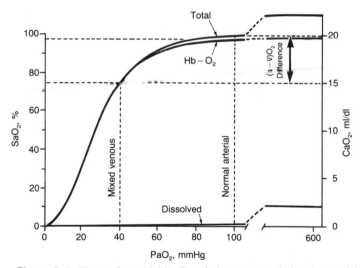

Figure 2–4. The oxyhemoglobin dissociation curve, relating the partial pressure of oxygen in arterial blood (PaO_2), in millimeters of mercury (mmHg); to arterial O_2 saturation (SaO_2) in per cent; and to the O_2 content of arterial blood (CaO_2) and assuming a normal hemoglobin concentration in milliliters per deciliter (ml/dl). The curve descends steeply below PaO_2 values of 50 mmHg, indicating severely reduced O_2-carrying capacity by hemoglobin below this PaO_2. The lower line represents O_2 in solution in the blood; the middle line depicts O_2 bound to hemoglobin at that PaO_2; the upper line shows O_2 bound to hemoglobin plus O_2 dissolved. Note that dissolved O_2 contributes little to CaO_2 at a PaO_2 in the normal range.

and O_2-enriched air reaches the alveoli to at least partially saturate the capillary blood. Many diseases that depress the PaO_2 are actually a combination of shunt and low $\dot{V}A/\dot{Q}$ mismatch. Indeed, shunt is merely an extreme form of mismatching. Its presence can be readily confirmed only by documenting the effects of breathing 100 per cent O_2, which should significantly improve the PaO_2 owing to pure low $\dot{V}A/\dot{Q}$ mismatching but not that caused by pure shunt.

Dead Space Ventilation. At the opposite end of the spectrum from shunt is dead space ventilation, discussed previously, in which ventilation is adequate but perfusion is lacking in the capillaries surrounding certain alveoli. This is often called high $\dot{V}A/\dot{Q}$ mismatching. Since CO_2 can be excreted only when the alveoli are exposed to capillary blood, dead space ventilation might be expected to alter the equilibration of CO_2. This does occur in some patients, but normal individuals increase $\dot{V}A$ in response to a rising $PaCO_2$. This not only returns the $PaCO_2$ to normal but also increases the PaO_2 because the augmented $\dot{V}A$ increases the amount of inspired air from which O_2 can be removed.

Hypoxemia and Its Causes

A decrease in the O_2 tension in any location in or outside of the body is referred to as hypoxia. A decrease in the PaO_2 is called hypoxemia. Thus, hypoxemia is arterial hypoxia. Hypoxemia can be caused by any or all of five conditions. The first three are low $\dot{V}A/\dot{Q}$ mismatching, shunt, and diffusion limitation, the last-named of which is unlikely to cause clinical hypoxemia for the reasons given in Diffusion Across the Alveolar-Capillary Membrane. The fourth reason is a decrease in the PIO_2, as occurs at high altitudes (see Fig. 1–1) or during a fire. The fifth cause of hypoxemia is hypoventilation, which is defined by an increase in $PaCO_2$; this independently lowers the PaO_2 because of a decrease in $\dot{V}A$. Of these five conditions, only the first three will increase the $P(A-a)O_2$. Their relationship to the hypoxemia of a given patient can best be appreciated by using the alveolar gas equation.

Alveolar Gas Equation

As noted above, $PACO_2$ and $PaCO_2$ depend only upon the ratio between $\dot{V}CO_2$ and $\dot{V}A$. This relationship is symbolized in the alveolar ventilation equation mentioned earlier and allows the $PaCO_2$ to be used in assessing the adequacy of ventilation. The PAO_2 and PaO_2 also are affected by $\dot{V}A$, but these values cannot be used directly for ventilatory assessment, first, because they are not equal, and second, because PAO_2 is influenced by PIO_2 as well as by tissue $\dot{V}O_2$. The actual relationship of these several factors is spelled out in the equation $PAO_2 = PIO_2$ corrected for water vapor $- \dot{V}O_2/\dot{V}A$. Inasmuch as $\dot{V}O_2$ and $\dot{V}CO_2$ are already related (they are equal if R, the respiratory exchange ratio discussed in Chapter 1, is 1), this equation can be combined with the alveolar ventilation equation to yield the alveolar gas equation: $PAO_2 = PIO_2$ corrected for water vapor $- PaCO_2/R$. The clinician can determine whether the $P(A-a)O_2$ is increased above its normal amount (10 mmHg when the subject is breathing ambient air at sea level) in a given arterial blood gas sample by using the alveolar gas equation. This information in turn narrows the possible causes of hypoxemia.

For example, assume for a particular patient breathing at one atmosphere that $R = 0.8$, the PIO_2 corrected for water vapor is 150 mmHg, and the normal PAO_2 is 100 mmHg. If the PaO_2 in a sample of arterial blood taken at sea level is 90 mmHg and the $PaCO_2$ is 40 mmHg, a normal $P(A-a)O_2$ of 10 mmHg is present, and the PaO_2 and $PaCO_2$ are normal. However, if the PaO_2 is 50 mmHg and the $PaCO_2$ is 40 mmHg, the $P(A-a)O_2$ is 50 mmHg. Hypoventilation is not present (the $PaCO_2$ is normal), and the patient is breathing at sea level, so the hypoxemia can be due only to $\dot{V}A/\dot{Q}$ mismatch, shunt, or diffusion limitation (the last of which is unlikely). Whether shunt is entirely responsible for the hypoxemia can be determined only by giving the patient 100 per cent O_2 and seeing if the PaO_2 improves, which would indicate low $\dot{V}A/\dot{Q}$ mismatch. As a third example, if the arterial blood gases revealed a PaO_2 of 50 mmHg and a $PaCO_2$ of 60 mmHg, the hypoxemia would be due in part to hypoventilation ($PaCO_2 = 60$ mmHg), but not entirely so, since the $P(A-a)O_2$ is greater than 10 mmHg. This tells the clinician that the patient's hypoxemia will not be corrected completely by normalizing the $PaCO_2$.

GAS TRANSPORT AND UPTAKE

Oxygen-Hemoglobin Interaction

Most of the O_2 transported in blood is in chemical combination with hemoglobin, a complex protein possessing four sites for the binding of O_2. These sites are almost filled to capacity under normal conditions, so the hemoglobin molecule is all but fully saturated. The relationship between PaO_2 and saturation is depicted graphically as the O_2-hemoglobin dissociation curve (see Fig. 2–4). Several consequences result from the S-shape of this curve. In the normal range of PaO_2 the curve is nearly flat, so small decreases in the PaO_2 cause only minor decrements in the SaO_2 and O_2 content. However, as the PaO_2 falls below 50 mmHg, the curve becomes steeper and the SaO_2 and O_2 content fall more rapidly. This is potentially dangerous, but the situation can be reversed if the PaO_2 is increased by only a small amount. This is accomplished by having the patient breathe supplemental O_2. Oxygen-hemoglobin interaction is discussed further in Chapters 7 and 14.

Arterial Oxygen Content

The actual amount of O_2 bound to hemoglobin and dissolved is called the O_2 content. The carrying capacity of hemoglobin is 1.34 ml O_2 per gram (gm) of hemoglobin. Normal arterial blood has a hemoglobin concentration of 15 gm/100 ml blood and thus carries 15 gm/100 ml × 1.34 ml/100 ml blood × a normal SaO_2 of 97 per cent; this equals 20 ml O_2/100 ml blood. Oxygen has a solubility of only 0.003 ml/100 ml blood/PaO_2 at a body temperature of 37° C, so the content of O_2 in solution at a normal PaO_2 is 0.003 ml × 100 ml blood × 90 mmHg or 0.3 ml O_2/100 ml blood. Adding these amounts yields an arterial O_2 content (CaO_2) of 20.3 ml/100 ml blood. The CaO_2 can be decreased if the hemoglobin concentration is reduced, as occurs in anemia, or if the PaO_2 and SaO_2 fall. The CaO_2 can be increased if the hemoglobin concentration is restored or if the PaO_2 is raised markedly. Increasing the PaO_2 to supernormal levels can be achieved in hyperbaric chambers, in which patients are exposed to O_2 at pressures greater than one atmosphere.

Oxygen Transport

Although the CaO_2 is a reliable indicator of the amount of O_2 carried in the blood, it does not necessarily reflect the O_2 actually delivered to the tissues. This is because tissue O_2 delivery depends not only on the CaO_2 but also on the total blood flow to the tissues, which is the same as the left ventricular or cardiac output ($\dot{Q}T$). Since $\dot{Q} = P/R$ in any hydraulic system, the normal left ventricular output of 5 L/min can be calculated by dividing the 100 mmHg pressure drop across the systemic circulation (mean arterial pressure [MAP] of 105 mmHg; mean right atrial pressure of 5 mmHg) by the SVR of 20 mmHg/L/min. From this relationship, it follows that left ventricular output will fall if MAP decreases or SVR increases without a reciprocal change in the other variable. Cardiac output also equals the amount of blood ejected by the left ventricle in a single contraction, or stroke volume (SV), multiplied by the number of contractions per minute, or heart rate (HR). Thus, $\dot{Q}T$ will fall if either the SV or the HR decreases.

Since $\dot{Q}T$ equals 5 L/min in health, the normal O_2 transport is approximately 20 ml/100 ml blood × 5 L/min, or approximately 1 L O_2/min. The actual O_2 transport can be calculated for clinical purposes by multiplying the CaO_2 by the $\dot{Q}T$, which can be measured by the indicator dilution technique discussed in Chapter 16.

Tissue Oxygen Extraction

Oxygen extraction by the peripheral tissues depends on three factors. One is the PO_2 in capillary blood, which must be 20 mmHg or higher for O_2 to diffuse into cells (the capillary PO_2 cannot be measured directly, but the PO_2 in mixed venous blood—the $P\bar{v}O_2$—provides an approximation). Another is the readiness of hemoglobin to release O_2 to the tissues; this is expressed by the position of the O_2-hemoglobin dissociation curve and by the partial pressure of O_2 at which half the hemoglobin is saturated, the P_{50}. The O_2-hemoglobin dissociation curve shifts to the right and the P_{50} increases when the temperature and PCO_2 rise and the pH declines, as occurs in and around actively metabolizing tissues. The dissociation curve shifts to the left and the P_{50} decreases when the temperature and PCO_2 fall and the pH rises, as occurs when tissue metabolism is low. The third factor governing O_2 uptake is the $\dot{V}O_2$ during aerobic metabolism. The relationship between O_2 extraction and transport is expressed in the Fick equation.

The Fick Equation

The Fick equation holds that the body's O_2 consumption is the product of the cardiac output and the difference in O_2 content between arterial and mixed venous blood, which is the same as O_2 extraction. The mixed venous O_2 content is symbolized as $C\bar{v}O_2$. Thus, according to the Fick equation, $\dot{V}O_2 = \dot{Q}_T \times (CaO_2 - C\bar{v}O_2)$, or $C(a-\bar{v})O_2$. Since $\dot{V}O_2 = 250$ ml/min, $\dot{Q}_T = 5$ L/min, and $CaO_2 = 20$ ml/100 ml blood, $C\bar{v}O_2$ is 15 ml/100 ml blood and $C(a-\bar{v})O_2$ is 5 ml/100 ml under normal conditions. Since only 5 ml of O_2 per 100 ml blood is being extracted under these conditions, a great reservoir of O_2 remains in the blood.

Relationship Between Oxygen Supply and Demand

Normally it is assumed that O_2 supply is determined by O_2 demand, so that $\dot{V}O_2$ regulates $\dot{Q}_T$ and $C(a-\bar{v})O_2$ reflects the adequacy of the heart to deliver O_2 to the tissues. In keeping with this assumption, the $C(a-\bar{v})O_2$ should increase above 5 ml/100 ml if $\dot{V}O_2$ rises and $\dot{Q}_T$ remains constant or if $\dot{Q}_T$ falls while $\dot{V}O_2$ remains the same. The $P\bar{v}O_2$ is a component of the $C\bar{v}O_2$, just as PaO_2 is a component of CaO_2. Thus, the $P\bar{v}O_2$ should fall below the normal level of 40 mmHg if O_2 transport and, particularly, $\dot{Q}_T$ decline. Some clinicians use the $P\bar{v}O_2$, which can be obtained from pulmonary arterial blood with a special catheter, to estimate the adequacy of O_2 transport. Alternatively, other clinicians use the saturation of O_2 in mixed venous blood ($S\bar{v}O_2$). Although this is appropriate in many patients, it does not apply to those with the adult respiratory distress syndrome (ARDS) or with states of very low $\dot{Q}_T$ in which O_2 demand appears to be regulated by supply rather than vice versa. This topic is discussed further in Chapter 16.

Shunt Equation

Shunt, as described above, involves the mixing of venous and arterialized blood in the left side of the heart prior to its distribution to the systemic circulation. The amount of shunted blood, $\dot{Q}s$, relative to the cardiac output, $\dot{Q}T$, may be calculated from the shunt equation:

$$\dot{Q}s/\dot{Q}T = \frac{CcO_2 - CaO_2}{CcO_2 - C\bar{v}O_2}$$

where CaO_2 and $C\bar{v}O_2$ are measured from the appropriate blood samples and the O_2 content of pulmonary capillary blood (CcO_2) is obtained by assuming that $PcO_2 = PaO_2$ calculated from the alveolar gas equation on 100 per cent O_2. Measurements made on less than 100 per cent O_2 yield a value for venous admixture because they reflect low $\dot{V}A/\dot{Q}$ mismatching in addition to shunt.

Carbon Dioxide Transport

Like O_2, CO_2 exists in physical solution and in chemical combination with hemoglobin in the blood. However, by far the greatest amount of CO_2 in the blood is in the form of bicarbonate ion (HCO_3^-). Carbon dioxide entering the blood from the tissues rapidly combines with water to form carbonic acid (H_2CO_3); in the presence of the enzyme carbonic anhydrase (CA), the carbonic acid dissociates to form hydrogen ion (H^+) and HCO_3^-. This reaction is written:

$$CO_2 + H_2O \rightleftarrows H_2CO_3 \overset{CA}{\rightleftarrows} H^+ + HCO_3^-$$

Because 90 per cent of the arterial CO_2 content can exist as HCO_3^- and need not be bound to hemoglobin, more CO_2 than O_2 is transported in the blood. The body stores of CO_2 also are greater, so the $PaCO_2$ changes much more slowly than PaO_2 with a change in $\dot{V}A$, even though the $PaCO_2$ is used to interpret ventilatory adequacy.

REGULATION OF VENTILATION

Control of Body pH

As noted in Chapter 1, ventilation is regulated in large part by central chemoreceptors in the medulla oblongata of the brain stem. The major stimulus to the receptors is the pH of brain extracellular fluid. Cells surrounding blood vessels in the brain allow free passage of CO_2 from the blood into the brain extracellular space but are relatively impermeable to H^+ and HCO_3^-. Because of the action of this functional blood-brain barrier, ventilation is affected immediately by changes in $PaCO_2$ that alter brain extracellular pH by the equation above. Equilibration of H^+ and HCO_3^- across the blood-brain barrier requires several hours, however, so the ventilatory response to changes in these ions in the blood is much slower. Nevertheless, the result of both processes is to maintain the body's pH within the normal range.

Control of PaO_2

Since blood flow in the carotid bodies is extremely high relative to their size, the peripheral chemoreceptors are exposed to a very small difference in arterial to venous PO_2 and PCO_2. This allows a rapid response in ventilation when the PaO_2 falls or $PaCO_2$ rises. Although the peripheral chemoreceptors respond to $PaCO_2$ changes, their primary function seems to be augmenting ventilation when the PaO_2 decreases below the level of approximately 60 mmHg. This rarely occurs in normal people except at high altitude, so the $PaCO_2$ usually determines $\dot{V}E$. However, the drive to breathe is regulated in large part by PaO_2 in chronically hypoxemic patients, including those with lung disease.

RECOMMENDED READING

1. Berger AJ.: Control of breathing. *In* Murray JF, and Nadel JA (eds.): *Textbook of Respiratory Medicine.* Philadelphia, W. B. Saunders Co., 1988, pp 140 166.
2. Cain SM: Assessment of tissue oxygenation. *Crit Care Clin*, 2:537–550, 1986.
3. Cain SM: Peripheral oxygen uptake and delivery in health and disease. *Clin Chest Med*, 4:39–48, 1983.
4. Collett PW, Roussos C, Macklem PJ: Respiratory mechanics. *In* Murray JF, and Nadel JA (eds.): *Textbook of Respiratory Medicine.* Philadelphia, W. B. Saunders Co., 1988, pp. 85–128.
5. Comroe JH: *Physiology of Respiration,* 2nd ed. Chicago, Year Book Medical Publishers, 1974.
6. Culver BH (ed.): *The Respiratory Systems: Syllabus for Human Biology 540.* Seattle, University of Washington, Lecture Notes, 1982.
7. Luce JM, and Culver BH: Respiratory muscle function in health and disease. *Chest*, 81:82–90, 1982.
8. Murray JF: *The Normal Lung,* 2nd ed. Philadelphia, W. B. Saunders Co., 1986.
9. Shapiro BA, et al.: *Clinical Application of Respiratory Care,* 2nd ed. Chicago, Year Book Medical Publishers, 1979.
10. Shapiro BA, et al.: *Clinical Application of Blood Gases,* 3rd ed. Chicago, Year Book Medical Publishers, 1982.
11. West JB: *Respiratory Physiology.* Baltimore, Williams & Wilkins, 1974.
12. West JB: Ventilation, blood flow, and gas exchanges. *In* Murray JF, and Nadel JA (eds.): *Textbook of Respiratory Medicine.* Philadelphia, W. B. Saunders Co., 1988, pp. 47–84.

3

WATER AND SOLUTE BALANCE

DISTRIBUTION OF WATER AND SOLUTES

_____

WATER

Body fluids contain water and dissolved substances called solutes. Water makes up 40 to 80 per cent of total body weight, depending on the amount of lean tissue present; lean tissue holds more water than fat does, so young, muscular individuals have the greatest quantity of water for a given amount of weight. Assuming an average of 60 per cent for water content, a 70-kg adult has 42 L of total body water.

SOLUTES

The body's normal solutes include electrolytes, sugars such as glucose, and urea, a product of protein metabolism that is toxic in high concentrations. The electrolytes consist of positively charged ions (cations), such as sodium (Na^+) and potassium (K^+), and negatively charged ions (anions), such as chloride (Cl^-) and bicarbonate (HCO_3^-). In solution these electrolytes are capable of conducting an electrical current. When electrolytes are combined chemically as salts, their electrical charges, or valences, are balanced and they do not possess a net charge. The electrolyte concentration of body fluids is expressed in terms of milliequivalents per liter (mEq/L) of a solution, usually water. An mEq is one one-thousandth of the molecular weight of a substance in grams divided by its valence. Electrolyte concentrations also may be expressed as millimols per liter (mmol/L), 1 mmol being one one-thousandth of the molecular weight of a substance.

OSMOLALITY

The semipermeable membranes that surround cells allow free passage of water but are relatively impermeable to the passage of solutes and large molecules such as proteins. When a solute to which a membrane is impermeable is placed on one side of the membrane, water flows to the side on which the solute is more concentrated until the original concentration difference or gradient no longer exists. The power of this gradient to attract water, which is proportional to the number of particles in solution, is called osmolality and is expressed in milliosmols per kilogram of water (mOsm/kg H_2O).

BODY COMPARTMENTS

Electrolytes are the most numerous and therefore the most osmotically active particles in the body. They are distributed preferentially within or outside cells because of the permeability of the cell membranes and because the electrolytes are transported across the membranes by ion pumps to maintain the electrical milieu inside and outside the cells. Na^+ and Cl^- are the major cation and anion respectively in extracellular fluid (ECF); their counterparts in intracellular fluid (ICF) are K^+ and anionic protons. These fluid spaces are also called body compartments.

The extracellular compartment contains the interstitial space, which is made up of lymphatics, connective tissue, and bone, and the intravascular space, which is filled with blood (Fig. 3–1). The

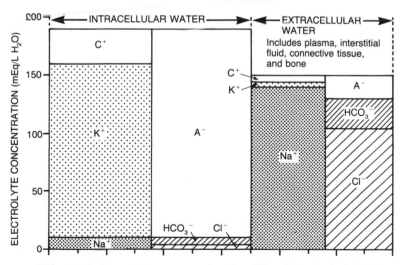

Figure 3–1. Electrolyte concentration, in milliequivalents per liter of water (mEq/L H_2O), in the body's two major water compartments. C^+ = unmeasured cations; K^+ = potassium; Na^+ = sodium; A^- = unmeasured anions; HCO_3^- = bicarbonate; Cl^- = chloride.

water portion of blood from which red and white blood cells have been separated is called plasma; serum is plasma from which platelets and clotting factors also have been removed. Since water passes freely across cell membranes, the amount in one compartment or another depends on their electrolyte concentrations. Normally, two thirds of body water is found in cells, and the remaining one third is extracellular and therefore either interstitial or intravascular. Two thirds of the normal 42 L of total body water, 28 L, is in the form of ICF. One third of the 42 L of total body water, 14 L, is in the form of ICF. Blood volume is approximately one third of the ECF, or 5 L. Because the normal hematocrit is 40 to 45 per cent, plasma volume is approximately 3 L. At the same time, the total volume of formed blood elements, mainly red blood cells, is 2 L.

WATER MOVEMENT BETWEEN COMPARTMENTS

Water content in the two body compartments will be altered if the concentration of electrolytes within the compartments changes. When Na^+ or some other solute that is confined to the ECF is added to the body, it attracts water osmotically from the intracellular compartment in proportion to the amount added. This results in an increase in ECF volume at the expense of the ICF. Preservation of ECF volume is essential, because the ECF includes the intravascular fluid necessary for organ perfusion. Indeed, the body defends ECF volume over osmolality in most instances.

WATER MOVEMENT ACROSS CAPILLARIES

General Principles

Albumin and Other Protein. Albumin and other proteins contribute less to serum or plasma osmolality than Na^+ and other electrolytes. They normally are present in far lower concentrations. Nevertheless, they may exert a pressure of 30 mmHg or greater inside the capillaries that contain them. This pressure, which is called oncotic pressure to distinguish it from the greater osmotic pressure generated by electrolytes, is offset by the hydrostatic pressure of water within the capillaries. The capillaries in turn are surrounded by the interstitium, which exerts oncotic and hydrostatic pressures of its own.

Fluid Exchange or Flux. Fluid movement into and out of a given capillary depends on a balance between these pressures and is summarized in the modified Starling equation: $F = K (Pc - Pi) - \sigma (\pi c - \pi i)$, where F is the net flux of the capillary; K is a permeability factor describing how readily water traverses the capillary membrane; Pc is capillary hydrostatic pressure; Pi is interstitial hydrostatic pressure; σ is a reflection coefficient describing how well the capillary membrane keeps proteins on one side; πc is capillary oncotic pressure; and πi is interstitial oncotic pressure. Assuming that capillary membrane integrity is intact and K stays constant, fluid normally passes out of the capillary at its arteriolar end, where Pc is higher than πc, and re-enters the capillary at its venular end, where the situation is reversed (Fig. 3–2). Although the net effect of the Starling forces is to keep fluid within the intravascular space, tissues in the body that contain capillaries, which most tissues do, are never truly dry. Furthermore, an unbalancing of the Starling forces, as would occur with a greatly increased Pc, a greatly decreased πc, or an increase in K, can greatly increase fluid flux out of the capillary. Extravascular interstitial fluid of this sort is called edema. Capillary hydrostatic pressure can be increased when total body Na^+ and ECF volume are increased, as occurs in congestive heart failure. Conversely, capillary oncotic pressure decreases in cirrhosis and nephrosis because protein production or conservation is inadequate. Increased capillary permeability occurs in certain conditions and diseases that cause inflammation and disruption of the capillary

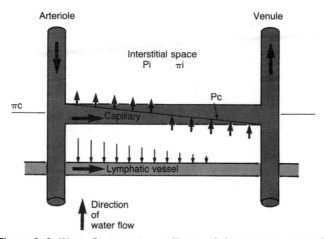

Figure 3–2. Water flow across a capillary and the pressures responsible for this flow. Interstitial hydrostatic (Pi) and oncotic (πi) pressures and capillary oncotic (πc) pressure are assumed to remain constant, as is capillary permeability. However, capillary hydrostatic pressure (Pc) decreases from arteriole to venule. Water therefore leaves the capillary at its arteriolar end and reenters at the venular end. Excess extravascular water is removed by lymphatic vessels located at or near the capillary. Unbalancing of the forces (as with increased Pc, decreased πc, or increased capillary permeability) or damage to the lymphatics would increase the flux of fluid out of the capillary.

endothelium, such as in burn cases and in neonatal or adult respiratory distress syndromes.

Since the capillary membrane is permeable to water but not protein when Pc or πc only is affected, the edema fluid that collects outside the capillary has a low specific gravity and a protein concentration less than half that of plasma or serum. This fluid generally looks thin and clear and is called a transudate. In contrast to this situation, when K is affected, the capillary membrane is permeable to protein as well as water, so the edema fluid has a high specific gravity and a protein concentration similar to that of serum. This fluid generally looks thicker and more opaque and is called an exudate. Although differentiating transudates from exudates is sometimes difficult, the distinction between the two types of edema fluid assists the clinician in determining how the fluid was formed.

Pulmonary Edema

Pulmonary edema fluid can be of the hydrostatic (pressure-related) or the increased permeability variety or can be a combination of the two, which shows that pulmonary edema occurs primarily because capillary hydrostatic pressure is increased or because permeability is altered. The terms "cardiogenic" and "noncardiogenic" also are used because hydrostatic edema occurs in the presence, and increased permeability edema in the absence, of elevated left ventricular filling pressures as approximated by pulmonary artery wedge pressure recordings. Normal hydrostatic pressure in the pulmonary capillaries is approximately 10 mmHg; this is exceeded by the serum oncotic pressure, so there is a net flux of water into the capillaries in the lung. However, the hydrostatic pressure may increase when pressure rises in the left ventricle during congestive heart failure or when left atrial pressure climbs independently, as in mitral stenosis. Pulmonary capillary hydrostatic pressures then exceed capillary oncotic pressure, especially if oncotic pressure is reduced to begin with, and transudation out of the capillaries begins.

The opposite situation is seen in the respiratory distress syndromes, in which damage to the pulmonary capillary membrane allows the exudation of protein and water regardless of capillary hydrostatic or oncotic pressure. When this happens, the presence of proteins in the interstitial space reverses the previous oncotic gradient (when Pc was greater than πc) and draws more water from the capillaries. In both hydrostatic edema and increased permeability edema, the excess extravascular water fills the interstitium. If interstitial lymphatics located around the bronchi and the branches of the pulmonary arteries cannot drain the water, it floods the alveolar spaces, impairing their ability to participate in gas exchange and producing the picture of pulmonary edema.

Pleural Effusion

Edema in the pleural space is called pleural effusion. The pleural space normally contains a small amount of fluid that lubricates the parietal pleura on the inside of the chest wall and the visceral pleura that envelops the lung. The fluid formerly was thought to come from capillaries supplying the parietal pleura, but it is now believed that the fluid seeps from capillaries supplying the visceral pleura as well. Once formed, the fluid normally is reabsorbed by lymphatics. Pleural effusions may collect if capillary hydrostatic pressure increases, if capillary oncotic pressure decreases, if lymphatic drainage is compromised (because of obstruction of the lymphatics by tumor, for example), or if the capillary membranes are inflamed. Large transudative pleural effusions are common in congestive heart failure, when pleural capillary pressure is increased. They also occur in cirrhosis and nephrosis, in which the capillary oncotic pressure is reduced. Exudative pleural effusions accumulate most commonly in pneumonia and in carcinomatous involvement of the pleura. This topic is discussed at length in Chapter 19.

Peripheral Edema

Peripheral edema is the name given to fluid that collects in dependent regions, such as the ankles. When present in the abdomen, the edema is termed ascites. A condition called anasarca exists if the entire body is swollen with fluid. Although peripheral edema may result from low oncotic pressure or from obstruction of venous flow, it most commonly occurs secondary to elevated venous pressure in the right atrium. The edema begins in the lower extremities, because venous pressure is greatest there owing to gravity. Total body Na^+ is always increased when edema is present, inasmuch as the kidneys retain Na^+ because renal perfusion is low, and they sense an inadequate arterial volume, either because of low cardiac output, as in congestive heart failure, or because arterial vasodilation causes decreased vascular filling, as in cirrhosis.

ESTIMATION OF EXTRACELLULAR FLUID VOLUME

As noted before, ECF volume depends on the amount of Na^+ in the ECF; thus, Na^+ depletion causes ECF volume depletion and Na^+ excess causes ECF volume excess. The most sensitive sign of ECF volume depletion is a decreased intravascular volume, which is called hypovolemia. Normally, when a person changes from a lying to a sitting position with the legs dangling, or when he stands, his pulse and systolic blood pressure change little and his diastolic blood pressure increases by 5 to 10 mmHg. However, if intravascular volume is reduced by only 10 per cent, the pulse will rise by 10 beats per minute and the diastolic pressure will fall by 10 mmHg; the systolic pressure may also fall slightly. Orthostatic changes of this sort also can occur in patients who are bedridden and lack autonomic nervous system tone, so other signs of intravascular volume inadequacy must be sought.

Intravascular venous deficiency is suggested by a lack of distension of the internal jugular veins above the sternal angle when patients are sitting at a 45 degree angle. Jugular venous distension should be present if intravascular volume is excessive, however, and patients will lack orthostatic changes and may even be hypertensive. In addition, they may manifest pulmonary or peripheral edema. Volume assessment by physical examination may be difficult in patients whose Na^+ status varies from day to day. Daily records of weight gain or loss and Na^+ and water intake and loss are essential in such patients. Some patients also require direct measurement of right atrial pressure by central venous pressure catheters or of pulmonary artery wedge pressure by catheterization. These techniques are discussed in Chapter 16.

ESTIMATION OF EXTRACELLULAR FLUID OSMOLALITY

Because Na^+ is the major ECF cation and must be balanced by Cl^- and HCO_3^- for the ECF to remain electrically neutral, ECF osmolality can be approximated by doubling the serum or plasma Na^+ concentration and adding the smaller contribution of other solutes. Thus, osmolality equals $2 \times Na^+$ concentration + glucose concentration/18 + blood urea nitrogen (BUN) concentration/2.8. The normal serum Na^+ concentration is 140 mEq/L; glucose is approximately 100 milligrams per deciliter (mg/dl), and the BUN is 10 mg/dl. Serum osmolality normally is 285 mOsm/kg H_2O, with a range of 280 to 295 mOsm/kg H_2O.

Osmolality also can be measured in the laboratory by the freezing point depression and change in water vapor methods. If the measured osmolality exceeds the estimated osmolality, an osmolar gap is said to be present and the clinician should be alerted to the presence of other unmeasured osmols. These might come from alcohols such as ethanol (osmolar contribution equals ethanol concentration divided by 4.6); mannitol or glycerol, substances given intravenously to patients with cerebral edema or glaucoma (osmolar contribution equals mannitol concentration divided by 18 *or* glycerol concentration divided by 9); or sorbitol, a sugar contained in certain medications (osmolar contribution equals sorbitol concentration divided by 18).

TONICITY

Tonicity is a term used to describe the osmotic equivalence of fluids. Isotonic fluids have the same osmolality as serum or plasma;

hypotonic fluids have less; hypertonic fluids have more. (The tonicity of common intravenous fluid preparations is given in Table 3–1.) Hypotonicity results when the concentration of ECF solutes, in most cases Na^+, decreases and causes net ICF volume excess. By contrast, hypertonicity occurs when ECF solutes increase and cause net ICF volume depletion. Most solutes that cause hypertonicity, including Na^+ and glucose, also cause hyperosmolality. However, the terms are not always interchangeable; high levels of urea or ethanol raise serum osmolality but do not cause hypertonicity, because they produce no lasting osmotic gradient across cell membranes and therefore do not cause water to shift between body compartments.

REGULATION OF WATER AND SOLUTE BALANCE

DAILY LOSSES

The body loses fixed amounts of water and solutes each day. For example, to rid itself of urea and other metabolic waste products, the kidney daily excretes 1500 ml of water containing 50 mEq Na^+, 40 mEq K^+, and 90 mEq Cl^-. Approximately 1000 ml of pure water per day is lost through the skin as sweat and through the lungs as water vapor. This amount can rise markedly as the ambient temperature increases, particularly if the air is poorly humidified. Water also leaves the body in stool and in gastrointestinal fluids that vary in their solute content (Table 3–2). To preserve ECF volume and maintain osmolality, the body must either compensate for these irreversible losses by increasing its intake of water and solutes, especially Na^+, or invoke mechanisms to conserve them.

REGULATION OF INTAKE

When plasma osmolality increases because water is lost and the Na^+ concentration increases, thirst receptors in the hypothalamus of the brain are stimulated, producing the desire to drink water until the normal Na^+ concentration is restored. The loss of blood volume that occurs in massive bleeding is an even greater stimulus to thirst, inasmuch as the body preserves ECF volume more avidly than osmolality. Thus, although their serum or plasma osmolality may be normal, bleeding patients will drink water to maintain their intravascular volume even though they dilute their Na^+ concentra-

Table 3–1. INTRAVENOUS SOLUTIONS AND ADDITIVES USED TO MAINTAIN WATER AND SOLUTE BALANCE

SOLUTION	TONICITY			GLUCOSE CONCENTRATION (mEq/L or per Ampule)	ELECTROLYTE CONCENTRATION (mEq/L or per Ampule)					
	Hypotonic	Isotonic	Hypertonic		Na$^+$	Ca^{2+}	K$^+$	Cl$^-$	HCO$_3^-$	Lactate
5% D/W	x			50						
10% D/W	x			100						
20% D/W			x	200						
50% D/W			x	500						
5% D/0.45% NaCl	x			50	77			77		
5% D/0.9% NaCl		x		50	154			154		
0.45% NaCl	x				77			77		
0.9% NaCl		x			154			154		
3% NaCl			x		513			513		
Ringer's solution		x			148	4	4	156		
Ringer's lactate		x			130	3	4	109		28
7.5% NaHCO₃			x		44 in 50-ml ampule				44 in 50-ml ampule	
25% mannitol			x	*						
50% glucose			x	25 in 50-ml ampule						

KEY: D = dextrose, W = water, Na$^+$ = sodium, K$^+$ = potassium, Cl$^-$ = chloride, HCO$_3^-$ = bicarbonate, Ca^{2+} = calcium, NaCl = sodium chloride (saline), NaHCO$_3$ = sodium bicarbonate.
*Contains 12.5 gm mannitol per 50 ml ampule.

Table 3-2. DAILY VOLUMES AND CONCENTRATIONS OF MAJOR SOLUTES IN BODY FLUIDS

	AVERAGE VOLUME (L/day)	ELECTROLYTE CONCENTRATION (mEq/L)				
		Na+	K+	H+	Cl-	HCO3-
Saliva	1.5	30* (20–50)†	20 (16–23)	— —	31 (20–50)	15 (10–20)
Gastric juice	2.5	50 (30–90)	10 (5–10)	90 —	110 (50–130)	0 —
Bile	0.5	140 (120–170)	5 (5–10)	— —	105 (80–120)	40 (30–50)
Pancreatic juice	0.7	140 (110–150)	5 (5–10)	— —	60 (50–100)	90 (70–110)
Small intestine	1.5	120 (70–160)	5 (0–5)	— —	110 (70–130)	35 (20–40)
Diarrhea	1.0–10	130 (120–140)	10 (5–15)	— —	95 (90–100)	20 (15–30)
Sweat	0–3	50 (20–100)	5 (0–15)	— —	50 (20–100)	0 —

KEY: Na+ = sodium, K+ = potassium, H+ = hydrogen, Cl- = chloride, HCO3- = bicarbonate.
*Mean.
†Range.

tion in the process and become hypo-osmolar and hypotonic. Sodium intake also will increase when ECF volume decreases or when the kidneys perceive that ECF volume is low, although dietary factors more often dictate Na^+ consumption in normal people.

REGULATION OF OUTPUT

The body's major mechanism to conserve water and electrolytes involves retention of these substances by the kidney. Renal water regulation is mediated by antidiuretic hormone (ADH), or vasopressin, which is secreted by the posterior pituitary gland of the brain and increases renal reabsorption of water in response to increases in serum osmolality and decreases in volume. If serum osmolality rises as high as 295 mOsm/kg H_2O, urine osmolality may increase to the 800 to 1000 range. Conversely, urine osmolality of less than 100 mOsm/kg H_2O can be expected when serum osmolality falls to 280.

Decreasing intravascular volume also leads to a fall in arterial pressure and renal perfusion, factors that facilitate adrenergic nervous system stimulation, pituitary ADH release, and the renal retention of Na^+ and water. In addition, the cortex of the adrenal gland is stimulated by volume depletion to secrete mineralocorticoid hormones, including aldosterone, that increase Na^+ reabsorption in the distal tubules of the kidney, in exchange for K^+ and hydrogen ion (H^+). Although these latter mechanisms conserve Na^+ content to maintain ECF volume status, pure abnormalities in Na^+ concentration, that is, in plasma osmolality, are corrected by changes in water excretion and retention and not by changes in the amount of total body Na^+.

ADEQUACY OF WATER AND SOLUTE REGULATION

The regulating mechanisms just described can generally defend against the threats to volume and osmolality that occur with routine physiological perturbations, such as vigorous exercise on a hot, dry day. Nevertheless, these defenses can be overwhelmed if body losses of water and solutes are severe, if intake of these substances cannot be increased, or if output cannot be controlled. Patients may lose large quantities of water and solute in sweat, for example, or through protracted vomiting or diarrhea. Patients who are unconscious or lack access to water and solutes cannot compensate for these losses, especially if their kidneys are diseased or if the glands that secrete ADH and aldosterone are damaged. If hospitalized, they are at the mercy of clinicians administering water and solutes to them.

WATER AND SOLUTE IMBALANCES AND THEIR THERAPY

HYPOVOLEMIA

As noted previously, the effects of intravascular volume loss and hyperperfusion are so deleterious that ECF volume is defended even to the detriment of ECF osmolality in the presence of hypovolemia. Hypovolemia occurs when the rate of Na^+ and water intake is less than the rate of loss of these substances on a short- or long-term basis. Total body water always is decreased during volume depletion. Total body Na^+ usually is decreased as well, but hypovolemia can occur with any Na^+ concentration. This is because the Na^+ concentration represents only the relative amounts of Na^+ and water in serum or plasma and not the total amount of these substances in the body.

The most common clinical cause of hypovolemia is hemorrhage, which represents isotonic fluid loss. With loss of gastrointestinal fluid, the ECF can be either isotonic or hypotonic, depending on the site of loss. Central diabetes insipidus (DI), caused by a deficiency in the pituitary secretion of ADH, and nephrogenic DI, in which the kidneys cannot concentrate urine in response to the hormone, cause hypotonic fluid loss. The ultimate manifestation of hypovolemic inadequate tissue perfusion is called shock. The treatment is to restore the fluid loss at the appropriate tonicity.

HYPERVOLEMIA

Intravascular volume expansion, or hypervolemia, is a state in which ECF volume is increased either acutely or chronically. Hypervolemia occurs when the rate of Na^+ and water intake is greater than the rate of loss of these substances. Total body water always is increased during volume expansion. Total body Na^+ usually is increased as well, but hypervolemia can occur at any Na^+ concentration. This is because the Na^+ concentration represents only the relative amounts of Na^+ and water in serum or plasma and not the total amount of these substances in the body.

Hypervolemia occurs in edematous conditions such as congestive heart failure, in which a low cardiac output stimulates adrenergic nervous system activity, ADH secretion, aldosterone release, and Na^+ and water retention; and cirrhosis, in which arterial vasodilation stimulates Na^+ and water retention by similar mechanisms. Another cause of hypervolemia is impaired renal excretion of Na^+ and water, as may be seen with renal failure. Hypervolemia is treated by removing the excess fluid, for example, with diuretics or renal dialysis.

HYPOTONICITY

General Principles

As noted previously, hypotonicity occurs when ECF solutes are decreased relative to water, so that serum osmolality falls and water shifts to the ICF. For practical purposes, this is reflected in a decrease in the serum Na^+ concentration to 135 mEq/L or less. The water excess that exists in this situation can be calculated from the formula

$$\text{Water excess in L} = \frac{140 - \text{serum } Na^+ \text{ concentration}}{140} \times (0.6 \times \text{body weight in kg})$$

Although the low Na^+ concentration is referred to as hyponatremia, this term does not necessarily indicate the body's Na^+ content. In fact, hypotonicity may exist when the Na^+ content is normal, decreased, or increased. The major symptom caused by hypotonicity is water intoxication, which is characterized by apathy and a decline in mental concentration that may progress to generalized seizures. Water intoxication is caused by swelling of cells in the central nervous system, a condition called cerebral edema. Other symptoms associated with hypotonicity reflect concomitant abnormalities of Na^+ content and ECF volume.

Hypotonicity With a Normal Na⁺ Content

Hypotonicity with a normal Na^+ content and ECF volume is seen when ADH or ADH-like material is inappropriately secreted in patients with lung or brain tumors. The diagnosis of the syndrome of inappropriate ADH, as this condition is called, is suggested by the combination of serum hypo-osmolality, urine hyperosmolality, a urine Na^+ concentration of greater than 50 mEq/L, and a normal intravascular volume as suggested by a lack of orthostatic changes. Usually, the hypotonicity is not severe; patients may be asymptomatic and require either no treatment or mild water restriction. If the hypotonicity is severe (serum Na^+ concentration = 110 mEq/L or less), if the patient is convulsing, or if both circumstances exist, a combination of hypertonic fluids rich in Na^+ should be given, along with furosemide or other diuretics that cause the kidneys to excrete hypotonic urine with a lower Na^+ content.

Hypotonicity With a Decreased Na⁺ Content

Hypotonicity with decreased Na^+ content and ECF volume is seen for the most part in patients who lose large amounts of Na^+ and water from their kidneys, gastrointestinal tract, or bloodstream and replace only the water they have lost. The water is retained because the body releases ADH to maintain ECF volume. However, the water equilibrates in the intracellular and extracellular compartments, and ECF volume is not restored. The inadequate intravascular volume in such patients may cause postural changes in blood pressure and symptoms of poor organ perfusion. The urine Na^+ should be less than 20 mEq/L, and urine osmolality will be greater than serum osmolality. Very severe volume depletion should be treated with hypertonic fluids. Isotonic NaCl is sufficient for patients when volume depletion is not so severe.

Hypotonicity With an Increased Na^+ Content

Hypotonicity with an increased Na^+ content and ECF volume occurs primarily in patients with congestive heart failure, cirrhosis, or nephrosis. Although intravascular volume is increased in all three conditions, it is not interpreted as being adequate by the kidneys, which retain Na^+ because renal blood flow is reduced and aldosterone secretion by the adrenal glands is raised. The kidneys also retain water because the posterior pituitary liberates ADH. In cirrhosis and nephrosis, the apparent intravascular volume inadequacy is related in part to an insufficiency of serum proteins caused by decreased protein synthesis by the liver in the former condition and by increased protein loss by the kidneys in the latter. Osmolality may be normalized in some patients with hypotonicity and Na^+ excess if they are given diuretics followed by hypertonic fluids. However, Na^+ repletion of this sort usually worsens edema and other manifestations of Na^+ excess without improving the serum Na^+ concentration, because the body retains more water to restore osmolality and perhaps also because it still senses that the ECF volume is low. Therefore most patients do best with a combination of Na^+ *and* water restriction.

HYPERTONICITY

General Principles

Hypertonicity occurs when ECF solutes increase relative to water so that serum osmolality rises and water shifts from the ICF. In most but not all situations, Na^+ is the solute in excess, and the serum Na^+ is 145 mEq/L or more. The water deficit that exists in this situation can be calculated from the formula

$$\text{Water deficit in L} = \frac{\text{serum } Na^+ \text{ concentration} - 140}{140} \times (0.6 \times \text{body weight in kg})$$

Although the high Na^+ concentration is referred to as hypernatremia, total body Na^+ content may be normal, low, or high.

The major clinical sign of hypertonicity is thirst, assuming patients can communicate. The major clinical symptoms are lethargy and obtundation caused by the depleted water content of cells in the central nervous system, a condition called cerebral dehydration. Presumably because of their vulnerability to dehydration, brain cells can protect themselves by gradually generating intracellular solutes, or "idiogenic osmols," that attract extra water in the face of overall ICF water depletion. Thus, returning serum osmolality to normal too rapidly in hypertonic patients may cause rebound cerebral edema and water intoxication. Other symptoms of hypertonicity relate to associated abnormalities in Na^+ content and ECF volume or to the effects of solutes other than Na^+.

Hypertonicity With a Normal Na^+ Content

Hypertonicity with a normal Na^+ content and ECF volume, or pure water depletion, is seen either in patients who lack access to water or in those who lose it from the respiratory tract because of a greatly increased minute ventilation or because they are breathing unhumidified gases. This condition can be corrected with water administration.

Hypertonicity With a Decreased Na^+ Content

Hypertonicity with a decreased Na^+ content and ECF volume is seen in patients who lose water and Na^+ and cannot replace their losses. Such losses may occur through the skin in patients who sweat profusely, since sweat is hypotonic. They also may originate (1) from the gastrointestinal tract in patients with severe vomiting or diarrhea or (2) from the kidneys, either when the presence of osmotically active substances like glucose or mannitol draw water and Na^+ from the body or when there is a deficiency in production and release of ADH (central diabetes insipidus) or a deficiency in the renal response to the hormone (nephrogenic diabetes insipidus).

Central diabetes insipidus may follow injury to the hypothalamus or pituitary following head trauma or neurosurgery. Nephrogenic diabetes insipidus may result from renal disease or from the administration of certain drugs. The urine Na^+ should be greater than 50 mEq/L in both forms of diabetes insipidus unless volume depletion is severe, and the urine osmolality should be less than that of serum. Patients with central diabetes insipidus usually increase urine osmolality and correct hypertonicity when given exogenous vasopressin, whereas patients with nephrogenic diabetes insipidus do not. Acute hypertonicity with symptoms of intravascular volume inadequacy should be treated with isotonic fluids. Once the ECF has been restored, the abnormality in osmolality can be treated by water administration. Water should be given orally or intravenously as dextrose in water at a rate of less than 500 ml/hour if possible to avoid rebound water intoxication.

Hypertonicity With an Increased Na+ Content

Hypertonicity with an increased Na^+ content and ECF volume is seen in patients given large amounts of Na^+ in the form of NaCl tablets, sodium bicarbonate ($NaHCO_3$), or hypertonic fluids. Total ECF solute content is approximately 4000 mOsm in 70-kg adults. The ECF solute content of a patient given 20 ampules of $NaHCO_3$, each containing 44 mEq Na^+, during cardiopulmonary resuscitation will increase by 1760 mOsm. The serum Na^+ concentration will rise from 140 to 160 mEq/L, and 4000 ml of water will shift from the ICF to the ECF. This ECF overload in turn might cause sudden pulmonary edema and severe cerebral dehydration. The brain cells will not have enough time to generate idiogenic osmols. Insults of this sort require rapid treatment with furosemide to induce renal Na^+ and water loss, and with water, usually given intravenously, to correct osmolality. Patients whose serum Na^+ exceeds 180 mEq/L may require hemodialysis to restore water and solute balance.

Hypertonicity Due to Hyperglycemia

Hyperglycemia, an increase in the serum glucose concentration, may occur immediately in patients receiving hyperalimentation fluids rich in carbohydrates. Although hypertonicity will occur in this situation, total body Na^+ and water will not be affected. Alternatively, hyperglycemia may develop gradually in patients with diabetic ketoacidosis and those with hyperosmolar nonketotic coma, conditions characterized by lack of insulin or by a decreased tissue responsiveness to the hormone. These patients may experience profound renal Na^+ and water losses and may not replace their losses adequately. Hyperglycemia attracts water from the ICF to the ECF and artifactually lowers the serum Na^+ concentration in all circumstances, so the rise in Na^+ concentration seen in hypertonicity due to Na^+ alone may or may not be present, depending on whether more Na^+ or water has been lost.

The serum Na^+ concentration can be expected to fall by 1.6 mEq/L for every 100 mg/dl rise in the glucose concentration over its normal level of approximately 100 mg/dl. Calculation of the true Na^+ concentration by this method should tell the clinician what the patient's Na^+ concentration will be after hyperglycemia is corrected by insulin. Since total body Na^+ is likely to be low unless hyperglycemia is acute, regardless of the true serum Na^+ concentration, water should not be given initially to correct the hyperosmolality caused by glucose. Instead, the patient should receive isotonic fluids to insure intravascular volume adequacy.

Once intravascular volume is restored, the patient may be given water to correct hypertonicity due to an increased Na^+ concentration, if it exists. The rapidity of water administration should reflect its rate of loss when hyperglycemia was present. Overly aggressive rehydration during correction of hyperglycemia is particularly hazardous in patients with hyperosmolar nonketotic coma. In such patients, water once held in the ECF by its high glucose concentration, which may approach 2000 mg/dl, shifts rapidly into the ICF and may cause water intoxication as it enters cerebral cells.

Hypertonicity Due to Solutes Other Than Na^+ and Glucose

Hypertonicity also may result from the presence of mannitol, glycerol, sorbitol, and other solutes in the ECF. These substances may cause a sodium and water diuresis and may also artifactually lower the serum Na^+ concentration by diluting the ECF, as glucose does. Treatment of hypertonicity due to these solutes is similar to that for hyperglycemia, in that attention is focused first on ECF volume protection and then on correction of hyperosmolality.

RECOMMENDED READING

1. Andreoli TE: Disorders of fluid volume, electrolyte, and acid-base balance. *In* Wyngaarden JB, and Smith LH (eds.): *Cecil's Textbook of Medicine*, 17th ed. Philadelphia, W. B. Saunders Co., 1985, pp. 515–543.
2. Arieff AI: Hyponatremia, convulsions, respiratory arrest, and permanent brain damage after elective surgery in healthy women. *N Engl J Med*, 314:1529–1534, 1987.
3. Berl T, et al.: Clinical disorders of water metabolism. *Kidney Int*, 10:117–132, 1976.
4. Fieg PU, and McCurdy DK: The hypertonic state. *New Engl J Med*, 297:1444–1454, 1977.
5. Pitts RF: *Physiology of the Kidney and Body Fluids*, 3rd ed. Chicago, Year Book Medical Publishers, 1974.
6. Schrier RW: New treatments for hyponatremia. *New Engl J Med*, 298:214–220, 1978.
7. Schrier RW (ed.): *Renal and Electrolyte Disorders*, 2nd ed. Boston, Little, Brown & Co., 1980.
8. Schrier RW: Pathogenesis of sodium and water retention in high-output cardiac failure, nephrotic syndrome, cirrhosis, and pregnancy. *N Engl J Med*, 319:1065–1072, 1127–1134, 1988.
9. Schrier RW: Body fluid volume regulation in health and disease: A unifying hypothesis. *Ann Intern Med*, 113:155–159, 1991.
10. Staub NC: The pathogenesis of pulmonary edema. *Prog Cardiovasc Dis*, 23:53–74, 1980.

4

ACID-BASE BALANCE

ACID-BASE PHYSIOLOGY

pH AND ACID-BASE BALANCE

When the body is in normal acid-base balance, its intracellular and extracellular fluids are neither excessively acidic nor alkaline. Acid-base status may be quantified in terms of either the serum or plasma concentration of hydrogen ions (H^+) or the negative logarithm of that concentration, pH. Using a log scale not only is conventional but also allows relatively small changes in pH units to express large changes in the availability of H^+. The pH of arterial blood, which ideally is 7.4 (slightly more alkaline than water [pH = 7.0]), normally ranges from 7.38 to 7.42. However, it may range from 6.8 to 7.7 during certain derangements, which will be discussed.

ACIDS, BASES, AND BUFFERS

Acids are defined as substances that donate H^+, whereas bases are substances that accept them. For the reaction $HA \rightleftarrows H^+ + A^-$, HA is the acid and A^- is its conjugate base. The strength of the acid HA depends on the extent to which it forms H^+ and A^- in water, that is, its degree of dissociation. The tendency of an acid to dissociate in water is quantified in the Henderson-Hasselbalch equation:

$$pH = pK + \log \frac{\text{base concentration}}{\text{acid concentration}}$$

where pK is a constant that reflects the strength of a given acid. The combination of a weak acid or base and its salt is a buffer. This is a substance that resists change in H^+ concentration upon addition of a stronger acid or base.

THE CARBONIC ACID BUFFERING SYSTEM

Carbonic acid (H_2CO_3) is formed by the hydration of CO_2 in the presence of the enzyme carbonic anhydrase (CA) by the reaction

$$CO_2 + H_2O \overset{CA}{\rightleftarrows} H_2CO_3 \rightleftarrows H^+ + HCO_3^-$$

Carbonic acid is a weak acid from a chemical standpoint, because its dissociation into H^+ and bicarbonate ion (HCO_3^-) is incomplete in comparison with strong acids, such as hydrochloric acid (HCl). The Henderson-Hasselbalch equation for carbonic acid is

$$pH = 6.1 + \log \frac{HCO_3^- \text{ concentration}}{CO_2 \text{ concentration}}$$

Since the CO_2 concentration is linearly related to the partial pressure of CO_2 in arterial blood ($PaCO_2$) by a solubility constant, the equation can be rewritten

$$pH = 6.1 + \log \frac{HCO_3^- \text{ concentration}}{0.3 \times PaCO_2}$$

This equation is useful in assessing acid-base status, first because its components can be measured in an arterial blood gas sample, and second because the $PaCO_2$ reflects the respiratory component of the acid-base balance and the HCO_3^- concentration reflects the metabolic component.

The usefulness of the HCO_3^- concentration can be seen in an example of carbonic acid buffering. If HCl is added to a solution containing sodium bicarbonate ($NaHCO_3$), the major salt of carbonic acid in extracellular fluid, the following reaction takes place:

$$\begin{array}{c} CO_2 + H_2O \\ \Updownarrow \text{ CA} \\ HCl + NaHCO_3 \rightleftarrows H_2CO_3 + NaCl \\ \Updownarrow \\ H^+ + HCO_3^- \end{array}$$

The H^+ produced by the dissociation of H_2CO_3 is less than that which might result from the direct dissociation of H_2CO_3 and is less than that which might result from the direct dissociation of HCl, first because H_2CO_3 dissociates less than HCl (chemical buffering) and second because H_2CO_3 also forms CO_2, which escapes the body through the lungs (physical buffering).

The respiratory contribution of CO_2 is assumed to be held constant in this equation, so that all the CO_2 comes directly from H_2CO_3. In fact, the ready escape of CO_2 drives the reaction toward the CO_2 side so much that very little H^+ is ultimately produced. That which is produced reacts with HCO_3^- to generate CO_2, so the change in HCO_3^- concentration can be used as an index of metabolic alterations in acid-base status.

OTHER BUFFERING SYSTEMS

Strictly speaking, the use of a change in HCO_3^- concentration as a reflection of the amount of H^+ added to or subtracted from a solution is valid only when carbonic acid and its salts are the only buffers in the solution. Yet many noncarbonic buffers are found throughout the body. For example, hemoglobin, which exists within red blood cells as a weak acid and its potassium salt, shares in the extracellular buffering of a metabolic acid or an alkali load. Because of this, the change in HCO_3^- concentration in extracellular fluid (ECF) is not equal to the metabolic acid or base added, as it would be in a pure carbonic acid solution, but is slightly less, approximately 1 milliequivalent per liter (mEq/L) per 0.1 pH unit, or ten times the change in pH. The HCO_3^- changes in the same direction and by a similar amount when $PaCO_2$ changes, for when CO_2 is added to or subtracted from the blood, more or less HCO_3^- is formed.

These changes in HCO_3^- concentration in ECF are not so dissimilar from those that would occur in a carbonic acid solution that they would render the HCO_3^- concentration useless in assessing acid-base status. Indeed, the HCO_3^- concentration offers a good approximation of the direction and magnitude of metabolic disturbance when it has increased or decreased from a normal level of 24 mEq/L by 2 mEq/L or more. Nevertheless, more precise quantification of metabolic disorders, especially when smaller changes in HCO_3^- concentration are present, necessitates that the base excess be calculated. This calculation will not be described here, because it is seldom required in clinical medicine.

ACID-BASE IMBALANCES AND THEIR THERAPY

CHARACTERIZATION OF ACID-BASE STATUS

The relative acidity of blood with a pH of less than 7.35 or so is called acidemia, whereas the relative alkalinity of blood with a pH of 7.45 or greater is called alkalemia. These terms are preferable to the words acidosis and alkalosis, which are used to describe the processes through which acidemia and alkalemia occur. Respiratory acidosis results from an increase in $PaCO_2$; this increase is called hypoventilation because alveolar ventilation ($\dot{V}A$) is decreased. Respiratory alkalosis results from a decrease in $PaCO_2$; this decrease is called hyperventilation inasmuch as $\dot{V}A$ is increased. Metabolic acidosis results from a decrease in HCO_3^- concentration or an increase in H^+ concentration. Respiratory and metabolic acidosis and alkalosis often occur together, either as secondary compensation for one another or as unrelated primary processes. The pH that results may be high, low, or normal, depending on the nature and extent of the processes involved.

CONSEQUENCES OF ACID-BASE IMBALANCE

Regardless of the processes that underlie it, an excess acidity of body fluids, that is, an increase in H^+ and a low pH, generally depresses organ function. This is especially true of the heart, which pumps less effectively. The heart may also lose its inherent rhythmicity and develop a potentially lethal pattern called ventricular fibrillation. Vascular smooth muscle relaxes in the presence of H^+, so blood vessels dilate and become unresponsive to drugs that would otherwise alter their caliber. In acidemia of a respiratory nature, the high CO_2 concentration further dilates cerebral blood vessels and increases blood flow through them. Excess alkalinity, that is, a decrease in H^+ concentration and a high pH, also depresses organ function, and in addition it may lead to a neuromuscular excitability that can precipitate severe cardiac dysrhythmias. Given these possible consequences, it is fortunate that the body defends itself against acid-base imbalance in several ways.

DEFENSES AGAINST ACID-BASE IMBALANCE

Primary disorders of acidosis or alkalosis will produce acidemia or alkalemia, unless defense mechanisms are invoked and homeostasis—in this case, a nearly normal pH—is restored. The initial defense involves the carbonic and noncarbonic buffers described previously and takes minutes to occur. The second defense is called secondary compensation and occurs over several hours to days. In secondary compensation, the ratio of HCO_3^- concentration to $PaCO_2$, contained in the Henderson-Hasselbalch equation for the dissociation of H_2CO_3, is brought toward normal by altering whichever of the two variables was unchanged primarily. Thus, a metabolic acidosis that causes a decrease in HCO_3^- will be compensated for by a respiratory alkalosis that causes a decrease in the $PaCO_2$, and vice versa.

Changes in the HCO_3^- concentration not resulting from carbonic and noncarbonic buffering are controlled by the kidneys, which excrete or retain HCO_3^-, whereas the lungs control $PaCO_2$. Because of this, the Henderson-Hasselbalch equation for H_2CO_3 can be rewritten as

$$pH = pK + \log \frac{kidneys}{lungs}$$

to conceptualize how compensation occurs. Although the $PaCO_2$ can change quickly, the relatively slow process of renal HCO_3^- adjustment accounts for the time required for secondary metabolic compensation. Such compensation rarely is complete, so the pH usually does not return to or overshoot normal. The third and final defense against acid-base imbalance is correction of the primary abnormality if such is possible. An example would be increasing

$\dot{V}A$ in response to a respiratory acidosis related to an increase in $PaCO_2$.

COMMON ACID-BASE DISORDERS AND THEIR TREATMENT

Respiratory Acidosis

This disorder, as noted previously, is caused by alveolar hypo-ventilation and by definition can be present only when the $PaCO_2$ exceeds approximately 45 mmHg. This elevation in $PaCO_2$ is also called hypercapnia. Acute respiratory acidosis usually is a primary disorder seen in sedative drug overdosage, respiratory arrest, or exacerbations of obstructive and restrictive lung disease. Respiratory acidosis also may serve as compensation for metabolic alka-losis, although a $PaCO_2$ over 50 mmHg for purely compensatory reasons is unusual. Although the acidemia of uncompensated respiratory acidosis generally depresses cardiovascular and cerebral function, hypercapnia may increase cardiac irritability through activation of the sympathetic nervous system. It also increases cerebral blood flow: Since CO_2 crosses the blood-brain barrier, acute hypercapnia is a potent stimulus of ventilation in persons who are physically able to breathe.

Acute respiratory acidosis is defended against by buffering and eventually by a renal retention of HCO_3^-, that is, by metabolic alkalosis. Although acute respiratory acidosis can be treated by administration of alkali, this is neither indicated nor necessary if the $PaCO_2$ can be lowered by increasing $\dot{V}A$. If the patient cannot achieve this increase spontaneously, mechanical ventilation may be required. If uncorrected, acute respiratory acidosis may progress to the chronic respiratory acidosis seen in patients with severe obstructive or restrictive lung disease. Such patients become adjusted to the high $PaCO_2$ associated with this condition, and because the pH is near-normal, aggressive therapy of the acid-base disorder is not required. However, intervention often is mandated by the superimposition of acute respiratory acidosis upon chronic respiratory acidosis, as frequently occurs when pulmonary patients develop bronchitis or pneumonia and experience acute hypercapnic respiratory failure. Respiratory failure is discussed in greater detail in Chapter 7.

Respiratory Alkalosis

Respiratory alkalosis results from alveolar hyperventilation and is characterized by a decrease in the $PaCO_2$ to below 35 mmHg. This decrease is also called hypocapnia. Acute respiratory alkalosis may result from anxiety in patients with the acute hyperventilation syndrome. Nonetheless, because a decreased $PaCO_2$ also may accompany shock, sepsis, salicylate intoxication, or overvigorous mechanical ventilation, the diagnosis of hyperventilation syndrome should be one of exclusion. Respiratory alkalosis also may serve as compensation for metabolic acidosis and in such circumstances may be quite profound. The alkalemia associated with uncompensated respiratory alkalosis increases cardiac and cerebral irritability. In addition, hypocapnia decreases cerebral blood flow, and the exchange of extracellular potassium and calcium for intracellular H^+ increases neuromuscular irritability. As a result, cardiac dysrhythmias and seizures may occur in patients with this disorder.

The treatment of acute respiratory alkalosis usually is aimed at its underlying cause. This includes reduction of the minute ventilation of alkalemic patients on mechanical ventilators; correction with metabolic acids such as dilute HCl is rarely required. Chronic respiratory alkalosis is seen in individuals living at high altitudes who are stimulated to hyperventilate by the low ambient-inspired oxygen fraction, patients with restrictive lung disease, and persons undergoing long-term mechanical ventilation. Since the pH is near-normal in such situations, treatment of the acid-base disorder is not required.

Metabolic Acidosis

Metabolic acidosis results from either the loss of HCO_3^- or the addition of H^+ to the body. It is characterized by reduced HCO_3^- concentration. Metabolic acidosis may be divided into one of two types, depending whether or not an anion gap is present. As discussed in Chapter 3, the total number of cations—sodium (Na^+) and potassium (K^+)—and anions—chloride (Cl^-), HCO_3^-, and small amounts of phosphate, sulfate, and other metabolic salts—must be equal for serum or plasma to maintain electrical neutrality. A 10 mEq/L difference between Na^+ and (Cl^- + HCO_3^-) is usually reported in serum samples sent to the laboratory, however, because phosphates, sulfates, and other anions are not measured.

Although HCO_3^- concentration is generally reduced in all forms of metabolic acidosis, the concentration of Cl^- increases when exogenous acids like HCl are ingested, when metabolic acidosis is a compensation for respiratory alkalosis, or in renal tubular acidosis. In these instances, the anion difference or gap does not increase. However, in other disorders the fall in HCO_3^- concentration is balanced by a rise not in Cl^- concentration but instead in the concentrations of other unmeasured anions, and an anion gap greater than 10 mEq/L occurs (Fig. 4–1). In addition to phosphate and sulfate, which may accumulate in renal failure, these unmeasured anions include lactate, the result of anaerobic metabolism; acetate and other products of the breakdown of ketones that occurs during starvation and in diabetes, in which glucose is not metabolized; and certain acidic compounds such as salicylates (Table 4–1). Acute metabolic acidosis with an anion gap due to lactate accumulation is particularly common in patients with poor tissue perfusion, respiratory failure, or both (see Chapter 7).

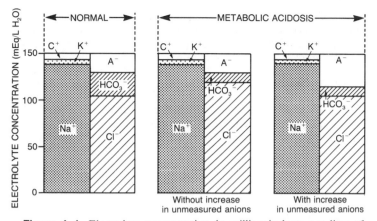

Figure 4–1. Electrolyte concentration in milliequivalents per liter of water (mEq/L H_2O) under normal conditions and during metabolic acidosis, with or without an increase in unmeasured anions. C^+ = unmeasured cations; K^+ = potassium; Na^+ = sodium; A^- = unmeasured anions; HCO_3^- = bicarbonate; Cl^- = chloride.

Whatever its cause, acute metabolic acidosis is a severe acid-base disturbance because pH falls precipitously and body stores of HCO_3^- are depleted. Respiratory alkalosis may provide some compensation, but many patients with lung disease cannot hyperventilate for prolonged periods. Therapy for acute metabolic acidosis is aimed at the underlying disorder, such as the prevention

Table 4–1. CAUSES OF METABOLIC ACIDOSIS

WITH AN INCREASED ANION GAP
Uncontrolled diabetes mellitus
Renal failure
Lactic acidosis
Ingestion of
    Ethyl alcohol, with starvation and production of keto acids
    Salicylate
    Methyl alcohol
    Paraldehyde
    Ethylene glycol
WITH A NORMAL ANION GAP
Diarrhea or loss of other gastrointestinal fluids with high HCO_3^-
    concentrations
Renal tubular acidosis
Ureterosigmoidostomy
Administration of
    HCl
    NH_4Cl
    Carbonic anhydrase inhibitors

KEY: HCO_3^- = bicarbonate, HCl = hydrochloric acid, NH_4Cl = ammonium chloride.

of anaerobic metabolism and excess lactic acid production by increasing blood supply to a patient's tissues or the prevention of ketone metabolism by supplying a diabetic patient with insulin. When this will not suffice, or when the pH is below 7.0 or the HCO_3^- concentration is below 5 mEq/L, HCO_3^- (in the form of $NaHCO_3$) should be given.

The dose of HCO_3^- in mEq/L may be calculated by the following formula: HCO_3^- mEq needed = (normal HCO_3^- concentration of 24 mEq/L − observed HCO_3^- concentration) × (0.4 × body weight in kg). For practical purposes, however, and to avoid giving too much HCO_3^-, $NaHCO_3$ usually is given in one-ampule (44 mEq) boluses, and the pH and serum HCO_3^- concentration are followed closely to avoid overcompensation and the creation of metabolic alkalosis. The patient's intravascular volume status also must be monitored, because the Na^+ administered in $NaHCO_3$ remains in the ECF and attracts water from the intracellular fluid (ICF); this latter action may cause coma, owing to hypertonicity of cells in the central nervous system (see Chapter 3). Chronic metabolic acidosis, as may occur in patients with chronic diarrhea or renal failure, may also require supplemental HCO_3^- to replenish body HCO_3^- stores and to prevent the dissolution of bone, which serves as a buffer when HCO_3^- concentration is low. Clinicians should bear in mind that HCO_3^- ultimately will be converted into CO_2 and cause respiratory acidosis unless the CO_2 can be eliminated by the lungs.

Metabolic Alkalosis

Metabolic alkalosis results from the loss of H^+ or the addition of HCO_3^- to the body. It is usually generated by the loss of H^+, Na^+, and K^+, either from the gastrointestinal tract during vomiting or nasogastric suctioning or from the kidneys in patients taking diuretics, such as thiazides, that block the renal reabsorption of Cl^-. Extracellular fluid volume is decreased in all these situations, so the metabolic alkalosis is maintained by enhanced renal reabsorption of $NaHCO_3$ in an effort to support ECF volume. Total body Cl^- stores also are reduced, since Cl^- is the major anion for the cations lost from the body, and the urinary Cl^- concentration should be less than 10 mEq/L. This indicates that the alkalosis should be chloride-responsive; that is, it should be correctable with Cl^-. Metabolic alkalosis can also occur with a normal or high ECF volume in patients with severe K^+ depletion and hyperaldosteronism, in which case the urinary Cl^- concentration should be greater than 10 mEq/L. This indicates that the alkalosis may not respond to only Cl^-.

The formula used above to determine HCO_3^- depletion may be used to estimate Cl^- depletion by substituting Cl^- for the final calculated HCO_3^-, since a reciprocal relationship exists between HCO_3^- and Cl^-. For practical purposes, Cl^- is usually given as

NaCl while serum electrolytes are monitored. Supplemental K^+ is needed for patients who are not chloride-responsive; it can usually be given as KCl. In fact, some clinicians give KCl to all patients with metabolic alkalosis without worrying about why it has occurred. Patients whose ECF volume is normal or increased or in whom metabolic and respiratory alkalosis coexist may be treated with dilute HCl, although this is seldom necessary.

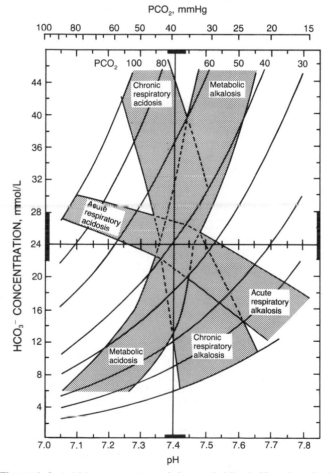

Figure 4–2. Acid-base nomogram of changes in blood pH, carbon dioxide tension (PCO_2) in millimeters of mercury (mmHg), and bicarbonate (HCO_3^-) concentration in millimols per liter (mmol/L). The acid-base disturbance can be named by finding the point at which these variables intersect on the nomogram.

Combined Acid-Base Disorders

Combinations of the above disorders occur commonly and are particularly severe if the respiratory and metabolic processes are in the same direction, as in the case of combined respiratory and metabolic alkalosis just cited. When this occurs, the blood pH is so alkalemic (or acidemic, in the case of combined respiratory and metabolic acidosis) that the question of whether one process is compensatory for the other is rarely raised. This question does come up, however, when the processes oppose each other and the possibility that one is primary exists. One approach to this problem is to use empirically developed nomograms that plot changes in pH and $PaCO_2$ and HCO_3^- concentrations in various states (Fig. 4–2). Another approach is to remember that because secondary compensation rarely returns the pH to normal and never overshoots in the opposite direction, the primary process is likely to be reflected in the pH.

When three acid-base disturbances may be present, the following approach is advised. First, the anion gap should be calculated; if it is greater than 10 mEq/L, a primary anion gap metabolic acidosis must exist because compensating metabolic acidosis is of the non-anion gap variety. Next, the excess anion gap, which is the difference between the measured anion gap and the normal gap of 10 mEq/L, should be calculated and added to the measured HCO_3^- concentration. This will yield the HCO_3^- concentration that was present before the most recent acid-base disturbance occurred. If the sum is greater than 22 mEq/L, an underlying metabolic alkalosis must be present; if the sum is less than 22 mEq/L, an underlying non–anion gap metabolic acidosis must exist.

RECOMMENDED READING

1. Andreoli TE: Disorders of fluid volume, electrolyte, and acid-base balance. *In* Wyngaarden JB, and Smith LH (eds.): *Cecil's Textbook of Medicine,* 17th ed. Philadelphia, W.B. Saunders Co., 1985, pp. 515–543.
2. Culver BH (ed.): *The Respiratory System: Syllabus for Human Biology 540.* Seattle, University of Washington, Lecture Notes, 1982.
3. Emmett M, and Narins RC: Clinical use of the anion gap. *Medicine* (Baltimore), 56:38–54, 1977.
4. Gabow PA, et al.: Diagnostic importance of an increased anion gap. *N Engl J Med,* 303:854–858, 1980.
5. Haber RJ: A practical approach to acid-base disorders. *West J Med,* 155:146–151, 1991.
6. Kreisberg M: Lactate homeostasis and lactic acidosis. *Ann Intern Med,* 92:227–237, 1980.
7. Ott SM, and Luce JM: Acid-base disturbances. *In* Luce JM, and Peirson DJ (eds.): *Critical Care Medicine.* Philadelphia, W.B. Saunders Co., 1988, pp. 271–283.
8. Pitts RF: *Physiology of the Kidney and Body Fluids,* 3rd ed. Chicago, Year Book Medical Publishers, 1974.

9. Schrier RW: *Renal and Electrolyte Disorders,* 2nd ed. Boston, Little, Brown & Co., 1980.

10. Seldin DW, and Rector FC: Symposium on acid-base homeostasis: the generation and maintenance of metabolic alkalosis. *Kidney Int,* 1:306–312, 1972.

11. Shapiro BA, et al.: *Clinical Application of Blood Gases,* 3rd ed. Chicago, Year Book Medical Publishers, 1982.

5

A PHYSIOLOGICAL APPROACH TO RESPIRATORY DISEASE

CATEGORIZATION OF RESPIRATORY DISEASES

OVERVIEW

Respiratory diseases may be categorized in terms of anatomical position or pathology, etiology, or epidemiology. Another approach is to organize them into four types on the basis of their underlying pathophysiology. Respiratory diseases involving gas exchange in the lung include obstructive diseases that reduce airflow, restrictive diseases that limit lung volumes, vascular diseases that diminish the alveolar-capillary membrane, and disorders of ventilatory regulation.

OBSTRUCTIVE PULMONARY DISEASES

GENERAL PRINCIPLES

Factors Affecting Airflow

Obstructive pulmonary diseases are so named because they slow the rate of airflow into and out of the lungs. Airflow between the atmosphere and the alveoli depends on the pressure gradient and the resistance between the two as expressed in the formula for flow in any hydraulic system: flow $(\dot{Q})$ = pressure (P)/resistance (R). Thus, the rate of airflow can be limited by a decrease in P, an increase in R, or a combination of the two. The pressure gradient required for airflow is the difference between atmospheric pressure at the mouth and pressure in the alveoli or whatever part of the airway causes flow limitation, if it exists. At the same time, the driving pressure for airflow is the difference between alveolar and pleural pressures, which is called the transpulmonary pressure. During passive expiration, the transpulmonary pressure is the recoil pressure of the lung, as the respiratory muscles are not actively contracting. Because of this relationship, obstructive diseases that decrease recoil pressure reduce airflow.

Inspiration

Resistance to airflow depends on the viscosity of gas and the length and caliber of the conducting airways. Airway caliber is related to position of the airways in the tracheobronchial tree, bronchial smooth muscle tone, mucus secretions, pressure across the airway wall, and lung volume. Atmospheric pressure is greater than the pressure in the lumen of the upper airway outside the thorax during inspiration, so the upper airway tends to collapse. This situation is reversed in the intrathoracic airways, which are held open because their intraluminal pressure exceeds the surrounding pleural pressure. Patients with upper airway obstruction may have difficult and noisy breathing, called stridor, during inspiration. Airflow obstruction can be measured in such patients by flow-volume loops or spirometry; these techniques are described in Chapter 6.

Expiration

During expiration the pressure inside the upper airway is greater than atmospheric pressure, so the extrathoracic airway is held open. However, since pleural pressure is more positive than that inside the intrathoracic airways, they tend to collapse. All but the most peripheral airways remain open in normal people so that air is evacuated from the lungs during expiration at a normal rate. By contrast, patients with lower airways obstruction frequently exhibit slow flow rates on spirometry and trap air in their lungs, increasing their residual volume (RV). This situation is worsened by forced expiration involving respiratory muscle contraction. In this situation, the pleural pressure becomes even more positive and causes a greater degree of dynamic airway compression, especially if the tissue surrounding the airways is weakened by a disease such as emphysema (Fig. 5–1). Attempts to overcome this compression by generating greater expiratory muscle force are fruitless and merely increase the already high work of breathing that characterizes airway obstruction.

Gas Exchange Abnormalities in Obstruction

Obstructive pulmonary disease usually is associated with hypoxemia related to ventilation-perfusion ($\dot{V}A/\dot{Q}$) mismatching. Hypo-

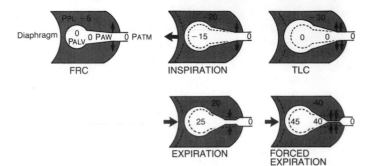

Figure 5–1. Dynamic expansion of airways during inspiration from functional residual capacity (FRC) to total lung capacity (TLC) and compression of airways during passive and forced expiration to residual volume (RV). The driving pressure for airflow is the difference between pleural pressure (PPL) and alveolar pressure (PALV), which is called the transpulmonary pressure. The pressure gradient required for airflow is the difference between atmospheric pressure at the mouth (PATM) and the pressure in the alveoli (or pressure at any part of the airway, PAW, that causes flow limitation). During passive expiration, the transpulmonary pressure reflects only the recoil pressure of the lung because the respiratory muscles are not active. During forced expiration, when the respiratory muscles are active, the highly positive pleural pressure collapses intrathoracic airways near the mouth, especially when the airways are weakened by disease. Because of this, increased muscular effort does not increase airflow. Arrows indicate direction of motion of diaphragm.

ventilation, reflected in an elevated arterial carbon dioxide tension ($PaCO_2$), may be caused late in the course of disease by an increased alveolar dead space due to ventilation of poorly perfused areas of the lung. The patients have an inability, because of severely disordered ventilatory mechanics or abnormal ventilatory regulation, to compensate for this dead space by augmenting minute ventilation.

UPPER AIRWAY OBSTRUCTION

Obstructive Sleep Apnea

Sleep apnea may be defined as cessation of airflow at the nose and mouth for ten seconds or longer during sleep. Clinically significant sleep apnea is present if the patient averages five or more such episodes per hour over several hours of sleep. Three forms of sleep apnea have been distinguished: central apnea, in which the cessation of airflow is accompanied by a lack of respiratory muscle movement, indicating a disorder of ventilatory regulation; upper airway obstructive apnea, in which airflow is absent despite respiratory muscle movement; and mixed apnea, in which an episode of cessation of airflow is associated initially with lack of muscle movement and later by resumption of unsuccessful ventilatory efforts.

Upper airway obstructive sleep apnea was first noted in children with jaw deformities or hypertrophied tonsils and adenoids. It subsequently has been reported in patients, many of them obese men, with extreme relaxation of the pharyngeal muscles during sleep. Some patients with sleep apnea are asymptomatic; others suffer from daytime somnolence and sequelae of nocturnal hypoxemia and hypercapnia, such as headaches. The treatment of obstructive apnea involves removal of the obstruction; this includes weight loss in the obese. Permanent tracheostomy may be indicated if these measures fail. Continuous positive airway pressure applied nasally also may be quite effective (see Chapter 17). Central sleep apnea may be treated with the drugs progesterone and protriptyline.

LOWER AIRWAY OBSTRUCTION

Asthma

Asthma, which also may be thought of as reversible obstructive pulmonary disease, is a disorder in which the lower airways narrow in response to various stimuli and then usually widen spontaneously or after treatment. Narrowing is due to contraction of bronchial smooth muscle, thickening of the bronchial walls with swelling and hyperplasia of mucus-secreting cells, and plugging of the airways with secretions. The causes of this condition are many; some patients respond to specific allergens, such as pollen or animal dander, whereas attacks in others are triggered by cigarette smoke and other irritants, emotional stress, upper respiratory infections, or exercise. Some patients, usually children with a history of allergic reactions and positive skin tests, are said to have extrinsic asthma. Others, usually adults in whom specific allergens cannot be identified, are said to have the intrinsic form of the disease. Many of the latter are cigarette smokers with chronic bronchitis and emphysema. Airway inflammation probably is present in all patients with asthma.

Asthmatic patients of both types manifest decreased airflow rates and increased lung volumes, especially RV, due to air trapping during acute attacks. They are generally hypoxemic because of low $\dot{V}_A/\dot{Q}$ mismatching. The $PaCO_2$ is low in the early stages of an acute attack, when $\dot{V}_A$ is more than adequate; an increased $PaCO_2$ suggests that the patients are tiring and that emergency intubation and mechanical ventilation may be necessary. Fortunately, most asthma attacks can be reversed by the drugs discussed in Chapter 11. These include beta-adrenergic agonists, such as isoproterenol;

theophylline; and corticosteroids. Asthma attacks can be prevented in some patients by the regular inhalation of metaproterenol corticosteroids or cromolyn sodium, both of which reduce airway inflammation.

Chronic Bronchitis

Chronic bronchitis is a clinical diagnosis given to patients with cough productive of sputum on most days for at least three months per year during two successive years. The sputum production results from bronchial mucous glands that hypertrophy and increase in number in response to chronic irritation. These excessive secretions increase airflow obstruction and low $\dot{V}A/\dot{Q}$ mismatching in some, but not all, patients. A few individuals with profound hypoxemia also develop right ventricular enlargement and cor pulmonale. In the United States, chronic bronchitis is seen almost exclusively in cigarette smokers, as is emphysema. Treatment includes cessation of smoking and the administration of antibiotics, such as ampicillin, that are thought to decrease the amount of bacteria, including *Streptococcus pneumoniae* and *Haemophilus influenzae*, that colonize the lower airways.

Emphysema

Emphysema is a pathological diagnosis that describes the distention and destruction of alveolar walls. This decrease in functional lung tissue causes airflow obstruction primarily by reducing elastic recoil. The airways also tend to collapse because they are no longer held open by adjacent tissue. In many patients, alveolar destruction is accompanied by a loss of capillaries that leads to an overall decrease in size of the alveolar-capillary membrane; this can be identified by a diminution in diffusing capacity. Ventilation and perfusion may decrease by equal amounts in this circumstance, so that $\dot{V}A/\dot{Q}$ mismatch and the hypoxemia that would result from it do not occur. Nevertheless, hypoxemia is usually present in the late stages of the disease, especially if chronic bronchitis also exists. Cigarette smoking is linked to emphysema by unknown mechanisms. A genetic predisposition to this disorder is seen in patients with alpha$_1$-antitrypsin deficiency. Inasmuch as emphysema is irreversible, no treatment is available for the disease. However, respiratory muscle endurance training is tried in some patients (see Chapter 17). Furthermore, patients who stop smoking may prevent further destruction of their lungs.

What Is Chronic Obstructive Pulmonary Disease?

Strictly speaking, chronic obstructive pulmonary disease (COPD) could refer to any longstanding obstructive process. Yet the term is generally used to describe the lesion in patients, most of them cigarette smokers, who exhibit either chronic bronchitis, emphysema, or a combination of the two. Some of these patients also manifest intrinsic asthma and therefore are said to have a reversible component of airflow obstruction. Patients with COPD generally are not divided into clinical subsets but are instead treated empirically as if they had all three components. Thus, they may receive antibiotic therapy for presumed chronic bronchitis, bronchodilator therapy for asthma, respiratory muscle training for emphysema, and supplemental O_2 for cor pulmonale.

Bronchiectasis

Bronchiectasis is a permanent dilatation of one or more large bronchi caused by destruction of the elastic and muscular components of the bronchial wall due to chronic infection. Sputum production becomes excessive. This disease occurs in patients with recurrent severe respiratory infections, especially in youth, and in patients with tuberculosis, cystic fibrosis, or ciliary dyskinesia.

Cystic Fibrosis

Cystic fibrosis is a chronic obstructive disease complicated by bronchiectasis that is associated with dysfunction of the pancreas and liver. It is transmitted genetically (autosomal recessive) and affects one in 2000 white infants. The pulmonary manifestations of cystic fibrosis usually begin in childhood with the secretion of thick mucus. The larger airways become infected by mucoid strains of *Pseudomonas aeruginosa* and *Escherichia coli*; mucus then becomes purulent. Cystic fibrosis is diagnosed by documenting a high sodium (Na^+) concentration in sweat. Treatment is aimed at replacing losses in addition to thinning secretions with hydration and antibiotics and removing them with chest clapping, postural drainage, and coughing. Pancreatic enzymes are given to patients with concurrent malabsorption due to pancreatic insufficiency.

RESTRICTIVE PULMONARY DISEASES

GENERAL PRINCIPLES

Restrictive pulmonary diseases are characterized by a reduction in lung volumes. They are caused by disorders that limit the normal amount or the expansion of lung tissue: abnormalities of the thoracic cage, respiratory muscle dysfunction, diseases occupying lung space, and diseases occupying the pleural space. To enlarge the thoracic cage and to expand the lung during inspiration, the respiratory muscles must generate a pressure greater than the recoil pressure of the lung. The ratio of volume change in inspiration per unit change in recoil pressure is called respiratory system compliance (CRS). Compliance is decreased in all restrictive diseases, just as airflow resistance is increased in obstructive diseases. The work of breathing is also increased as CRS decreases, inasmuch as more muscle contraction is required to generate the pressure needed to increase the volume of the lungs.

Restrictive disease is diagnosed by a decrease in lung volumes, particularly in total lung capacity (TLC). Flow rates are normal or even high in this condition because the airways may be held open by the stiff lungs. The PaO_2 usually is low due to $\dot{V}A/\dot{Q}$ mismatching. The $PaCO_2$ may be low early in the course of illness, presumably because of mechanical reflexes that stimulate ventilation, but will increase if the restriction becomes too severe.

ABNORMALITIES OF THE THORACIC CAGE

Obesity

The respiratory complications of obesity relate primarily to obese patients' heavy lower thorax and abdomen, which severely reduce lung volumes, especially in the supine position. This reduction is most marked in functional residual capacity (FRC), the point at which the outward force of the thoracic cage and the inward recoil pressure of the lungs are balanced. If FRC is reduced enough, the distal airways and alveoli at the bases are closed and no longer participate in gas exchange. This condition, which is called atelectasis, can be duplicated by confining a normal person in a tight corset or cast. Since ventilation at the bases is poor but blood flow is preferentially distributed there owing to gravity, $\dot{V}A/\dot{Q}$ mismatching and hypoxemia result. The hypoxemia may be worse at night if the patients also suffer from obstructive sleep apnea.

Some obese patients also are hypercapnic, probably because of a combination of severe mechanical limitations, CO_2 retention at night, and abnormal ventilatory regulation. Obese patients with hypoxemia, hypercapnia, daytime somnolence, cor pulmonale, and polycythemia (an increase in the amount of red blood cells to compensate for hypoxemia) are said to have the obesity-hypoventilation syndrome, or pickwickian syndrome. Most of the respiratory complications of obesity, including the obesity-hypoventilation syndrome, are reversible upon weight loss.

RESPIRATORY MUSCLE DYSFUNCTION

Generalized Neuromuscular Weakness

Restrictive pulmonary disease can result from a variety of neuromuscular disorders, including poliomyelitis, Guillain-Barré syndrome, myasthenia gravis, tetanus, botulism, and muscular dystrophy. It also may be seen in electrolyte disturbances that affect muscle function, such as severe hypokalemia. Although most of these disorders cause diffuse muscle weakness, ventilatory performance is severely compromised only if the diaphragm is involved.

Cervical Cord Injury

Cervical spinal cord trauma, spinal artery infarction, or cord compression by tumor may cause two different types of quadriplegia. Severe damage at or above cord segments C-3 to C-5 involves the phrenic nerves and causes partial or complete bilateral diaphragmatic paralysis. Because the hemidiaphragms cannot contract effectively, the lower ribcage does not expand laterally during inspiration. In addition, intercostal muscle paralysis caudal to the lesion limits lateral extension of the middle and upper ribcage. Sternocleidomastoid, scalene, and trapezoid activity persists in high cord injuries, but contraction of these muscles causes an increase primarily in the anterior-posterior dimensions of the upper ribcage and pulls the hemidiaphragms toward the head. Abdominal paradox, in which the abdominal wall is sucked in by the negative intra-abdominal pressure as the hemidiaphragms ascend, is a sign of diaphragmatic dysfunction in patients who inspire only with their accessory muscles (Fig. 5–2).

As a result of their profound respiratory muscle dysfunction, patients with high cervical quadriplegia are unable to generate an adequate vital capacity (VC) during inspiration. They therefore manifest high $PaCO_2$ and low PaO_2. The hypoxemia of these patients results both from hypoventilation and from microatelectasis that occurs because of retained secretions and because the inward recoil of the lungs is no longer affected by the outward recoil of the chest wall. Hypercapnia and hypoxemia frequently worsen when the patients breathe spontaneously in the supine position and their abdominal contents force the hemidiaphragms cephalad. Alveolar hypoventilation is even more pronounced during sleep, a phenomenon that has been ascribed to diminished CO_2 responsiveness, but more likely results from inhibition of intercostal and accessory muscle activity.

Quadriplegic patients with lesions in the lower cervical cord, whose phrenic nerve nuclei are completely or partially intact, can contract their hemidiaphragms to a greater or lesser extent. Nevertheless, they lack the intercostal muscle activity necessary to stabilize the ribcage so that the hemidiaphragms can function properly. Diaphragmatic contraction therefore results in paradoxical inward motion of the upper and middle ribcage during inspiration until the chest wall stiffens because of spasticity or fibrosis of muscles, as it eventually does in most patients with chronic neuromuscular disease. Furthermore, because these patients lack

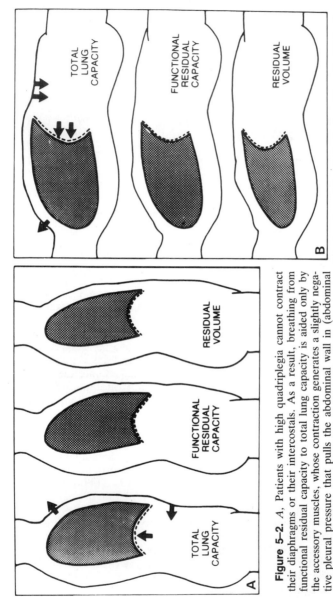

Figure 5–2. *A*, Patients with high quadriplegia cannot contract their diaphragms or their intercostals. As a result, breathing from functional residual capacity to total lung capacity is aided only by the accessory muscles, whose contraction generates a slightly negative pleural pressure that pulls the abdominal wall in (abdominal paradox). Expiration to residual volume cannot be achieved because of dysfunction of the abdominal muscles. *B*, Although patients with high quadriplegia are capable of minimal inspiration when upright, their diaphragms are displaced even more toward the head as a result of gravity when they are supine. This results in an even smaller inspiratory volume. (From Luce JM, and Pierson DJ (eds.): *Critical Care Medicine*. Philadelphia, W. B. Saunders Co., 1988, p. 438.)

abdominal muscle tone, their hemidiaphragms cannot contract from the steeply domed position in which their fiber length-tension relationship is optimized. Thus, their VC and TLC are diminished. This diminution is most pronounced when the patients sit up and the hemidiaphragms are not supported by their abdominal contents; it is minimized when they are supine (Fig. 5–3).

The other major problem in patients with cervical cord lesions at any level is that they cannot exhale forcefully to RV. This is primarily because they have lost the use of their abdominal and other expiratory muscles. At the same time, the patients cannot inhale to TLC because of inspiratory muscle dysfunction. The combination of expiratory and inspiratory weakness prevents them from coughing and clearing secretions. Recent studies have demonstrated that some quadriplegics use the clavicular portion of their pectoralis major muscles to reduce RV toward normal and have suggested that patients might cough more effectively by training these muscles. Nevertheless, many patients do not use their muscles in this fashion and therefore are at high risk of respiratory tract infections, including pneumonia.

Unilateral Diaphragmatic Paralysis

Unilateral diaphragmatic paralysis most often results from involvement of a phrenic nerve by tumor, trauma, or infection. It induces immobility of the ipsilateral abdominal wall and a lag in the upward movement of the thoracic cage over the involved hemidiaphragm during inspiration to TLC (Fig. 5–4). Yet this frequently is obscured by the proper functioning of the contralateral hemidiaphragm, and adult patients usually can tolerate the slight drop in PaO_2 seen in this disorder. Nevertheless, ventilatory failure has been observed in infants following disruption of the phrenic nerve at surgery.

DISEASES AFFECTING LUNG TISSUE

Pneumonia

Pneumonia refers to any pulmonary infection that involves alveolar tissue, in contrast to interstitial disease. Viral, fungal, parasitic, mycobacterial (tuberculous), and protozoal *(Pneumocystis carinii)* pneumonias occur, especially in patients with severely impaired defense mechanisms, but bacterial pneumonia is most common in otherwise normal individuals. The airways should be sterile below the larynx, although the airways of patients with chronic bronchitis, bronchiectasis, or cystic fibrosis are colonized with bacteria there. In other persons, bacteria can reach the lungs by aspiration of oropharyngeal contents, by means of the bloodstream, or by aerosolization in gases inhaled from contaminated

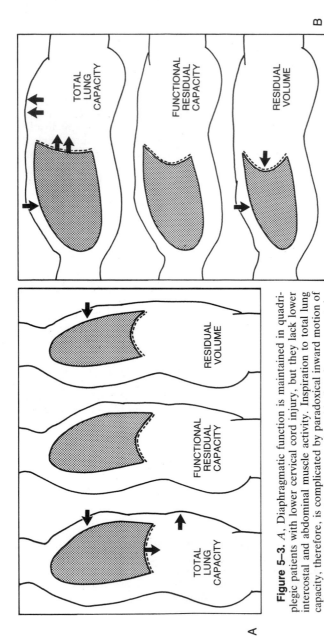

Figure 5–3. *A,* Diaphragmatic function is maintained in quadriplegic patients with lower cervical cord injury, but they lack lower intercostal and abdominal muscle activity. Inspiration to total lung capacity, therefore, is complicated by paradoxical inward motion of the upper thorax, whereas normal residual volume cannot be achieved in expiration because of abdominal muscle dysfunction. The slight inward movement of the chest wall in expiration is accomplished by contraction of the pectoralis major muscle. *B,* Lower quadriplegic patients are more comfortable in the supine position, in which the abdominal viscera push up to the diaphragm and enhance its activity. Arrows indicate direction of movement, not muscular force applied. (From Luce JM, and Culver BH: Respiratory muscle function in health and disease. *Chest,* 81:82–90, 1982.)

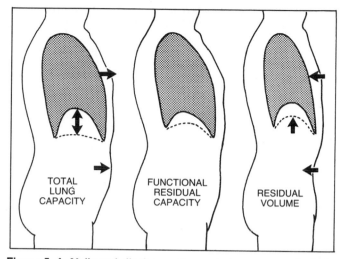

Figure 5–4. Unilateral diaphragmatic paralysis causes paradoxical upward displacement of the involved hemidiaphragm during inspiration to total lung capacity. The paralyzed hemidiaphragm usually rides higher in the chest at functional residual capacity. Arrows indicate direction of movement, not force applied. (From Luce JM, and Culver BH: Respiratory muscle function in health and disease. *Chest,* 81:82–90, 1982. Reprinted by permission of the publisher.)

respiratory therapy equipment. If the bacteria are not cleared by alveolar macrophages, an intense inflammatory reaction occurs. Symptoms of this reaction include fever, cough productive of purulent sputum, and chest pain. Hypoxemia is caused by low $\dot{V}_A/\dot{Q}$ mismatching and shunt. Pneumonia that is successfully treated by the appropriate antimicrobial drugs usually results in complete resolution of symptoms and restoration of lung architecture.

Lung Tumors

Benign or malignant tumors in the lung can cause pain, hemoptysis, and a host of other symptoms. Their major physiological effect is to decrease lung volume and to cause hypoxemia through $\dot{V}_A/\dot{Q}$ mismatching. Some tumors also obstruct airways and limit airflow. Their public health impact is much more striking than the physiological abnormalities they cause.

Interstitial Diseases

Interstitial diseases primarily involve the supporting structures of the lung rather than the airspaces, although overlap often occurs.

These disorders are legion: they include reactions to organic and inorganic dust, neoplastic infiltrates, sarcoidosis, and idiopathic pulmonary fibrosis. Restriction is due to infiltration of the interstitium with inflammatory cells and, as the disease progresses, scar tissue. Symptoms include dry cough and breathlessness that is related in part to hypoxemia and in part to mechanical reflexes from the lung. Treatment is aimed at the underlying process; corticosteroids are often used.

Neonatal and Adult Respiratory Distress Syndromes

The distress syndromes are a common cause of respiratory failure. They are covered in Chapter 7.

DISEASES AFFECTING PLEURAL SPACE

Collections of air (pneumothorax) or fluid (pleural effusion) in the pleural space interfere with the mechanics of ventilation and may seriously compromise lung function. These diseases are discussed in Chapter 19.

PULMONARY VASCULAR DISEASES

GENERAL PRINCIPLES

Pulmonary vascular diseases diminish the surface area of the alveolar-capillary membrane. This reduction is most commonly due to generalized constriction of the smooth muscle of the blood vessels through the process of hypoxic pulmonary vasoconstriction (described in Chapter 2). Pulmonary vascular disease may also result from thromboemboli and infiltrative disorders that obliterate the vascular bed and from chronic left-sided heart failure that induces changes in the pulmonary vessels. Lung volumes usually are normal in vascular disease unless the concomitant infiltration of lung tissue is widespread. Airflow rates are also normal unless compression of the airways is caused by scar tissue or edema fluid. The $PaCO_2$ is generally low owing to hyperventilation; the PaO_2 also is low owing to $\dot{V}A/\dot{Q}$ mismatching. Most important, the dead space ventilation fraction (V_D/V_T) is increased because many areas of the lung are not perfused with blood, and the diffusion capacity is decreased because the surface area of the alveolar-capillary membrane is reduced. These abnormalities characteristically worsen with exercise.

PULMONARY HEART DISEASE

Right ventricular enlargement and elevated end-diastolic right ventricular pressures most commonly occur secondary to left heart failure but may also result from lung disease. The latter condition is called pulmonary heart disease, or cor pulmonale. Although its onset may be acute if the pulmonary circulation is blocked by emboli, cor pulmonale more often represents the end stage of severe restrictive or obstructive pulmonary disease. The major mechanism of cor pulmonale in these conditions is hypoxic pulmonary vasoconstriction.

Patients with cor pulmonale often show the signs of right heart failure: distended neck veins, liver enlarged by pooled venous blood, and peripheral edema. Large pulmonary arteries may be evident on the chest roentgenogram, and the electrocardiogram (ECG) reveals right atrial and right ventricular enlargement. Treatment is aimed at reversing alveolar hypoxia with bronchodilating drugs and antibiotics and by judiciously increasing the amount of inspired O_2. Diuretics may be used to reduce edema. Digitalis has little effect on the right ventricle and generally is reserved for patients with left ventricular disease.

PULMONARY THROMBOEMBOLISM

Thrombi are plugs in the heart or blood vessels that are composed of blood elements; emboli are sudden blockages of an artery by foreign material. Pulmonary thromboembolism results from passage of thrombi into the pulmonary artery. Clinically recognized pulmonary thromboembolism usually is an acute process involving large vessels in the lung, although recurrent embolization to small arteries may be overlooked until patients exhibit the symptoms of chronic pulmonary vascular disease. The thrombi originate in the right atrium or the right ventricle or, more commonly, in the deep veins of the thighs, prostate, or pelvis in persons predisposed to this condition by virtue of chronic heart failure, neoplasms, immobilization, surgery, or trauma. The thromboemboli cause ischemia of lung tissue deprived of pulmonary arterial blood, but infarction is rare because the bronchial circulation usually supplies blood to the affected area. Hemoptysis, the coughing up of blood, may occur if infarction is present; more common symptoms include dyspnea and chest pain. Hypoxemia usually occurs because of $\dot{V}A/\dot{Q}$ mismatching due to the release of bronchospastic substances. Although VD/VT rises, the $PaCO_2$ usually is reduced because alveolar ventilation increases in response to hypoxemia and to the thromboemboli themselves.

The diagnosis of pulmonary thromboembolism may be made by radionuclide lung scans, which reveal areas of normal ventilation where perfusion is lacking. Pulmonary arteriography may be necessary in patients, such as those with COPD, whose ventilation and perfusion are abnormal to begin with. The traditional treatment of pulmonary thromboembolism is designed to prevent further clot propagation and recurrent embolization by administration of the anticoagulants heparin and Coumadin, heparin immediately and Coumadin over subsequent weeks or months. A newer approach is to dissolve clots acutely with substances such as streptokinase and urokinase. This therapy is indicated primarily when thromboembolism causes severe hemodynamic compromise.

LEFT HEART FAILURE

Left heart failure may occur at the level of the left ventricle, after myocardial infarction, or of the left atrium, as with mitral valve stenosis. The elevated end-diastolic filling pressures in these chambers cause an increase in pulmonary venous pressure; pulmonary artery pressure must then increase to maintain cardiac output. The increase in pulmonary venous pressure unbalances the Starling forces (discussed in Chapter 3), so fluid transudes from the pulmonary capillaries into the interstitium and, ultimately, into the alveoli. This fluid may be bloody if red blood cells also leak from the capillaries.

Although airflow obstruction may occur owing to compression of the airways by edema, a restrictive defect is more common; thus, pulmonary edema may be classified as a restrictive pulmonary disease. Hypoxemia due to low $\dot{V}A/\dot{Q}$ mismatch and shunt is present. The $PaCO_2$ is usually low. Irreversible pulmonary vascular disease occurs acutely in very few instances, and the diffusing capacity may actually increase in response to an augmented intravascular volume. However, the diffusing capacity eventually decreases in chronic left heart failure as the pulmonary arteries and arterioles are altered by the high pulmonary artery pressures.

The symptoms of left heart failure are breathlessness, especially while the patient is recumbent at night, and fatigue, owing to a progressive decline in the cardiac output. Signs and symptoms of secondary right ventricular failure may occur with both acute and chronic left heart failure. Patients may have a large heart on chest roentgenogram. The ECG may show left atrial and left ventricular hypertrophy. The diagnosis of left heart failure frequently is made by demonstrating elevated left-sided pressures, including an increased pulmonary artery wedge tracing. Treatment involves increasing left ventricular contractility with digitalis, lowering systemic vascular resistance with vasodilating drugs, or repairing damaged valves.

DISORDERED VENTILATORY REGULATION

GENERAL PRINCIPLES

Disorders of ventilatory regulation cause hypoventilation or hyperventilation. Although these disorders may be due to primary dysfunction of the ventilatory control center or of the central or peripheral chemoreceptors, they generally are manifested only in patients with concurrent obstructive, restrictive, or pulmonary vascular disease. Disordered regulation may be suspected when ventilatory responses to hypercapnia or hypoxemia are inappropriate. The chronicity of these inappropriate responses is suggested by high or low bicarbonate concentration and base excess reflecting metabolic compensation for prolonged hypoventilation or hyperventilation. Assuming that mechanical limitations have been excluded, the diagnosis of disordered regulation is confirmed by observing an abnormal response to breathing low O_2 or high CO_2 mixtures in the laboratory.

HYPOVENTILATION

Central Hypoventilation

Hypoventilation may follow neurological damage to the ventilatory control center in the brainstem by infection, trauma, tumor, or vascular insufficiency. Central sleep apnea presumably is one manifestation of such damage. Another is Ondine's curse, in which patients with ventilatory center hyposensitivity breathe normally while awake but stop breathing entirely during sleep, when they lack higher cortical inputs.

Chemical Hypoventilation

Chemical depression of the ventilatory control center and the chemoreceptors is caused by narcotic and sedative-hypnotic drugs, especially in high concentrations. Patients with metabolic alkalosis also hypoventilate, as do those with hypothyroidism. In such patients with normal lungs, the alveolar-to-arterial PO_2 gradient $[P(A-a)O_2]$ should be normal. If it is increased, another cause of hypoxemia, such as $\dot{V}A/\dot{Q}$ mismatching produced by the aspiration of gastric contents, should be sought.

HYPERVENTILATION

Central Hyperventilation

Central neurogenic hyperventilation may result from injuries to the brainstem. Nevertheless, acute or chronic anxiety is the most common cause of hyperventilation. Although many people will overbreathe in response to pain and anticipated medical or surgical procedures, patients with the so-called hyperventilation syndrome have more persistent anxiety. Despite its common occurrence, the hyperventilation syndrome remains a diagnosis of exclusion, and it should not result in an abnormal $P(A-a)O_2$.

Chemical Hyperventilation

Many drugs, such as amphetamines, increase ventilation only by increasing CO_2 production and should not be considered ventilatory stimulants. Other agents, such as doxapram, stimulate ventilation more selectively but also are capable of generalized central nervous system stimulation. Progesterone, a hormone that increases during pregnancy and the luteal phase of the menstrual cycle, appears to stimulate ventilation without these other effects and is useful for chronic therapy in some situations. It is used in treating some patients with chronic hypoventilation, including those with central sleep apnea and the obesity-hypoventilation syndrome. Hyperventilation is also a response to metabolic acidosis and to hypoxemia.

RECOMMENDED READING

1. Boot TF: Cystic fibroses. In Murray JF, and Nadel JA (eds.): *Textbook of Respiratory Medicine*. Philadelphia, W.B. Saunders Co., 1988, pp. 1126–1152.
2. Culver BH (ed.): *The Respiratory System: Syllabus for Human Biology 540*. Seattle, University of Washington, Lecture Notes, 1982.
3. Estenne M, et al.: The effect of pectoralis muscle training in tetraplegic patients. *Am Rev Respir Dis*, 139:1218–1222, 1989.
4. Fishman AP: State of the art: Chronic cor pulmonale. *Am Rev Respir Dis*, 114:775–794, 1976.
5. Luce JM: Respiratory consequences of obesity. *Chest*, 78:626–631, 1980.
6. Luce JM, and Culver BH: Respiratory muscle function in health and disease. *Chest*, 81:82–90, 1982.
7. Luce JM: Medical management of spinal cord injury. *Crit Care Med*, 13:126–131, 1985.
8. Moser KM: Pulmonary embolism. *In* Murray JF, and Nadel JA (eds.): *Textbook of Respiratory Medicine*. Philadelphia, W. B. Saunders Co., 1988, pp. 1299–1327.
9. Phillipson EA: Sleep disorders. *In* Murray JF, and Nadel JA (eds.): *Textbook of Respiratory Medicine*. Philadelphia, W. B. Saunders Co., 1988, pp. 1841–1860.
10. Snider GL: Chronic bronchitis and emphysema. *In* Murray JF, and Nadel JA (eds.): *Textbook of Respiratory Medicine*. Philadelphia, W. B. Saunders Co., 1988, pp. 1069–1106.
11. Thurlbeck WM: *Chronic Airflow Obstruction in Lung Disease*. Philadelphia, W. B. Saunders Co., 1976.
12. Woolcock AJ: Asthma. *In* Murray JF, and Nadel JA (eds.): *Textbook of Respiratory Medicine*. Philadelphia, W. B. Saunders Co., 1988, pp. 1030–1068.

6

METHODS OF DIAGNOSING RESPIRATORY DISEASE

DIAGNOSTIC METHODS

ROUTINE DIAGNOSTIC METHODS

Historical Features of Respiratory Disease

Cough. Cough is a defense mechanism that clears material from the tracheobronchial tree. Persistent cough is never normal; its presence is indicative of excessive mucus, foreign particles, irritation from erosive lesions, or airway hyperreactivity. In patients with chronic bronchitis, morning cough appears first and progresses to more or less continuous coughing. In other nonsmoking patients, morning cough may result from nocturnal postnasal drainage. Interstitial lung diseases often cause a nonproductive cough, and asthma may present as cough in the absence of breathlessness or wheezing.

Sputum. Sputum or phlegm coughed up from the lungs is most often made up of clear, relatively thin mucus. A change in color or consistency means white blood cell accumulation and stasis but not necessarily infection. Patients with chronic bronchitis usually expectorate no more than a half cup of sputum daily. If more is present, bronchiectasis should be suspected. Feculent sputum is expectorated, often in large quantities, by patients with anaerobic lung infections, including lung abscesses.

Hemoptysis. The coughing up of blood is called hemoptysis. The site of bleeding may be anywhere in the upper or lower airways or in the lung parenchyma. Some patients thought to have hemoptysis actually vomit blood from the upper gastrointestinal tract but are unaware of its origin. Blood from the gastrointestinal tract is dark brown in color because of the action of gastric acid upon it. Blood from the respiratory tree most often comes from the bronchial circulation and is bright red because it has been oxygenated. It frequently is mixed with sputum. Although chronic bronchitis is the most common cause of hemoptysis in the United States, other causes, including cancer and tuberculosis, must be excluded.

Dyspnea. Dyspnea or breathlessness usually is experienced first with exertion and eventually at rest as the underlying disease progresses. It may stem from pulmonary or cardiac dysfunction and frequently represents a combination of the two. Dyspnea from chronic pulmonary disease most often evolves gradually unless the patient is undergoing an acute exacerbation. Dyspnea due to left ventricular failure is usually worsened by lying down (orthopnea), especially at night (paroxysmal nocturnal dyspnea), when intravascular volume increases with the reabsorption of fluid that was previously stored in the dependent extremities.

Chest Pain. The lung parenchyma contains no pain fibers, so respiratory diseases are generally painless unless they involve the airways, large blood vessels, or parietal pleura. Tracheal pain is common in viral infections, including influenza. Patients whose pulmonary arteries are dilated because of pulmonary hypertension sometimes experience central chest discomfort. Inflammation of the parietal pleura, or pleurisy, causes stabbing pain accentuated by coughing, inspiration, and other maneuvers in which the pleural surfaces rub together. This is seen in viral or bacterial infections of the pleural space. Irritation of the diaphragmatic pleura from subdiaphragmatic inflammation is referred to the ipsilateral shoulder owing to the dual innervation of the intercostal and phrenic nerves. The pain of myocardial ischemia or infarction is characteristically described as substernal pressure that may radiate to the left shoulder and arm.

Physical Examination of the Respiratory System

Breathing Patterns. Normal adults breathe 12 to 22 times per minute with a tidal volume (V_T) of 5 to 7 ml/kg of body weight. An increase in the ventilatory rate (f) is called tachypnea. A decrease in f is called bradypnea. The word hyperpnea describes an increase in V_T with a normal or increased f. Hyperpnea with large increases in V_T is referred to as Kussmaul breathing. Patients with obstructive pulmonary disease generally have a prolonged expiratory phase to offset their expiratory airflow obstruction. They also may exhale slowly through pursed lips, a maneuver called pursed lip breathing. Patients with restrictive pulmonary disease generally breathe with a small V_T, owing to decreased respiratory system compliance (C_{RS}). Bradypnea is seen in patients with disordered ventilatory regulation due to drugs or central nervous system dysfunction. Cheyne-Stokes breathing consists of a waxing and waning of ventilatory effort during sleep. It is thought to represent a resetting of an abnormally sensitive ventilatory regulation center when blood flow to the center is prolonged by left ventricular failure or cerebrovascular disease.

Cyanosis. Cyanosis is a blue coloration caused by the presence of desaturated hemoglobin in capillaries under skin or mucous membranes. When seen in the tongue and soft palate, where blood flow is high, cyanosis is indicative of hypoxemia. Cyanosis elsewhere, in the fingers for example, may merely reflect stagnant blood flow. Since hypoxemia may be present without cyanosis and cyanosis need not be due to hypoxemia, blood gases must be used in assessing the adequacy of arterial oxygenation.

Clubbing. Normally an angle less than 180 degrees exists between the base of the fingernail and the adjacent dorsal surface of the finger, and the circumference of the finger at that point is less than that at the distal phalangeal joint. Clubbing, a physical finding in lung cancer, suppurative pulmonary infections, certain liver disorders, and congenital cyanotic heart disease, causes an increase in the soft tissue underlying the terminal phalanx. This results in an increase in the normal angle and a reversal of the circumferential relationship. These changes are best appreciated when the finger is viewed from the side (Fig. 6–1).

Examination of the Chest. The thoracic cage should be examined

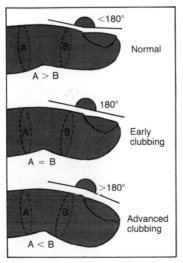

Figure 6–1. Lateral view of fingertip, showing normal nail bed angle and circumference compared with those seen in early and advanced finger clubbing.

for skeletal abnormalities and respiratory muscle activity. The normal lung emits a resonant, hollow sound when the chest wall is drummed upon with the tips of the fingers. Increased resonance is heard when the relative amount of air exceeds the amount of tissue in the thorax, as with emphysema or pneumothorax. Decreased percussion may be present when the alveoli or the pleural space is filled with fluid. Movement of air into and out of the thorax is best appreciated by listening to the posterior lung bases with a stethoscope. Generally only inspiration and the first part of expiration are audible; this is called vesicular breathing. Bronchial breathing, in which both expiration and inspiration are heard, occurs when lung tissue infiltrated by pneumonia or another consolidative process transmits airway sounds to the chest wall.

Breath sounds are diminished when fluid interferes with sound transmission or when little air is moving, as occurs when patients breathe with a small V_T. Adventitious sounds include wheezing, a high-pitched, musical noise generated by narrowed airways, as in patients with asthma; rales or crackles, discontinuous popping sounds that reflect the opening of small airways and alveoli in conditions like pulmonary edema; and rhonchi or gurgles, bubbling sounds that stem from intraluminal secretions and are common in patients with chronic bronchitis or pneumonia. Stridor, a loud "whooping" sound on inspiration, is caused by upper airway obstruction; it may be confused with wheezing in some individuals.

ARTERIAL BLOOD GASES

Technique

Although a test of pulmonary function, arterial blood gases are so important in assessing overall respiratory status that they are considered separately. This test involves obtaining a small (2 to 5 ml) sample of blood, usually from the radial artery in the wrist or the brachial artery at the elbow. A small (22- to 25-gauge) needle is passed through the skin at a 45-degree angle; blood will pump into the syringe when the artery is entered. The puncture site should be compressed for five minutes after the needle is removed to prevent hematoma formation. The blood gas syringe is heparinized to prevent clotting and transported in ice to retard the consumption of oxygen (O_2) and the production of carbon dioxide (CO_2) by cells in the blood.

Interpretation

The arterial pH, arterial CO_2 tension ($PaCO_2$), and arterial O_2 tension (PaO_2) are measured directly from an arterial blood gas sample. The arterial O_2 saturation (SaO_2), arterial O_2 content (CaO_2), and bicarbonate (HCO_3^-) concentration may be calculated from those measurements; the SaO$_2$ also can be measured directly by a process called oximetry.

As described in Chapter 4, the arterial pH is a measurement of the hydrogen ion concentration in blood and is a reflection of the body's acid-base balance. It may change for either metabolic or respiratory reasons and cannot be used by itself to differentiate betweeen them. Thus, an arterial pH of >7.45 represents alkalemia of either source, and a pH of <7.35 represents nonspecific acidemia.

As discussed in Chapter 2, the PaCO$_2$ reflects the adequacy of alveolar ventilation. Alveolar hypoventilation, which causes respiratory acidosis (not necessarily acidemia, which requires a pH change), is present with a PaCO$_2$ of >40 mmHg. Alveolar hyperventilation or respiratory alkalosis is a PaCO$_2$ of <40 mmHg. Since the pH usually changes in a direction opposite to the PaCO$_2$ when the latter changes acutely, the combination of a low pH and a high PaCO$_2$ signifies acute respiratory acidosis (and acidemia), whereas a high pH and a low PaCO$_2$ signify acute respiratory alkalosis (and alkalemia). Conversely, a normal pH in the setting of a high or low PaCO$_2$ generally means that the acidosis or alkalosis is chronic. The base excess, discussed in Chapter 4, is increased in metabolic alkalosis and decreased in metabolic acidosis.

The PaO$_2$ is a measure of the dissolved O$_2$ tension at a given fraction of inspired O$_2$ (FiO$_2$). Hypoxemia, a reduction in the PaO$_2$ below the normal level of approximately 90 mmHg in a young adult, may be due to inhalation of O$_2$ at a low FiO$_2$, alveolar hypoventilation, ventilation-perfusion mismatching, right-to-left intrapulmonary shunt or, rarely, diffusion limitation. Determining which of these factors is or are responsible for hypoxemia is discussed in Chapter 2. Because the SaO$_2$ normally parallels the PaO$_2$, a calculated SaO$_2$ is appropriate in most clinical situations. This relationship does not hold in the presence of carbon monoxide (CO) poisoning, however, when most of the hemoglobin in blood is bound to CO rather than O$_2$. As a result, the SaO$_2$ and a carboxyhemoglobin level should be measured directly in CO poisoning.

The PaO$_2$ is one component of the CaO$_2$, which is calculated from the SaO$_2$, the amount of hemoglobin capable of being saturated, and the solubility of O$_2$ in blood multiplied by the PaO$_2$. Since the amount of O$_2$ going to the peripheral tissue is the product of the CaO$_2$ and the left ventricular output ($\dot{Q}$T), the PaO$_2$ does not necessarily reflect the adequacy of tissue oxygenation. It may be normal or nearly normal in the early stage of shock, for example, even though the patient has poor regional blood flow to the brain and other organs. Patients poisoned with cyanide (CN), which interferes with intracellular respiration, may have a normal PaO$_2$, SaO$_2$, and CaO$_2$, yet their cells will die because they cannot extract O$_2$ from the blood.

Indications

Arterial blood gas determinations are indicated whenever abnormalities in the pH, $PaCO_2$, and PaO_2 might be expected. Their frequency relates to the rate of expected changes in patient status, ventilator settings, and other factors; they usually are determined at least once daily in patients with respiratory disorders in the Intensive Care Unit (ICU). As cited above, the SaO_2 should be measured directly whenever CO poisoning is suspected.

PULSE OXIMETRY

Technique

Although most clinicians rely on the PaO_2 to determine the adequacy of arterial oxygenation, the SaO_2 better reflects the amount of O_2 traveling to the tissues. Systemic arterial oxygen saturation can be calculated from the PaO_2 using the ideal O_2-hemoglobin dissociation wave. Alternatively, it can be measured directly by oximetry, in which light of certain wavelengths is passed through a blood sample and the rate of saturated to desaturated hemoglobin is determined. Pulse oximeters are devices with miniaturized sensors that attach to an ear lobe or a digit and estimate per cent of SaO_2 from measurements of changes in light absorption associated with systolic pulsations of blood flow.

Interpretation

One major disadvantage of pulse oximetry is that it does not determine what other species of hemoglobin, such as methemoglobin or carboxyhemoglobin, may be present in addition to oxyhemoglobin. Another is that SaO_2 measurements are relatively insensitive in detecting significant changes in PaO_2 at high levels of oxygenation or when the SaO_2 is less than 90 per cent, because of the shape of the O_2-hemoglobin dissociation curve. This means that pulse oximetry is most useful in patients who have near-normal SaO_2 but are at danger of desaturation. Such patients might include those being monitored during or immediately after surgery.

Indications

Pulse oximetry may be used to monitor patients in all medical settings provided that its limitations are kept in mind. Monitoring may be either periodic or continuous. Determination of SaO_2 usually cannot substitute for the PaO_2 in determining the advisability of long-term O_2 therapy.

CHEST ROENTGENOLOGY

Chest Roentgenographic Techniques

When x-rays hit photographic film after passing unimpeded through air structures, the film turns black. In contrast, x-rays that are absorbed by solid structures do not blacken the film, and the structures that have impeded their progress appear white. Thus, the air-filled (air-dense) lungs look black on a chest roentgenogram, the solid (calcium-dense) bones appear white, and the less solid (fat- or water-dense) heart and mediastinal tissues are gray. Since x-rays are emitted from an x-ray tube in a fan-shaped pattern, they are spread more if a relatively great distance exists between the tube and the photographic film. If the thorax being x-rayed is close to the film, the scatter around the thorax will be less and the resultant film image will be smaller than would occur if the thorax were far from the film.

Routine chest roentgenograms are taken with the patient facing and touching the film cassette with the x-rays passing from a posterior to anterior direction at a tube-to-patient distance of six feet; this is called a PA view. Portable roentgenograms, including those in the ICU, are taken in an anterior to posterior direction with the patient sitting upright or lying supine on the film cassette and facing the tube, which usually is some feet away. The heart and other structures appear wider on an AP than on a PA film as a result, and cardiac enlargement may be misdiagnosed unless attention is paid to how the film was taken.

Other radiographic techniques include fluoroscopy, in which the x-rays are emitted continuously while body tissues are observed in motion; tomography, in which the x-ray tube and film are moved about the patient so that a desired structure, such as a mass lesion in the lung, is in the plane of focus and the surrounding tissues are blurred; and computed tomography (CT), in which a number of tubes surrounding the patient are operated simultaneously to provide a series of "cuts" through the transverse axis of the body that are integrated by a computer.

Common Chest Roentgenographic Patterns

Normal. Routine PA and lateral roentgenograms of the normal chest reveal the lungs, heart, and mediastinal structures encompassed by the ribs and bony skeleton (Fig. 6–2). The upper abdomen is also visible. The heart occupies a midposition in the chest, and its lateral dimension is less than half that of the chest itself. Although the air-filled trachea and major bronchi may be visible, smaller airways cannot be seen because their walls are too thin to stand out from surrounding alveoli. The aorta, pulmonary arteries, and some pulmonary veins are visible at the hilum; smaller generations of vessels may be distinguished out to the periphery of the lungs. The lung parenchyma itself usually is not visible, although lobar fissures may be apparent if they lie perpendicular to the x-ray beam.

Consolidation. When alveoli are filled with fluid or inflammatory cells from pulmonary edema or pneumonia, areas of consolidation appear white against the surrounding alveoli. Fluid-filled airways also may be visible. Air-filled airways coursing through consolidated lung tissue appear as tubular structures; these are called air bronchograms. When a consolidated area abuts another tissue of similar radiographic density, such as the heart, visual separation at the border of the two structures is obscured. This phenomenon is called the silhouette sign, even though a lack of silhouette is present.

Atelectasis. Atelectasis signifies the collapse or loss of volume of normally air-filled tissue in alveoli, segments, lobes, or entire lungs. Small areas of alveolar collapse may appear as linear streaks at the lung bases. Larger amounts may resemble consolidation and be manifested as a few air bronchograms. However, they can be differentiated from parenchymal infiltrates, which usually cause the volume of the involved area to increase, by displacement of lobar fissures or loss of volume in the affected lung.

PULMONARY FUNCTION TESTS

General Principles

Pulmonary function tests objectively quantify lung function and dysfunction. They are useful in detecting mild abnormalities, defining the type of abnormality present, identifying patients at

---

Figure 6–2. Structures visualized on routine *(A)* posteroanterior and *(B)* lateral chest roentgenograms.

In part *A,* the numbers refer to anatomical structures as follows: (1) trachea; (2) right main bronchus; (3) left main bronchus; (4) left pulmonary artery; (5) right upper lobe pulmonary vein; (6) right interlobar artery; (7) right lower and middle lobe vein; (8) aortic knob; (9) superior vena cava; (10) aortic arch.

In part *B,* the structures identified are as follows: (1) tracheal air column; (2) right intermediate bronchus; (3) left upper lobe bronchus; (4) right upper lobe bronchus; (5) left interlobar artery; (6) right interlobar artery; (7) confluence of pulmonary veins; (8) aortic arch; (9) brachiocephalic vessels. (From Fraser RG, and Paré JAP: *Diagnosis of Diseases of the Chest*, 2nd ed. Philadelphia, W. B. Saunders Co., 1977, Vol. 1.)

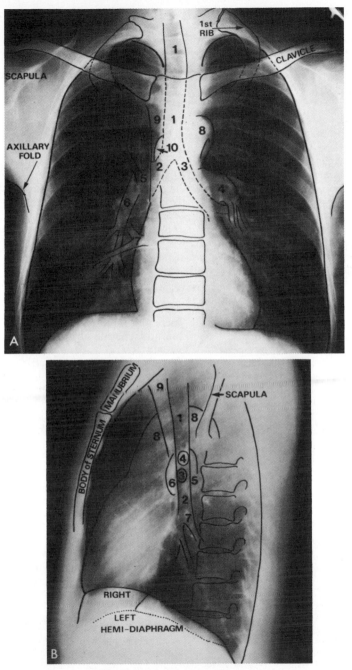

Figure 6–2 *See legend on opposite page*

high risk of respiratory complications following surgery or other stresses, documenting the degree of disability, and assessing the results of treatment.

Tests of Ventilatory Mechanics

Spirometry. Ventilatory mechanics are most commonly measured by spirometry (Fig. 6–3). In this test, patients breathe in their regular fashion until instructed to take the deepest possible inspiration to total lung capacity (TLC) and then to exhale the air to residual volume (RV). The volume of air exhaled as quickly as possible is the forced vital capacity (FVC), whereas that portion of the FVC exhaled in the first second is the forced expiratory volume in one second (FEV_1) (Fig. 6–4). The FVC reflects the patient's ability to breathe deeply and to cough and should be well in excess of 15 ml/kg. It is reduced by obstructive lung diseases that increase RV and by restrictive diseases that decrease TLC. The ratio FEV_1/FVC is reduced by obstruction but is normal or increased in restrictive processes.

Although FVC can be reduced by both obstruction and restriction, TLC and RV are usually increased in the former situation and reduced in the latter. Therefore, to separate obstruction from restriction, measurement of TLC and RV may be necessary in certain patients. This cannot be accomplished by spirometry because gas remains in the lungs after reaching RV, so the tests of lung volume described below must be performed. However, the inspiratory and expiratory reserve volumes (IRV and ERV) can be measured by spirometry. The inspired vital capacity and the forced inspiratory volume in one second also can be determined.

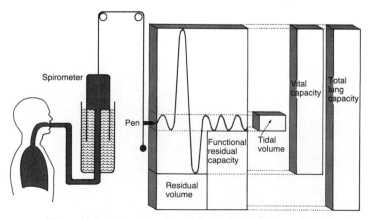

Figure 6–3. Unforced spirometric tracing and lung volumes.

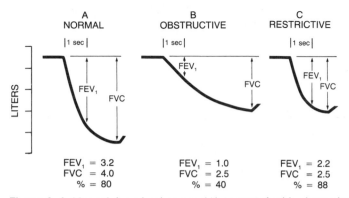

Figure 6–4. Normal forced spirogram *(A)* compared with obstructive *(B)* and restrictive *(C)* spirograms. FEV$_1$ = forced expiratory volume in one second; FVC = forced vital capacity.

Another parameter is flow over the middle half of the FVC, the forced expiratory flow between 25 and 75 per cent of the FVC (FEF$_{25-75}$), which may be abnormal in small airways disease.

Flow Volume Curves. Instead of measuring the volume of air exhaled or inhaled over time, as is the case with spirometry, flow-volume curves measure the rate of airflow over lung volume as patients exhale quickly from TLC to RV or inhale from RV to TLC. The curves reveal expiratory airflow obstruction if flow is diminished, especially at low lung volumes. Flow-volume curves also may detect inspiratory airflow obstruction in disorders of the upper airway. In this situation, expiratory flow may be normal, but inspiratory flow will reach a plateau as the airway collapses because atmospheric pressure exceeds intraluminal pressure in the extrathoracic trachea. Illustrative flow-volume curves are provided in Figure 6–5.

Tests of Lung Volume

Total lung capacity may be derived by measuring functional residual capacity (FRC), the resting point of the lungs and thoracic cage that generally is reproducible from moment to moment, and adding the IRV obtained by spirometry. Residual volume equals TLC minus VC. Functional residual capacity may be measured by observing the dilution of inert gases like helium (He) that are not absorbed into the bloodstream as they fill the lungs. Starting from FRC, patients breathe in a known volume of He and O$_2$ from a spirometer; the fractional concentrations of He are measured before and after the gas equilibrates between the spirometer and the lungs, and FRC is calculated by multiplying the original volume

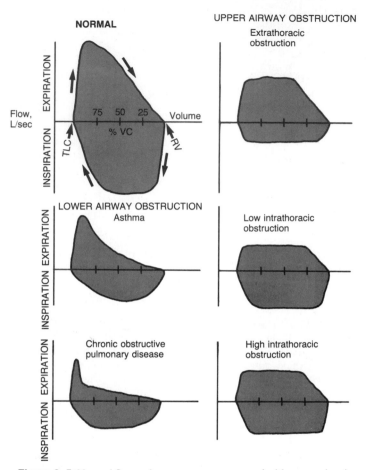

Figure 6–5. Normal flow-volume curve, as compared with curves showing lower and upper airway obstruction. Flow is measured in liters per second (L/sec). Volume is measured as the subject inhales a vital capacity (VC) breath from residual volume (RV) to total lung capacity (TLC) and then exhales.

of gas and the ratio of the fraction of He before and after equilibration. In the nitrogen (N_2) washout method, N_2 is collected over 7 minutes from the lungs of patients starting at FRC and breathing in 100 per cent O_2. The fraction of expired N_2 is measured at the mouth, and when it is zero, signifying that all the N_2 has left the lungs, the collected volume of N_2 is equal to 79 per cent of its normal concentration in air, times the FRC.

Tests of Ventilatory Uniformity

In the N_2 washout described in the preceding paragraph, patients breathe 100 per cent O_2 while the fraction of expired N_2 is measured at the mouth. The N_2 in expired gas will fall smoothly toward zero if ventilation is normal; the rate of fall is slower if ventilation is nonuniform due to airflow obstruction, so the slope of the N_2 fraction over time is decreased. In the single-breath N_2 plateau test, patients breathe 100 per cent O_2 from RV to TLC and then exhale slowly while N_2 is measured at the mouth. Initially the N_2 fraction is zero because only the just inhaled O_2 is present in the anatomical dead space. The N_2 fraction rises quickly when alveolar gas reaches the mouth and then reaches a plateau. This plateau has a gradual slope as N_2 leaves areas that O_2 could penetrate. The slope is increased when airflow obstruction is present.

Diffusing Capacity

The diffusing capacity primarily reflects the surface area of the alveolar-capillary membrane and not its thickness, as once was thought. Measurement of the diffusing capacity of O_2 is difficult because that gas is already present in blood. Carbon monoxide, which is normally not present in the body and is taken up by red blood cells even more avidly than O_2, is therefore used as the test gas. In the single-breath method of measuring the diffusing capacity of carbon monoxide (DLCO), the patient inhales a mixture of 0.39 per cent CO, O_2, and a small amount of an inert gas such as He in a single breath from RV to TLC. The patient then holds the breath for ten seconds and exhales. The fraction of CO in a sample of gas collected late in exhalation is considered the same as the alveolar fraction. The difference between this fraction and the fraction of CO in the inhaled gas is used to calculate the uptake of CO, and hence the diffusing capacity. The DLCO most often is corrected for the hemoglobin concentration and for lung volume, which is measured by the dilution of the inert gas included in the inspired sample. The DLCO is reduced whenever the surface area of the alveolar-capillary membrane is diminished, as occurs in emphysema and pulmonary vascular disease.

Carbon Dioxide Production and O_2 Consumption

The CO_2 production ($\dot{V}CO_2$) and O_2 consumption ($\dot{V}O_2$) can be determined by measuring the concentrations of the two gases in inspired and expired samples that are collected over several minutes to provide full equilibration. Since CO_2 is not present in the inspired gas, the $\dot{V}CO_2$ in liters per minute (L/min) equals the amount of CO_2 collected divided by the number of minutes, usually three, over which gas is collected. Oxygen is present in both inspired and expired samples; the difference between the two samples equals $\dot{V}O_2$. The $\dot{V}CO_2$ and $\dot{V}O_2$ are increased by processes such as fever and hyperthyroidism that increase metabolism.

Minute Ventilation

As discussed in Chapter 2, minute ventilation ($\dot{V}E$) is the product of VT and f. These values may be taken directly from a spirometric tracing. The spirogram also can be used to determine the maximum minute ventilation (MVV), the greatest amount of air patients can inhale and exhale in one minute (the volume usually is collected over 12 seconds and then multiplied by 5). The $\dot{V}E$ also can be measured at the bedside by determining VT with portable devices and counting f, as can the MVV. Normal and abnormal values of VT and f are discussed above.

Minute ventilation normally is 5 to 10 L/min in adults. This amount decreases when ventilatory needs are small or when patients hypoventilate owing to mechanical factors or improper ventilatory regulation. An increased $\dot{V}E$ is observed with large ventilatory demands due to a rise in dead space ($\dot{V}D$), $\dot{V}CO_2$, or both, and with hyperventilation. Measurement of $\dot{V}E$ in combination with arterial blood gases therefore provides important information about both the needs and the adequacy of ventilation. Generally speaking, patients require mechanical ventilation if their $\dot{V}E$ is substantially out of the normal range, their blood gases also are abnormal, and they cannot double their $\dot{V}E$ on demand and thereby improve their blood gases.

Dead Space Fraction

The dead space fraction (VD/VT) is the amount of VT used to ventilate areas of anatomical and alveolar VD that do not participate in gas exchange. Together, these areas are called physiological dead space. Anatomical VD is about 2 ml/kg of body weight. Alveolar VD is insignificant in health but increases in pulmonary vascular disease. Since CO_2 is virtually absent in inspired gas, expired gas coming from areas of dead space contains no CO_2. Thus, the difference between alveolar CO_2 ($PACO_2$) and the expired CO_2 ($PECO_2$) reveals the relative amount of VT supplying areas of VD. Arterial PCO_2 as measured in a blood gas sample may be substituted for $PACO_2$ because the gas is assumed to be in equilibrium across the alveolar-capillary membrane. Expired PCO_2 is measured directly over several minutes as part of the determination of $\dot{V}CO_2$. The ratio VD/VT equals $PaCO_2 - PECO_2/PaCO_2$. This ratio normally is 0.4 or less. It should decrease during exercise as pulmonary artery pressure increases somewhat and pulmonary capillaries not normally perfused with blood, such as those at the lung apices, are recruited for gas exchange. The dead space fraction increases with pulmonary vascular disease on exercise and, eventually, at rest if the disease progresses. Values of VD/VT in excess of 0.6 generally are indications for mechanical ventilation.

Exercise Testing

Exercise testing simulates the clinical condition in which many patients first feel dyspneic, and it often indicates what physiological abnormalities underlie this complaint. It can be used to diagnose pulmonary vascular disease, document early disability in persons whose pulmonary function tests are otherwise unremarkable, and differentiate between cardiac and pulmonary disorders. In most protocols, $\dot{V}E$, $\dot{V}O_2$, heart rate, blood pressure, and arterial blood gases are measured as patients exercise as strenuously as possible on a treadmill or stationary bicycle. Normal individuals increase $\dot{V}E$ and heart rate and decrease blood pressure and VD/VT as they exercise. Their PaO_2 remains constant, and their $PaCO_2$ falls as they hyperventilate in response to the lactic acid produced by anaerobic metabolism during the later stages of exercise. Patients with heart disease often increase blood pressure and heart rate more than normal and cannot reach high values of $\dot{V}O_2$ because their cardiac output is insufficient. Patients with severe obstructive or restrictive pulmonary diseases characteristically cannot increase $\dot{V}E$ to meet the demands of exercise, although their VD/VT and $PaCO_2$ may fall as expected. By contrast, pulmonary vascular diseases often cause an increase in VD/VT and $PaCO_2$. The PaO_2 also may fall.

Negative Inspiratory Pressure

The respiratory muscles must generate a negative inspiratory pressure of -20 centimeters of water (cmH_2O) or greater to maintain a normal VC. Measurement of negative pressure with a manometer applied to the mouth or the inspiratory tubing of a mechanical ventilator provides a good assessment of muscle function. It should be used when dysfunction is suspected and during weaning from mechanical ventilation.

Tests of Ventilatory Regulation

Assuming that mechanical limitations have been ruled out, impaired ventilatory regulation is suggested by a failure to augment $\dot{V}E$ in response to hypercapnia, hypoxemia, or a combination of the two. Such inappropriate responses can be quantitated in the laboratory by measuring $\dot{V}E$ and arterial blood gases as patients breathe high CO_2 or low O_2 mixtures.

Sleep Studies

Recent research has demonstrated that many respiratory patients and some otherwise normal people decrease their arterial saturation and PaO_2 during sleep, especially the rapid eye movement phase, owing to upper airway obstruction, central sleep apnea, or both.

Certain individuals also may experience an increase in $PaCO_2$ during apneic episodes. Sleep studies may be helpful in documenting such abnormalities and in suggesting the need for further treatment, including progesterone or protriptyline for ventilatory stimulation, surgical procedures to overcome anatomical airway obstruction, or supplemental O_2. These studies are generally conducted at night or over several daytime hours in special chambers or in a quiet corner of the ICU. Electroencephalography is used to monitor sleep phases, and electrocardiographic monitoring provides information about dysrhythmias during sleep. Ear oximetry offers a noninvasive way of monitoring O_2 saturation; alternatively, an indwelling arterial catheter may be used to obtain arterial blood gases. By simultaneously measuring respiratory muscle activity and airflow across the nose and mouth, the clinician can determine whether sleep apnea is of the obstructive type, in which airflow is absent despite muscle activity; the central type, in which there is a lack of muscle activity as well as of airflow; or a combination of the two.

SPECIMEN COLLECTION AND BIOPSY PROCEDURES

Sputum Collection

Expectorated sputum samples are generally adequate for cytological and bacteriological analysis, although some patients cannot raise sputum spontaneously. Sputum samples can generally be obtained in such patients by gentle nasotracheal suctioning.

Sputum Induction

Sputum samples may be induced by inhalation of hypertonic (3 per cent) saline, which is irritative to the airways. Samples obtained in this fashion are likely to reflect alveolar contents and to not be contaminated by upper respiratory secretions, particularly if the teeth and buccal mucosa are brushed and the mouth is rinsed before induction. Thus samples may be analyzed for a variety of alveolar pathogens, including *Mycobacterium tuberculosis* and *Pneumocystis carinii*.

Transthoracic Needle Aspiration

If sputum cannot be obtained easily but secretions from the lungs are urgently needed, the lung parenchyma may be penetrated directly with a thin (18- to 25-gauge) spinal needle under sterile conditions. The needle is directed, often under fluoroscopic guidance, toward the area of densest consolidation; a small amount of saline is injected into the area and aspirated into a syringe. Alternatively, when information is being sought about a peripheral lung mass, the needle may be carefully inserted into the mass for aspiration of material for culture and cytological analysis. Pneumothorax and intrapulmonary bleeding are the major complications of transthoracic aspiration, and pursuit of mass lesions generally requires a conscious and cooperative patient.

Thoracentesis and Pleural Biopsy

During thoracentesis, a patient's skin and parietal pleura are anesthetized under sterile conditions, and a short, thin (18- to 25-gauge) needle is introduced into the pleural space. A small quantity of pleural fluid is aspirated for determination of its red and white blood cell count and protein concentration and for bacterial culture, among other studies. This procedure may be followed by pleural biopsy, in which a larger needle with a cutting edge and collection chamber is introduced for biopsy of the parietal pleura. Thoracentesis should be performed in all patients with unexplained pleural effusions, especially when empyema, which requires prompt and complete drainage, is suspected. Pleural biopsy is generally reserved for patients with suspected carcinomatous or tuberculous involvement of the pleura. Pneumothorax is a major complication and should be looked for on a postprocedure chest roentgenogram.

Fiberoptic Bronchoscopy with Bronchoalveolar Lavage and Transbronchial Biopsy

Equipment. The fiberoptic bronchoscope is a thin, flexible instrument that is used to visualize the lower airways up to the level of the subsegmental bronchi. Most bronchoscopes have channels through which saline can be introduced, directed into the smaller airways and alveoli, and then retrieved; this procedure is called bronchoalveolar lavage (BAL). Many bronchoscopes also allow the passage of catheters with retractable inner chambers that permit the collection of lower airway and lung secretions without contamination. Small forceps also may be advanced through the bronchoscope for biopsy of intraluminal lesions. In addition, the forceps may be passed into the lung periphery under fluoroscopic guidance for transbronchial biopsy (TBB) of parenchymal infiltrates or mass lesions.

Procedure. TBB yields specimens large enough to be examined by a pathologist, whereas BAL provides material for culture and cytological analysis. The bronchoscope may be introduced across the larynx, either directly through the nose or mouth, via an endotracheal tube, or through a tracheostomy tube. Placement through a special adaptor allows patients receiving mechanical ventilation to undergo the procedure without a prohibitive loss of airway pressure. Patients generally receive parenteral atropine to decrease secretions and prevent reflex bradycardia during the bronchoscopy, and their nasopharynx or oropharynx is anesthetized with topical lidocaine. These drugs help most patients experience bronchoscopy with minimal discomfort, although some cannot tolerate the procedure, primarily owing to a heightened gag reflex.

Indications. Bronchoscopy is indicated in assessment of airway anatomy, removal of foreign bodies, determination of the origin of hemoptysis, collection of lavage fluid, and biopsy of accessible lesions. It lowers the PaO_2 and is therefore contraindicated in severely hypoxemic patients whose PaO_2 cannot be improved by supplemental O_2. Transbronchial biopsy is contraindicated when serious bleeding or pneumothorax is likely to result from the procedure, but BAL may be used in almost all patients who can tolerate bronchoscopy.

Open Lung Biopsy

Occasionally a diagnosis cannot be made by the aforementioned procedures, or a large specimen is required for pathological analysis. When this happens, open lung biopsy may be performed. This requires general anesthesia and an operation, called a thoracotomy, in which the chest is entered. Thoracotomy requires hospitalization and produces pain. Nevertheless, open lung biopsy may be necessary in some patients.

RECOMMENDED READING

1. Bowton DL, et al.: Pulse oximetry monitoring outside the Intensive Care Unit: Progress or problem. *Ann Intern Med,* 115:450–454, 1991.
2. Cherniack NS: Dyspnea. *In* Murray JF, and Nadel JA (eds.): *Textbook of Respiratory Medicine.* Philadelphia, W. B. Saunders Co., 1988, pp. 389–396.
3. Felson B: A new look at pattern recognition of diffuse pulmonary disease. *Am J Roentgenol,* 113:183–189, 1979.
4. Felson B: *Chest Roentgenology.* Philadelphia, W. B. Saunders Co., 1973.
5. Gold WM, and Boushey HA: Pulmonary function testing. *In* Murray JF, and Nadel JA (eds.): *Textbook of Respiratory Medicine.* Philadelphia, W. B. Saunders Co., 1988, pp. 611–682.
6. Greenspan RH, and Mann H: Radiographic techniques. *In* Murray JF, and Nadel JA (eds.): *Textbook of Respiratory Medicine.* Philadelphia, W. B. Saunders Co., 1988, pp. 478–534.
7. Petty TL (ed.): *Pulmonary Diagnostic Techniques.* Philadelphia, Lea & Febiger, 1975.
8. Reynolds HY: Bronchoalveolar lavage. *In* Murray JF, and Nadel JA (eds.): *Textbook of Respiratory Medicine.* Philadelphia, W. B. Saunders Co., 1988, pp. 597–610.
9. Sackner, MA.: State of the art: Bronchofiberoscopy. *Ann Rev Respir Dis,* 111:62–85, 1975.
10. Schnapp LM, and Cohen NA: Pulse oximetry: Uses and abuses. *Chest,* 98:1244–1250, 1990.

7

RESPIRATORY FAILURE, FAILURE OF OXYGEN TRANSPORT, AND FAILURE OF TISSUE OXYGEN EXTRACTION

RESPIRATION REVIEWED

GENERAL CONSIDERATIONS

Respiration was defined in Chapter 1 as the exchange of oxygen (O_2) and carbon dioxide (CO_2) between an organism, such as man, and its environment. In Chapter 2, human respiration was divided into five steps: (1) ventilation, the exchange of respiratory gases between the atmosphere and the lungs; (2) pulmonary perfusion, the flow of mixed venous blood through the pulmonary circulation to the alveolar capillaries and the return of arterialized blood from the capillaries to the left atrium; (3) pulmonary gas exchange, the transfer of O_2 and CO_2 across the alveolar-capillary membrane; (4) gas transport and uptake, the conveying of arterial blood from the left ventricle to the peripheral tissues, which extract O_2 and release CO_2 for transport back to the right atrium; and (5) regulation of ventilation, the control of arterial blood acidity-alkalinity and respiratory gas tensions by increasing or decreasing ventilation.

In theory, impairment in any or all of these steps could result in respiratory failure. However, the term *respiratory failure* customarily is reserved for disorders that result in abnormal arterial blood gases. Failure of O_2 transport and tissue extraction may accompany respiratory failure, but they are considered separately (Table 7–1).

Despite these arbitrary distinctions, the clinician should bear in mind that all severe impairments in respiration have the same result: inadequate oxygenation of vital organs such as the heart and the brain. These impairments are therefore commonly manifested by the same cardiovascular and neurological dysfunction. Because their clinical presentation is so similar, respiratory failure, failure of O_2 transport, and failure of tissue O_2 extraction are laboratory rather than clinical diagnoses.

Table 7-1. PATHOLOGICAL CONDITIONS IMPAIRING TISSUE OXYGENATION

CONDITION	DEFINITION	CLINICAL EXAMPLES	LABORATORY ABNORMALITIES
Respiratory failure	Abnormality in O_2 uptake, CO_2 elimination, or both, reflected in abnormal arterial blood gases	Severe asthma, chronic obstructive pulmonary disease, neonatal or adult respiratory distress syndrome	$PaCO_2 = 50$ mmHg or more, $PaO_2 = 50$ mmHg or less
Failure of O_2 transport	Limitation in O_2 delivery to peripheral tissues so that aerobic metabolism cannot be maintained	Anemia, carbon monoxide poisoning, cardiogenic shock	$P\bar{v}O_2 < 40$ mmHg, lactic acidosis
Failure of tissue O_2 extraction	Inability of cells to extract O_2 from blood and use it for aerobic metabolism	Cyanide poisoning, distributive shock (?)	$P\bar{v}O_2 > 40$ mmHg, lactic acidosis

KEY: O_2 = oxygen, CO_2 = carbon dioxide, PaO_2 = arterial O_2 tension, $PaCO_2$ = arterial CO_2 tension, $P\bar{v}O_2$ = mixed venous O_2 tension.

RESPIRATORY FAILURE

DEFINITION

Respiratory failure is an impairment in O_2 uptake, CO_2 elimination, or both that is reflected in abnormal arterial blood gases.

FAILURE OF VENTILATION AND FAILURE OF ARTERIAL OXYGENATION

Respiratory failure can be differentiated into failure of ventilation and failure of arterial oxygenation, although both kinds of failure often occur in the same individuals. Ventilatory failure is present when the arterial CO_2 tension ($PaCO_2$) significantly exceeds the normal level of approximately 45 mmHg; a $PaCO_2$ value of 50 mmHg or greater is required in most textbook definitions. Failure of arterial oxygenation is said to occur when the arterial O_2 tension (PaO_2), which normally is 90 mmHg in young adults at sea level, falls to 50 mmHg or less.

ACUTE AND CHRONIC RESPIRATORY FAILURE

Patients may have either acute or chronic forms of failure of ventilation, arterial oxygenation, or both. Superimposition of acute respiratory failure on chronic failure is common. Chronic failure usually causes organ damage that is not imminently life-threatening. Acute failure may be fatal if not treated immediately.

PATHOPHYSIOLOGY AND GENERAL MANAGEMENT OF FAILURE OF VENTILATION

Pathophysiology

Factors Affecting Arterial Carbon Dioxide Tension. As noted in Chapter 2, the alveolar ventilation equation states that the $PaCO_2$ is directly proportional to the body's CO_2 production ($\dot{V}CO_2$) and inversely proportional to alveolar ventilation ($\dot{V}A$). Alveolar ventilation is that amount of inspired gas that reaches the alveoli in the lungs. It is equal to minute ventilation ($\dot{V}E$), the total amount of gas passing through the mouth and the nose in a minute, minus dead space ventilation ($\dot{V}D$), the amount of gas that remains in the airways or in the alveoli that do not participate in gas exchange. Hypercapnia, an increase in $PaCO_2$ above normal, occurs (1) when $\dot{V}CO_2$ increases and $\dot{V}A$ does not, (2) when $\dot{V}A$ decreases even if

$\dot{V}CO_2$ does not increase, and (3) when $\dot{V}D$ increases without a concomitant increase in $\dot{V}A$.

Although $\dot{V}CO_2$ increases with fever, exercise, and other hypermetabolic states, most individuals, including those with respiratory disorders, can increase $\dot{V}E$ enough to maintain a normal $PaCO_2$. Nevertheless, patients who cannot increase their $\dot{V}E$ may develop respiratory failure that is caused by or, more commonly, compounded by a rise in $\dot{V}CO_2$. This occurs most often in patients with severe respiratory disorders, including upper and lower airway obstruction, especially asthma and chronic obstructive pulmonary disease (COPD); restrictive pulmonary diseases, including respiratory muscle dysfunction due to neuromuscular disorders; pulmonary vascular diseases, such as pulmonary thromboembolism, that occasionally raise $\dot{V}D$; and ventilatory regulation that is disturbed by depressant drugs or neurological disease.

Effect of Increasing Arterial Carbon Dioxide Tension. An acute rise in $PaCO_2$ of 10 mmHg or more will result in a change in pH from 7.4 to 7.3 or below that may severely depress cardiac function and trigger lethal arrhythmias. The rising $PaCO_2$ also dilates cerebral blood vessels, increases cerebral blood flow, and causes neurological disturbances ranging from restlessness and confusion to lethargy. If acute ventilatory failure of this sort does not result in death, or if the $PaCO_2$ reaches a plateau at 70 to 90 mmHg, the brain and body may adjust to the $PaCO_2$ elevation. Patients then may experience little more than headaches due to cerebral vasodilatation, so long as PaO_2 is maintained. Since the pH will return toward normal as the kidneys retain bicarbonate (HCO_3^-) to buffer CO_2, correcting the acid-base consequences of chronic ventilatory failure is not required.

Regardless of whether the rise in $PaCO_2$ is acute or chronic, however, patients with ventilatory failure also may have inadequate O_2 for gas exchange because of their reduced $\dot{V}A$. How this happens is spelled out in the alveolar gas equation introduced in Chapter 2. To reiterate, the alveolar O_2 tension (PAO_2) = (inspired O_2 tension [PIO_2] corrected for water vapor) − ($PaCO_2$/respiratory exchange ratio [R]). Assuming that R is 0.8, PIO_2 is 150 mmHg while the patient breathes humidified ambient air at sea level, and PAO_2 in normal lungs is 100 mmHg, the alveolar gas equation predicts that an increase in $PaCO_2$ from 40 to 80 mmHg will reduce the PAO_2 from 90 to 50 mmHg. If a normal 10 mmHg gradient exists between the alveolar and arterial PO_2 [$P(A − a)O_2$], the PaO_2 will be 40 mmHg. Thus hypoventilation is a cause of hypoxemia severe enough to be called respiratory failure. The $P(A − a)O_2$ will widen if the lungs are not normal, so the hypoxemia will be even more severe.

General Management

Ventilatory failure can be reversed only by altering those factors that determine the $PaCO_2$: $\dot{V}CO_2$ and $\dot{V}A$ ($\dot{V}A = \dot{V}E − \dot{V}D$). The body's CO_2 production can be returned to normal by using anti-pyretic drugs, such as aspirin and acetaminophen; by cooling blankets; by using antibiotics if infection is present; and by decreasing excessive muscle activity due to shivering or agitation. Alveolar hypoventilation can be treated by increasing $\dot{V}A$. In general, this can be accomplished by reducing airflow obstruction, overcoming lung restriction, or restoring normal ventilatory control. Intubation and mechanical ventilation may be necessary if these measures fail; this form of therapy to improve ventilation is discussed in Chapter 13. The patient's ventilatory status must be monitored, preferably in an intensive care unit (ICU), by means of arterial blood gas analysis and those methods discussed in Chapter 16. Patients whose ventilatory failure is complicated by failure of arterial oxygenation also may require hemodynamic monitoring.

PATHOPHYSIOLOGY AND GENERAL MANAGEMENT OF FAILURE OF ARTERIAL OXYGENATION

Pathophysiology

Hypoxemia
General Principles. As discussed in Chapter 2, hypoxemia may be related to low inspired P_{IO_2}, alveolar hypoventilation, low ventilation-perfusion ($\dot{V}A/\dot{Q}$) mismatching, shunt, or diffusion limitation. The first two causes are associated with a normal $P(A-a)O_2$ whereas the $P(A-a)O_2$ is increased in the latter three. Low P_{IO_2} as a cause of hypoxemia is common at high altitudes and during fires; it also occurs as a result of inadvertent interruption of O_2 administration in closed systems to hospitalized patients. Diffusion limitation, once taught as a major cause of hypoxemia, is currently not believed to contribute to clinical respiratory failure. Alveolar hypoventilation produces hypoxemia because less O_2 is available for gas exchange; this condition is diagnosed by a rise in $PaCO_2$ and is discussed above under the topic of failure of ventilation.
Ventilation-Perfusion Mismatching. Low ventilation-perfusion ($\dot{V}A/\dot{Q}$) mismatching, the most common cause of hypoxemia with an increased $P(A-a)O_2$, occurs when ventilation is not evenly matched with perfusion in certain areas of the lung. Venous blood returning from the peripheral tissues is not fully oxygenated as it passes by these areas before it mixes in the left atrium with oxygenated blood from better matched areas. The PaO_2 in this mixed effluent, which is the same as the PaO_2 drawn at the wrist, is determined by the mean O_2 content of these two streams, not by their partial pressures of O_2. As discussed in Chapter 2, the O_2 content of arterial blood (CaO_2) is equal to the number of grams of hemoglobin per 100 ml of blood times the O_2-carrying capacity of hemoglobin (1.34 ml O_2/gm) times the arterial O_2 saturation (SaO_2), plus the amount of O_2 dissolved in blood (0.003 ml/100 ml

blood times PaO_2). Because the CaO_2 depends upon the SaO_2, it is lowered by desaturated blood coming from areas of poor ventilation. However, because at least some ventilation is present even in the abnormal areas of the lung, the blood can be better saturated by raising the alveolar PO_2 in those areas.

Shunt. Shunt occurs when alveoli are collapsed or flooded with pus in pneumonia or flooded with edema fluid in left ventricular failure or the neonatal or adult respiratory distress syndrome. The pathophysiology of shunt is different from that of low $\dot{V}A/\dot{Q}$ mismatching. Absolutely no ventilation occurs in the abnormal lung areas in shunt, so venous blood perfusing the areas remains desaturated even when the PiO_2 is increased. The extra O_2 may improve saturation in normal lung areas from 97 to 100 per cent, but because the blood shunted by the abnormal areas retains a mixed venous saturation of only 75 per cent (or less in severe oxygenation failure), the CaO_2 is relatively unimproved. Shunt can be considered an extreme form of $\dot{V}A/\dot{Q}$ mismatching, and the two can be differentiated only by administering 100 per cent O_2; this will substantially improve $\dot{V}A/\dot{Q}$ mismatching but not shunt. The distinction between $\dot{V}A/\dot{Q}$ mismatching and shunt is important not only because these causes of hypoxemia occur in different diseases but also because their presence may dictate different measures to improve the PaO_2.

Effects of Decreasing Arterial Oxygen Tension. An acute fall in the PaO_2 from normal (90 mmHg in young adults) to 50 mmHg or less leads to impaired O_2 transport and generalized cellular hypoxia. This in turn compromises cerebral function, leading to agitation and eventually to coma, and may cause myocardial ischemia and left ventricular depression. Cardiac output declines, further impairing O_2 transport and stimulating anaerobic metabolism. The resulting lactic acidosis induces even more organ dysfunction. Although the brain and body may adjust to the chronic hypoxemia of altitude and certain cardiopulmonary diseases, pulmonary hypertension and cor pulmonale due to hypoxic pulmonary vasoconstriction usually are the price of this adaptation.

General Management

Failure of arterial oxygenation is treated by improving the PaO_2. This ultimately can be accomplished by reversing the process or processes responsible for hypoxemia in the first place. Thus, patients who are hypoxemic because they are exposed to the low PiO_2 of a high altitude or of smoke should have their PiO_2 increased. Hypoxemia due to hypoventilation will be improved by increasing $\dot{V}A$. The hypoxemia caused by $\dot{V}A/\dot{Q}$ mismatching in patients with asthma or COPD should respond to bronchodilator drugs and other therapy for those conditions. Treatment for pneumonia, left ventricular failure, or the neonatal or adult respiratory distress syndrome is aimed at decreasing shunt and improving the PaO_2.

While this is being accomplished, supplemental O_2 should be provided in one of two forms. Hypoxemia due to $\dot{V}A/\dot{Q}$ mismatching usually requires supplemental O_2 at an inspired O_2 fraction (FIO_2) of 0.50 or less, which is called low FIO_2 therapy. Low FIO_2 therapy is easy to administer by nasal prongs and other open systems in spontaneously breathing patients, although intubation and mechanical ventilation may be necessary if failure of ventilation is also present. It is also safe to give for many days because the risk of pulmonary O_2 toxicity is low (see Chapter 14).

On the other hand, hypoxemia due to shunt often requires supplemental O_2 at FIO_2 greater than 0.50. High FIO_2 therapy of this sort is difficult to achieve without a closed system that necessitates endotracheal intubation or a tightly fitting face mask. High FIO_2 therapy also may cause pulmonary O_2 toxicity if continued for longer than 24 to 48 hours. Because of this, positive end-expiratory pressure (PEEP) often is used to improve the PaO_2 in patients with shunt and thereby diminish their need for a high FIO_2. This topic is discussed further in Chapter 14.

RESPIRATORY FAILURE IN SPECIFIC DISEASES

Obstructive Pulmonary Disease

Lower Airway Obstruction

Asthma. Asthma that causes acute respiratory failure and does not respond to conventional therapy is called status asthmaticus. This condition may occur in those few patients who suffer from chronic hypoxemia and hypercapnia because their asthma is always uncontrollable but is more common in individuals whose pulmonary function is normal or near-normal between attacks. Hypoxemia in acute asthma is caused by $\dot{V}A/\dot{Q}$ mismatching and should improve with low FIO_2 therapy. Hypocapnia usually is the rule during an attack because ventilation is stimulated, presumably by pulmonary stretch receptors. Thus, the presence of a seemingly normal $PaCO_2$ in a patient who is not improving may be an ominous sign suggesting the onset of ventilatory failure.

Acute severe asthma is treated with bronchodilating drugs, including inhaled beta-adrenergic agonists, such as metaproterenol, intravenous theophylline, and corticosteroids. Oral or intravenous hydration also is essential in liquefying secretions and in compensating for the large amounts of water lost through the lungs. Most asthmatic patients respond to these measures and can avoid mechanical ventilation, which is associated with a high incidence of barotrauma in patients with status asthmaticus.

Despite these potential complications, mechanical ventilation should be initiated if the pH falls precipitously and clinical improvement is not expected soon.

Chronic Obstructive Pulmonary Disease. Chronic obstructive pulmonary disease (COPD), which includes chronic bronchitis and emphysema, is the most common cause of chronic hypoxemic and hypercapnic respiratory failure. Hypoxemia in patients with COPD usually results from $\dot{V}A/\dot{Q}$ mismatching. Hypoventilation, when present, is caused by severe airflow obstruction, respiratory muscle dysfunction, and perhaps a pre-existing or acquired abnormality of ventilatory regulation that allows some patients to decrease their work of breathing by increasing their $PaCO_2$ and excreting more CO_2 per breath. Although such patients tolerate chronic failure of ventilation, they and others whose $PaCO_2$ is usually normal may slip into acute ventilatory failure when bronchospasm, retained secretions from severe bronchitis or pneumonia, or further depression of ventilatory drives by drug therapy occurs.

Acute respiratory failure is usually treated in the same fashion in all patients with COPD regardless of their clinical subset. They should be given bronchodilators and corticosteroids with the assumption that they have reversible airflow obstruction, whether or not this has been demonstrated on pulmonary function testing. Pneumonia should be treated with appropriate antibiotics based on sputum examination and culture results. If only bronchitis is present, broad spectrum antibiotics such as trimethoprim-sulfamethoxazole should be given. Chest physiotherapy, including chest percussion and postural drainage, may be helpful in removing secretions (see Chapter 9). Oxygen should be given at a low FIO_2 to correct hypoxemia; high FIO_2 therapy is unnecessary and may cause hypoventilation. Patients with acute respiratory failure usually respond to this broad approach and seldom require intubation and mechanical ventilation, even though they require careful monitoring. The need for intubation and mechanical ventilation increases with worsening hypoxemia and falling pH and becomes unavoidable if patients are unresponsive to conservative measures.

Restrictive Pulmonary Disease

Respiratory Muscle Dysfunction

Both the acute and chronic forms of respiratory failure are common in patients with generalized neuromuscular weakness, cervical cord injury, or bilateral diaphragmatic paralysis. Sudden worsening of hypoxemia and hypercapnia may result from aspiration of gastric contents caused by difficulty in swallowing or a depressed gag reflex. It may also follow pneumonia or extensive atelectasis due to retained secretions in individuals who cannot take a deep breath or cough. In patients whose clinical status is unstable, these problems can be anticipated by monitoring gag reflex, swallowing ability, negative inspiratory force, and vital capacity on a daily basis. Aspiration can be lessened by proper positioning of patients during meals and by giving small meals orally or, when necessary, through feeding tubes. Pneumonia requires antibiotic therapy and improvement of airway clearance, as discussed in Chapter 9. Aids for lung inflation, discussed in Chapter 10, are helpful in preventing and treating atelectasis.

Most patients with severe neuromuscular disease require mechanical ventilation during episodes of acute respiratory failure. Patients with chronic failure may need ventilatory support with or without supplemental O_2 around the clock or during sleep, when they usually hypoventilate more. The negative pressure tank, or iron lung, may be used in stable patients who do not require frequent evaluation or nursing procedures that are difficult to perform inside the tank. However, most patients require intermittent positive-pressure ventilation.

Disease Limiting Lung Tissue

Neonatal Respiratory Distress Syndrome. The neonatal respiratory distress syndrome (NRDS) occurs in premature newborns who manifest immaturity of the alveolar Type II cells that normally produce and secrete surfactant. As discussed in Chapter 2, surfactant is a phospholipid that coats alveolar walls and reduces their surface tension in a volume-dependent manner, so that the surface tension is nearly abolished as the lungs deflate. The work needed to expand the lungs is reduced as a result of this action. The stability of the alveoli is also maintained; they collapse less at low volume, and their expansion helps to prevent pulmonary edema. The relative absence of surfactant in the lungs of premature infants with NRDS contributes to the diffuse atelectasis, pulmonary edema, intrapulmonary shunting, and profound hypoxemia seen in this disorder.

Because the pulmonary circulation is more sensitive to alveolar hypoxia and acidosis in newborns than in adults, marked pulmonary hypertension occurs in NRDS. This increases pulmonary vascular resistance, decreases right ventricular output, and forces desaturated blood to bypass the lungs through the foramen ovale and other extrapulmonary right-to-left fetal channels that normally close at birth. Left ventricular output also decreases, as does systemic vascular resistance, and patients may appear to be in shock. Although respiratory alkalosis occurs initially, usually in combination with an anion gap metabolic acidosis caused by lactic acid due to poor tissue perfusion with hypoxemic blood, respiratory acidosis may supervene and contribute to an extremely low pH.

The treatment of NRDS is aimed at improving oxygenation and thereby alleviating pulmonary hypertension, reducing pulmonary vascular resistance, closing extrapulmonary vascular channels, increasing pulmonary and systemic blood flow, and improving tissue perfusion. Cardiac output can also be assisted by the judicious use of intravascular volume expansion, and sodium bicarbonate ($NaHCO_3$) may be given to counteract metabolic acidosis if tissue perfusion is not improved. Because intrapulmonary shunt is present, oxygenation requires high FiO_2 treatment and PEEP or extracorporeal membrane oxygenation.

Adult Respiratory Distress Syndrome. The adult respiratory distress syndrome (ARDS) is characterized by severe dyspnea, hypoxemia, and decreased respiratory system compliance (Crs) and diffuse pulmonary infiltrates that follow massive acute lung injury from a variety of insults, including direct pulmonary trauma; aspiration of gastric contents; septic shock, often with gram-negative organisms; overwhelming viral, bacterial, fungal, or parasitic pneumonia; fat embolism after long bone fractures or surgery; radiation damage; respiratory burns and smoke inhalation; pancreatitis; and massive emergency transfusions. Oxygen toxicity causes an identical lesion in adults, making it difficult to separate the effects of ARDS from those of its therapy.

The pulmonary capillaries and Type I alveolar lining cells are damaged early in ARDS, as they are in NRDS. This causes an increase in permeability that leads to the accumulation of protein-rich interstitial fluid and alveolar flooding as lymphatic clearance mechanisms are overwhelmed. Type II cells and the surfactant they produce are assumed to be normal before the onset of ARDS. Nevertheless, proteinaceous edema fluid may damage the surfactant already present and interfere with its subsequent production by Type II cells. This results in extensive atelectasis that, in combination with alveolar flooding, causes intrapulmonary shunting and hypoxemia. Because of hyperventilation, the $PaCO_2$ is usually low in the initial stages of ARDS. Yet in some patients, especially those with burns or sepsis, extensive capillary damage and attendant intravascular coagulation eventually cause a marked increase in VD that causes the $PaCO_2$ to rise.

Although pulmonary hypertension due to alveolar hypoxia may occur in ARDS, it rarely is of the magnitude seen in NRDS, and its effects on right ventricular function are not so severe. Extrapulmonary diversion of desaturated blood also is uncommon in ARDS because most adults retain few remnants of the fetal circulation, and cardiac output is usually reduced only if primary left ventricular disease or hypovolemia is present. Nevertheless, management of the two conditions is similar because they both involve severe hypoxemia that is treated with high FiO_2 therapy and, usually, PEEP.

Although cardiac output can be enhanced by expanding intravascular volume with isotonic fluids, plasma, or albumin, the fluid and protein will leak through pulmonary capillaries and, in the case of protein, will worsen the oncotic forces that are already drawing water into the lung. For this reason, and because of their expense, plasma and albumin are used sparingly in ARDS, and isotonic fluids should be given only as needed to keep the pulmonary artery wedge pressure normal (10 to 15 mmHg) or low. Some clinicians optimize the wedge pressure by giving drugs to alter systemic vascular resistance and to enhance myocardial contractility. Antibiotics are indicated when infection is documented or suspected, and broad spectrum coverage should be initiated promptly when sepsis or overwhelming pneumonia attributable to as yet unidentified organisms is present.

Pulmonary Vascular Disease

Left Ventricular Failure. Acute hemodynamic pulmonary edema occasionally results from sudden left ventricular dysfunction such as that caused by myocardial ischemia or infarction. Decompensation of this sort also occurs in patients with chronic congestive heart failure whose intravascular volume is expanded because of sodium and water retention. Pulmonary artery catheterization may be necessary to differentiate hemodynamic pulmonary edema, which is caused by elevated left ventricular and left atrial end-diastolic pressures that are reflected in an increased pulmonary artery wedge pressure, from the increased permeability edema of ARDS, in which these pressures should be normal or low. The treatment of hemodynamic pulmonary edema in the setting of cardiogenic shock is discussed below.

Disordered Ventilatory Regulation

Chemical Hypoventilation. Ventilatory failure commonly results from central nervous system depression by drugs. Failure of oxygenation also may occur if hypoventilation is severe, if a process such as aspiration of gastric contents is also present, or if the drugs induce pulmonary edema by increasing capillary permeability. Measurement of arterial blood gases is essential in documenting the degree of hypoventilation and determining whether or not there is concurrent increase of the $P(A-a)O_2$. Protection of the airway and maintenance of adequate ventilation and oxygenation are the first priority in all patients with severely depressed consciousness. In addition to providing airway access, endotracheal tubes limit aspiration, which facilitates gastric lavage with saline and permits the administration of activated charcoal and cathartics via a nasogastric tube with greater safety. Pulmonary artery catheter monitoring is desirable in administering fluids to patients with hypotension or pulmonary edema induced by narcotics, salicylates, and other drugs.

FAILURE OF OXYGEN TRANSPORT

DEFINITION

Oxygen transport is said to fail when the amount of O_2 reaching the peripheral tissues is inadequate to support aerobic metabolism.

This generally is reflected in a low PO_2 of mixed venous blood ($P\bar{v}O_2$ less than 40 mmHg) caused in part by increased tissue O_2 extraction, or by lactic acidosis due to compensatory anaerobic metabolism, or by both.

PATHOPHYSIOLOGY AND GENERAL MANAGEMENT OF FAILURE OF OXYGEN TRANSPORT

Pathophysiology

Factors Governing Oxygen Transport. As discussed in Chapter 2, O_2 transport is the product of the amount of O_2 carried in arterial blood, the O_2 content (CaO_2), and the total blood flow to the tissues, the left ventricular output ($\dot{Q}T$). Left ventricular output may be calculated by multiplying the heart rate (HR) and the stroke volume (SV). It also is equal to the pressure gradient across the systemic circulation (mean arterial pressure [MAP] minus right atrial pressure) divided by the systemic vascular resistance (SVR). The SVR is composed of local resistances, arranged in parallel, that regulate regional blood flow.

According to the Fick equation, $\dot{Q}T$ also is equal to $\dot{V}O_2$, which represents the O_2 demands of the tissues, divided by the amount of O_2 extracted by the tissues, which is equal to the CaO_2 minus the mixed venous O_2 content ($C\bar{v}O_2$). Thus, $\dot{Q}T = \dot{V}O_2/C(a-\bar{v})O_2$.

Abnormalities of Oxygen Transport. Abnormalities in any or all of the above variables can alter O_2 transport. A common problem is a low CaO_2. One cause for this is hypoxemia, as seen in patients with asthma, COPD, and the respiratory distress syndromes. Tissue oxygenation also may be impaired in two situations in which the PaO_2 may be normal but the CaO_2 is reduced: anemia and carbon monoxide poisoning. Perhaps the most frequent abnormality of O_2 transport is an impairment in $\dot{Q}T$. This may result from a marked increase (tachydysrhythmia) or decrease (bradydysrhythmia) in HR or from an inadequate SV due to poor intravascular volume or left ventricular dysfunction. These problems will lower MAP unless SVR increases proportionately. Alternatively, a low $\dot{Q}T$ may occur because SVR is inappropriately high.

General Management

Failure of O_2 transport should prompt normalization of the abnormal variables outlined above. As previously mentioned, hypoxemic patients need O_2. The treatments of anemia and carbon monoxide poisoning are described below. Normalization of $\dot{Q}T$ may be a complex task. In general, it involves improving SV by optimizing intravascular volume, restoring HR if profound tachy- or bradydysrhythmias are present, and altering SVR and MAP with vasoactive drugs as discussed later.

FAILURE OF OXYGEN TRANSPORT IN SPECIFIC DISEASES

Anemia

Anemia is characterized by a low hemoglobin concentration. The PaO_2 and SaO_2 are normal in anemic patients with unimpaired lung function, and the $\dot{Q}T$ is often elevated as a compensatory mechanism to aid O_2 delivery. However, if the anemia is severe enough, lactic acidosis may be present. Patients with acute anemia usually require red blood cell transfusions; hyperbaric oxygenation has been used as a temporary measure to dissolve more O_2 in blood and improve O_2 transport in cases of uncorrectable anemia.

Carbon Monoxide Poisoning

Carbon monoxide (CO), which may be inhaled intentionally in a suicide attempt or unintentionally during a fire, forms a complex called carboxyhemoglobin that displaces O_2 from hemoglobin and reduces the CaO_2. Carbon monoxide also shifts the O_2 hemoglobin dissociation curve to the left and lowers the P_{50}, the partial pressure at which hemoglobin is one-half saturated with O_2, which limits the amount of O_2 released to the tissues. The PaO_2 remains normal in the early phases of CO poisoning; the carotid and aortic chemoreceptors are therefore not stimulated to augment ventilation. Ventilation is eventually increased, however, as cardiopulmonary dysfunction impairs the PaO_2.

The signs and symptoms of CO poisoning relate directly to the carboxyhemoglobin level, as outlined in Table 7–2. Because the SaO_2 routinely provided with arterial blood gas analysis is calculated from the PaO_2 and assumes a normal hemoglobin, a direct spectrophotometric O_2 saturation level, a carboxyhemoglobin level, or both should be requested whenever CO poisoning is suspected. Pulse oximetry is not helpful in the diagnosis of CO poisoning.

Table 7–2. CORRELATION BETWEEN CARBOXYHEMOGLOBIN LEVEL AND SIGNS AND SYMPTOMS OF CARBON MONOXIDE POISONING

% BLOOD SATURATION	SIGNS AND SYMPTOMS
0–10	None
10–20	Headache due to cerebral vasodilatation
20–30	Chest pain due to myocardial hypoxia
30–40	Severe headache, chest pain, weakness, nausea, vomiting
40–50	Same as preceding plus increased ventilation and heart rate
Greater than 50	Seizures, Cheyne-Stokes respiration, coma, death

Adapted from Goodman LS, et al.: *Goodman and Gilman's The Pharmacological Basis of Therapeutics*, 6th ed. New York, Macmillan, 1980.

Oxygen displaces CO from hemoglobin in direct proportion to the PaO_2. Therefore the treatment for CO poisoning is supplemental O_2 at as high an FiO_2 as possible. Hyperbaric oxygenation also may be used to improve the PaO_2 and dissolve more O_2.

Circulatory Shock

General Principles. Acute circulatory shock is characterized by ineffective general or regional blood flow and by tissue perfusion as manifested by lactic acidosis. Patients in shock need not be hypoxemic, although the PaO_2 may be low. Circulatory shock may be divided into the four categories listed in Table 7–3.

Hypovolemic Shock. Hypovolemia follows the loss of blood, plasma, electrolyte-containing fluids, or combinations thereof. This condition is especially common in trauma patients and in those who are bleeding from the gastrointestinal tract. Initially, cardiac output is inadequate owing only to decreased intravascular volume in patients without pre-existing heart disease, although myocardial function eventually may be depressed as a result of inadequate tissue oxygenation. Systemic vascular resistance usually increases in response to an outpouring of endogenous catecholamines. This may maintain MAP temporarily, but hypovolemic shock can be remedied only if intravascular volume is restored. Initial resuscitation usually involves large quantities of normal saline (NaCl) until blood or plasma can be replaced.

Cardiogenic Shock. Cardiogenic shock is caused by primary left ventricular dysfunction in the setting of myocardial infarction, congestive heart failure, or severe dysrhythmias. Such dysfunction affects O_2 transport in several ways. First, the rise in left ventricular end-diastolic filling pressure, owing to an increased volume in the ventricle (preload), causes water to transude from the pulmonary capillaries into the alveoli; the shunt that results from this edema

Table 7–3. **CLASSIFICATION OF CIRCULATORY SHOCK**

TYPE OF SHOCK	CHARACTERISTICS	CLINICAL EXAMPLES
Hypovolemic	Decreased intravascular volume	Blood loss due to hemorrhage, plasma loss due to burn, fluid and electrolyte loss due to diarrhea
Cardiogenic	Left ventricular dysfunction	Myocardial infarction, congestive heart failure
Distributive	Altered systemic or regional vascular resistance(s)	Bacterial sepsis, liver failure, inflammation
Obstructive	Anatomical obstruction to blood flow	Pulmonary embolism, cardiac tamponade, tension pneumothorax

Adapted from Weil MH, and Henning RJ.: New concepts in the diagnosis and fluid treatment of circulatory shock. *Anesth Analg,* 58:124–131, 1979.

reduces the PaO_2 and the CaO_2. The $P\bar{v}O_2$ and $C\bar{v}O_2$ also fall both because the amount of O_2 reaching the tissues is low and because poor peripheral perfusion increases tissue O_2 extraction. Since the decrease in $P\bar{v}O_2$ is greater than that in PaO_2, the $C(a-\bar{v})O_2$ usually widens. Although SVR increases and offsets the concurrent fall in MAP, this further compromises left ventricular function by increasing the afterload against which the ventricle must pump. It also increases myocardial $\dot{V}O_2$, a dangerous event during ischemia or infarction.

Cardiogenic shock is treated by manipulating the variable responsible for $\dot{Q}T$. Heart rate should be normalized whenever possible. Pulmonary artery catheterization is helpful in determining and optimizing pulmonary artery wedge pressure, a reflection of left ventricular end-diastolic pressure. Patients in cardiogenic shock often increase their $\dot{Q}T$ with a high wedge pressure (15 to 20 mmHg) because the increased preload lengthens the left ventricular muscle fibers and helps the ventricle pump more effectively; this is called the Frank-Starling mechanism. However, pulmonary edema will result if the wedge is too high. Left ventricular preload may be reduced by diuretics, which reduce intravascular volume, and by morphine sulfate or nitroglycerin compounds, which redistribute it to the venous capacitance vessels.

Alpha-adrenergic agonists such as high-dose dopamine or norepinephrine may be required to augment SVR and raise MAP in some patients; other patients may require reductions in SVR with nitroprusside and other arterial vasodilators. Beta agonists such as dobutamine are occasionally given to augment myocardial contractility, but this raises myocardial $\dot{V}O_2$. Impairment in arterial oxygenation is treated with supplemental O_2 at a high FiO_2.

Distributive Shock. Distributive shock results from changes in regional vascular resistance and blood flow. Venous capacitance also increases, diminishing the effective intravascular volume. These abnormalities occur during invasion of the bloodstream with bacteria and other microorganisms (sepsis), with liver failure, and with peritonitis and other inflammatory conditions.

Systemic vascular resistance generally is low during distributive shock; $\dot{Q}_T$ is high because resistance to left ventricular emptying (afterload) is diminished and because of circulating endogenous catecholamines. Distributive shock is treated with judicious use of saline to maintain preload while also avoiding transudation of fluid into the lung through pulmonary capillaries whose permeability often is increased. Alpha-adrenergic agents such as dopamine or norepinephrine may be necessary to raise SVR and support MAP, but care should be taken to ensure adequate renal perfusion; this may be aided by dopamine.

Patients with distributive shock who do not die of hypotension may go on to sustain the simultaneous or sequential dysfunction of several organ systems, especially the respiratory system; that is, they may develop ARDS. This syndrome, which is called multiple organ system failure (MOSF), has been attributed to poisoning of intracellular respiration or altered regional blood flow in the face of what would appear to be an adequate $\dot{Q}_T$. The end result is that patients develop a state of increased $P\bar{v}O_2$ and decreased $C(a-\bar{v})O_2$, as discussed under Failure of Tissue Oxygen Extraction.

Obstructive Shock. Obstructive shock results from anatomical impediments to blood flow. For example, pulmonary thromboembolism lowers $\dot{Q}_T$ by preventing blood in the right ventricle from reaching the left atrium. Tension pneumothorax compromises left ventricular filling, and hence SV, by compressing mediastinal structures, including the vena cava, which returns blood to the heart. Cardiac tamponade, which follows the influx of blood or fluid into the pericardial sac, also prevents left ventricular filling. Although temporary circulatory support may be achieved by increasing intravascular volume in selected patients, obstructive shock generally can be alleviated only if the obstruction is relieved.

FAILURE OF TISSUE OXYGEN EXTRACTION

DEFINITION

Inadequate tissue O_2 uptake results from the inability of cells to extract O_2 from the blood and use it for aerobic metabolism. This results in lactic acidosis and an increase in $P\bar{v}O_2$.

PATHOPHYSIOLOGY AND GENERAL MANAGEMENT OF FAILURE OF TISSUE OXYGEN UPTAKE

Pathophysiology

Factors Affecting Oxygen Uptake. Tissue O_2 extraction depends on three factors: the $\dot{V}O_2$ of the tissues, which determines their need for O_2; the $P\bar{v}O_2$, which usually must be 20 mmHg or greater for O_2 to diffuse into cells; and the readiness of hemoglobin to release O_2 to the tissues, as reflected in the position of the O_2-hemoglobin dissociation curve and the P_{50}. The P_{50} is affected by the temperature, PCO_2, and pH of the tissues. Severe alkalemia shifts the O_2-hemoglobin dissociation curve to the left, lowers the P_{50}, and impairs O_2 unloading. This also occurs with CO poisoning, as discussed previously.

General Management

Impaired tissue O_2 extraction is seen in cyanide poisoning and distributive shock, which are discussed in the following sections. As a general principle, severe alkalemia should be prevented to avoid compromising peripheral extraction.

FAILURE OF TISSUE OXYGEN UPTAKE IN SPECIFIC DISEASES

Cyanide Poisoning

Cyanide (CN) poisoning may occur during a suicide attempt or during smoke exposure in a fire that involved hydrocyanic acid. The CN ion released by the acid reacts with the iron in cytochrome oxidase, a key enzyme within cells, to form a complex that inhibits intracellular respiration. Although the PaO_2 is normal, intracellular hypoxia stimulates the carotid and aortic chemoreceptors; this markedly augments $\dot{V}A$ and may increase the PaO_2 above normal. Cardiac output and O_2 transport also increase until the myocardial cells succumb to hypoxia. Since $\dot{V}O_2$ is decreased and little or no O_2 is extracted by the tissues, the $P\bar{v}O_2$ increases and the $C(a-\bar{v})O_2$ narrows, the reverse of the situation in cardiogenic shock. The PO_2 in a venous sample obtained from a peripheral vein also may be greater than the normal level of approximately 40 mmHg.

Patients with CN poisoning do not respond to supplemental O_2. They will die of cardiopulmonary arrest unless given an antidote from the kit found in most emergency rooms. The kit contains sodium nitrite (0.3 to 0.5 gram dissolved in water and given intravenously), which frees cytochrome oxidase by combining with CN and hemoglobin to create cyanmethemoglobin. Sodium thiosulfate (12.5 grams in water given intravenously) then reacts with the CN to form thiocyanate, a relatively nontoxic substance that is excreted in the urine. The methemoglobin remaining from this reaction acts like CO in limiting O_2 transport, and the administration of another specific antidote, methylene blue, may be required.

Distributive Shock

As indicated earlier, patients with distributive shock may develop MOSF and demonstrate abnormalities of tissue oxygen extraction characterized by increased $P\bar{v}O_2$ and decreased $C(a-\bar{v})O_2$ in the face of apparently adequate $\dot{Q}T$. This situation has been attributed to abnormal intracellular respiration (because of its resemblance to CN poisoning) and altered regional blood flow. In the hope that the latter abnormality is present, some clinicians treat patients with distributive shock and MOSF with large saline infusions or intravenous dobutamine to increase $\dot{Q}T$ and thereby augment $\dot{V}O_2$. This approach has succeeded in increasing $\dot{V}O_2$ in some patients with sepsis and lactic acidosis, suggesting that their intracellular respiration is not poisoned. However, it has not been shown to affect the overall outcome of distributive shock or MOSF.

RECOMMENDED READING

1. Ashbaugh DG, et al.: Acute respiratory distress in adults. *Lancet*, 2:319–323, 1967.
2. Benowitz NL, et al.: Cardiopulmonary catastrophes in drug-overdosed patients. *Med Clin North Am*, 63:267–296, 1979.
3. Danek SJ, et al.: The dependence of oxygen uptake on oxygen delivery in the adult respiratory distress syndrome. *Am Rev Respir Dis,* 122:387–395, 1980.
4. Durinsky PM, and Gadek JE: Mechanisms of nonpulmonary oxygen failure in ARDS. *Chest* 96:885–892, 1989.
5. Gilbert EM, et al.: The effect of fluid loading, blood transfusion, and catecholamine infusion on oxygen delivery and consumption in patients with sepsis. *Am Rev Respir Dis* 134:873–879, 1986.
6. Goodman LS, et al.: *Goodman and Gilman's The Pharmacological Basis of Therapeutics,* 6th ed. New York, Macmillan, 1980.
7. Heffner JE, and Sahn SA: Salicylate-induced pulmonary edema. Clinical features and progress. *Ann Intern Med*, 95:405–409, 1981.
8. Hudson LD: Causes of the adult respiratory distress syndrome—clinical recognition. *Clin Chest Med*, 3:195–212, 1982.
9. Hudson LD: Ventilatory management of patients with adult respiratory distress syndrome. *Semin Respir Med*, 2:128–139, 1981.
10. Pierson DJ: Acute respiratory failure. *In* Sahn SA (ed.): *Pulmonary Emergencies.* New York, Churchill Livingstone, 1982, pp. 75–126.
11. Ralph D, and Robertson HT: Respiratory gas exchange in adult respiratory distress syndrome. *Semin Respir Med*, 2:114–122, 1981.
12. Shoemaker WC, et al.: Therapy of shock, based on pathophysiology, monitoring, and outcome prediction. *Crit Care Med* 18:519–525, 1980.

8

METHODS OF AIRWAY MAINTENANCE

ARTIFICIAL AIRWAYS

PHYSIOLOGICAL BASIS FOR THE USE OF ARTIFICIAL AIRWAYS

General Considerations

The free flow of gas into and out of the lungs is the goal of most aspects of respiratory care. Whenever disease or dysfunction compromises gas exchange, artificial airways are used (Fig. 8–1). These airways can be divided into those that occupy the nose or mouth, those that traverse the larynx (translaryngeal), and those that are placed directly in the trachea through a tracheostomy. The last two kinds of airways constitute endotracheal or transtracheal intubation and provide a secure airway. They often are preferable to those that merely occupy the nose or mouth, although all kinds are described in detail below.

Specific Indications

Prevention or Reversal of Upper Airway Obstruction. Potential or actual acute upper airway obstruction due to croup, epiglottitis, laryngeal tumors, or head and neck surgical trauma is usually managed by a transtracheal airway. An intermittent form of upper airway closure occurs during the obstructive sleep apnea syndrome, which is described in Chapter 5. In patients with this syndrome, relaxation of the oropharyngeal muscles during sleep causes a collapse of the pharyngeal walls and prolapse of the tongue to such an extent that the airway is completely closed. The obstruction is relieved only when the subjects awaken, which may occur hundreds of times during an eight-hour period of sleep. The low alveolar oxygen tension (PaO_2) that accompanies the apneic periods is sufficient to cause pulmonary artery hypertension and cor pulmonale in some individuals. The threat of sudden death because of dysrhythmias induced by hypoxemia also is real. Because of these factors, a permanent tracheostomy may be called for in patients who do not improve following weight reduction, nasal continuous

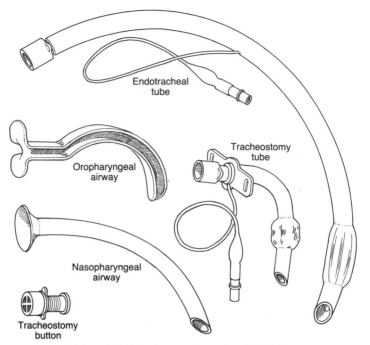

Figure 8–1. Five frequently used artificial airways.

positive airway pressure (CPAP), described in Chapter 13, or other forms of therapy. In certain cases a tracheostomy button (described later in the chapter) can be used in place of a standard tracheostomy tube.

Protection Against Aspiration. Translaryngeal airways or tracheostomy tubes with inflatable cuffs are frequently used to prevent aspiration of oropharyngeal or gastric contents. Although major aspiration can be prevented by this approach, it is important to recognize that the cuff does not provide absolute protection and that minor amounts of aspiration do occur. A cuff whose diameter is less than that of the tracheal lumen obviously permits continued aspiration, and a cuff whose resting diameter is larger than the lumen but whose wall has wrinkled may allow a thin trickle of fluid to pass (Fig. 8–2). If wrinkles are present, fluid may pass by the cuff when the pressure of the liquids above it exceeds the cuff-to-tracheal-wall pressure. Therefore, some clinicians suggest maintaining cuff pressures at approximately 15 cm H_2O as measured at end-exhalation.

Facilitating Tracheobronchial Toilet. Artificial airways are useful

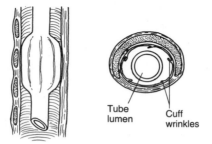

Tube lumen   Cuff wrinkles

Figure 8–2. Wrinkles are often present in low-pressure tracheal cuffs despite an airtight seal, because many cuffs are larger in diameter than the trachea. Secretions and oral or gastric feedings may trickle past a correctly inflated cuff through channels formed by the wrinkles.

whenever excessive or abnormal tracheobronchial secretions cannot be cleared by ciliary transport and cough. Patients without the normal ability or desire to move and change position frequently are also at risk for retention of secretions, particularly if they have concurrent respiratory disease. Transtracheal airways provide consistent access to the lower airways for repeated suctioning; however, the presence of excessive secretions should seldom be the only reason for selecting an artificial airway. Nasopharyngeal intubation, discussed under Kinds of Artificial Airways, is often successful in facilitating nasotracheal suctioning and is associated with minimal risk.

Providing a Closed System for Mechanical Ventilation. Patients who require mechanical support for respiratory failure (see Chapter 13) most often should be managed with endotracheal airways. Unconscious patients in particular are at high risk for aspiration as well because their gag reflexes are depressed, and they may also require frequent suctioning to remove tracheobronchial secretions. Although tightly fitting face or nasal masks are used to improve arterial oxygenation in some patients, including those with neonatal or adult respiratory distress syndromes (NRDS, ARDS), this approach is appropriate only in conscious, cooperative patients.

LIMITATIONS OF ARTIFICIAL AIRWAYS

Interference with Host Defenses

Artificial airways provide air to the lung that bypasses the normal air conditioning functions of the upper airway. The air is neither warmed nor humidified, and large particles are not scavenged by entrapment in nasal hairs. Ciliary motion is decreased in the area of the cuff when it is inflated, resulting in stasis of secretion transport at that level. This is probably of little clinical concern except in patients with excessive secretions.

Cough efficiency is also decreased by placement of transtracheal tubes because glottic and vocal cord closure is either ineffective because the stoma is below the larynx or impossible with a translaryngeal tube in place. Effective coughing depends on the ability to generate the high intrathoracic pressures necessary to achieve a high velocity of airflow. Glottic closure, large lung volumes, and expiratory (abdominal) muscle strength all are factors in determining the intrathoracic pressure. However, the importance of glottic closure is often overemphasized, as patients with normal muscular strength and cough reflexes regularly cough mucus from their tubes for considerable distances. For the same reasons, patients whose coughs are weak may not have a recovery of cough efficiency when their artificial airways are removed. Prediction of postextubation cough efficiency is best assessed by peak flow measured through the tube prior to extubation during a cough maneuver.

Interference with Nutrition and Communication

Compulsive attention to providing adequate protein and calories by other than the oral route is required in translaryngeal intubation. Oral feeding is prohibited by orotracheal tubes, although infants with nasotracheal tubes often can nurse from bottles. Adults can eat with such tubes in place only with difficulty. A major advantage of tracheostomies is that eating is possible. Communication, including the important aspect of emotional expression, is severely limited by all types of artificial airways although less so by tracheostomies. Providing a means of communication, particularly vocal communication, is essential for all conscious patients and is reason enough to perform a tracheostomy when long-term intubation is required. The sound of one's own voice is a powerful mood elevator and motivator and may make the difference in difficult-to-wean patients.

Increased Care and Expense

As foreign bodies, artificial airways require considerably more attention than the physiologic airway. Humidification of the inspired air by adding water vapor or aerosolized water to the inspired gas is required both to humidify the lower airways and to prevent crusting of secretions that collect in the lumen of the tube. Often, suctioning is also needed to remove mucous secretions or blood from the tube. Considerable time and effort must also be expended in keeping tubes in place. Careful taping and frequent repositioning are needed. Restraints are frequently required, as patients requiring airways are often confused and uncooperative. Unfortunately, these result in loss of mobility.

KINDS OF ARTIFICIAL AIRWAYS

Oropharyngeal Airway

Standard oropharyngeal (OP) airways (see Fig. 8–1) are designed and used to prevent obstruction of the airway by prolapse of the tongue. They also are used to prevent patients from biting the tongue, an oral endotracheal tube, or a fiberoptic bronchoscope. They are not intended for long-term airway management. Oropharyngeal airways are most appropriate in unconscious patients who lack a gag reflex or in patients whose own airway has been anesthetized, because the shape and placement of the airways elicit a marked gag response under normal conditions. Complications include dental and tongue trauma in addition to the potential for aspiration owing to gagging and vomiting. Particular care is necessary during cardiopulmonary resuscitation (CPR). The OP airway must be removed promptly when the victim begins to regain consciousness.

The OP airway is inserted by opening the jaw using the crossed finger technique, turning the airway sideways or upside down while placing it in the mouth and finally aligning it with the concave side against the tongue. This pulls the tongue forward and out of the oropharynx. The OP airway should not be taped in place unless the patient is under constant observation, since it is impossible to extrude the airway if vomiting occurs. Care must be taken when taping the airway not to entrap the tongue against the teeth or to apply pressure on the lips.

Nasopharyngeal Airway

The nasopharyngeal (NP) airway (see Fig. 8–1) also protects the upper airway by providing an unobstructed pathway past a relaxed tongue. It often is a better choice than the OP airway because it does not stimulate the gag reflex; however, its use is traditionally limited to the immediate postanesthetic period.

An additional use of the NP airway is to facilitate access to the trachea by a fiberoptic bronchoscope or a suction catheter. It is particularly useful in patients requiring repeated nasotracheal suctioning, as it both prevents trauma to the nasal mucous membrane and greatly increases the likelihood of intratracheal placement of the catheter. The latter result is due to the position of the distal end of the airway (Fig. 8–3) just above the glottic opening. The NP tube essentially guides the catheter directly to the trachea.

For prolonged nasopharyngeal intubation a soft latex tube should be chosen. Anesthetic sprays of the nares and the pharynx are used prior to insertion, and the tube is liberally lubricated with anesthetic jelly and inserted without force in a direction horizontal to the plane of the oral cavity (Fig. 8–3). Trauma and bleeding on insertion of any nasal tube are almost always due to the incorrect

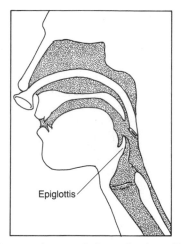

Epiglottis

Figure 8–3. The nasopharyngeal airway in place. Note that the distal end of the airway is just above the larynx, facilitating tracheal catheterization. In addition, the nasal mucosa is protected during repeated nasotracheal suctioning episodes.

insertion of the tube in an upward direction, which results in impaction on the turbinates. Pressure sores and erosion of nasal mucous membranes as well as sinusitis are possible complications, particularly if a too-large, stiff tube is used. If the tube does not have a generous flange at the proximal end, a large safety pin is inserted through the tube to prevent its migration. Taping is seldom necessary. The tube is well tolerated for as long as a week.

Endotracheal Tubes

Indications

Endotracheal (ET) tubes (see Fig. 8–1) are used whenever long-term (>1 to 2 hours) support of ventilation or arterial oxygenation, or both, are required. Persistent upper airway obstruction also requires a secure airway. Also, if secretion management is inadequate despite the use of the NP airway and the therapies described in Chapter 9, ET tubes may be the initial choice in preference to tracheostomy tubes because they can be rapidly placed and may eliminate a surgical procedure in what may turn out to be a relatively short-term problem.

Complications and Precautions

General complications of ET tubes include trauma to nasal and oral mucous membranes, teeth, tongue, larynx, and trachea during and after intubation. Intubation of the right and, less commonly, the left mainstem bronchus may cause degassing and atelectasis of the contralateral lung and occasionally, in the case of right mainstem catheterization, the right upper lobe. Infection of the ipsilateral sinuses and ear also occurs and should be suspected when unexplained fever occurs. Endotracheal tubes are foreign bodies, and an open conduit that bypasses natural host defenses; they also are uncomfortable. Thus, they should not be used just to make care "easier."

Insertion and Fixation
Oral Endotracheal Tube. Rapid insertion makes the oral ET tube (see Fig. 8–1) the tube of choice in emergency situations. In a nonemergency situation an alert cooperative patient should receive atropine, 0.8 mg intramuscularly, and lidocaine (4%) spray to the oropharynx. To shorten intubation time when hypoxia and ventilatory insufficiency are severe, a regimen such as thiopental, 25 to 100 mg intravenously, and succinylcholine, 1 mg/kg, is often used. The neck is flexed and the head extended in the sniff position with a thin pillow under the head only. The lower jaw should be held forward. A laryngoscope is usually used to expose the larynx, although blind intubation is sometimes possible with good positioning and cooperation. Difficult intubations due to limited head-neck mobility or abnormal anatomy are facilitated first by passing the fiberoptic laryngoscope or bronchoscope through the larynx and then by introducing the ET tube over the scope. This method also can be used during nasal intubation and tube changes.

An ET tube should be inserted until the cuff is approximately 3 to 5 cm past the vocal cords to allow for movement of the tube with flexion, extension, and lateral positioning of the head. Tube location is immediately assessed by hearing air movement during auscultation of both lung fields and observing bilateral expansion of the thorax. A chest roentgenogram confirms correct placement. Following this, any excess tube protruding from the mouth should be cut off. The remaining portion is measured from point of exit to the ET tube adapter so that major changes in tube position can be determined without the need for repeated chest roentgenograms.

Fixation of the oral ET tube is somewhat difficult because salivation is increased and a bite block or tube holder must be used. Alert patients will want to suction their own mouths, since swallowing is difficult. A strip of adhesive tape or occlusive dressing is placed on each cheek. Strips of tape are then placed on top of the first strips, and their free ends are split and wound around the tube and a bite block, which must be used to prevent the patient from biting and occluding the tube. The position of the tube and bite block should be changed from side to side every eight hours to relieve pressure on the lips and the tongue. Only the top adhesive strips are removed; the cheek strips remain in place to prevent repeated trauma from tape changes.

An advantage of the oral ET tube over the nasal ET tube is the larger size that can be passed. This reduces the work of breathing when the patient is breathing spontaneously and may permit fiberoptic bronchoscopy. However, larger-sized tubes are associated with increased laryngeal trauma and postextubation subglottic stenosis, particularly in women, whose larynxes generally are smaller than men's.

Nasal Endotracheal Tube. The nasal ET tube is preferred by many clinicians because of its relatively greater stability and ease of care, particularly with long-term intubation. However, nasal ET tubes kink more frequently and usually have a higher airflow resistance because a smaller size must be used. Blind intubation is an accepted technique when manipulation of the head and neck is prohibited by injury and visualization is difficult or impossible. Tongue extrusion is particularly helpful during blind nasal intubation because it lifts the epiglottis out of the way.

As with the oral ET tube, postintubation roentgenograms are necessary. Fixation is relatively easy, but care must be taken to prevent upward pressure of the tube on the nares (Fig. 8–4). Nasal necrosis can be avoided by anchoring the tube to the cheeks below the nose rather than snugly up to the tip of the nose. When facial burns are present, umbilical tape or tracheostomy ties are used instead of adhesive tape.

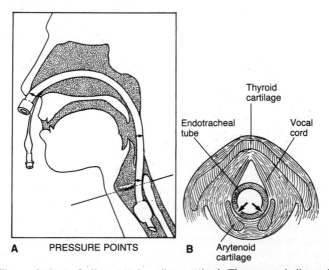

Figure 8–4. *A*, Cuff trauma is well recognized. The arrows indicate the direction of force and less well-known sites of pressure-induced trauma and necrosis seen with nasal endotracheal tubes. *B*, A cross-sectional view at the level of the line in *A* indicates areas within the larynx that are subject to pressure from both nasal and oral endotracheal tubes.

Tracheostomy Tubes

Indications. Tracheostomy tubes (see Fig. 8–1) provide a secure airway, may offer better access to copious secretions, and are much more comfortable than either the oral or the nasal ET tube. The tubes can be relatively large, so that airflow resistance is low, oral or nasal and laryngeal trauma is eliminated, and eating and talking are possible. However, tracheostomies usually are done only when acute upper airway obstruction prevents ET tube placement or when intubation is required for greater than three to four weeks, particularly if the patient is cooperative, relatively immobile, or both.

Changing to a tracheostomy from an ET tube may facilitate weaning in certain patients with chronic obstructive pulmonary disease (COPD). This is because airflow resistance through a tube relates to its length and radius, and a tracheostomy tube is shorter and often has a greater diameter than an ET tube. With the cuff of the tracheostomy tube deflated, total airway resistance may be sufficiently reduced to allow the patient to demonstrate an ability to ventilate spontaneously without tiring, which may be impossible through a higher-resistance ET tube. Deflating the cuff of an ET tube during weaning will not decrease overall resistance very much because the tube nearly fills the larynx. The use of pressure support (see Chapter 13) to conteract the additional work of breathing created by high-resistance ET tubes has eliminated some of these concerns.

Complications and Precautions. The rationale for extended ET tube use is the added cost, morbidity, and mortality associated with the tracheostomy procedure. Postextubation stenosis is also relatively frequent at the level of the tracheotomy incision, particularly if flaps are made instead of excision of the tracheal wall. Stenosis at the cuff level is no different from that seen with any other cuffed tube. There is evidence of increased bacterial infiltration of the larynx and therefore potential laryngeal damage and subglottic stenosis when tracheostomy follows translaryngeal intubation. The stoma site is the presumed source of bacterial contamination.

Insertion and Fixation. Cricothyroidotomy is the fastest procedure in acute upper airway obstruction when ET intubation is impossible; this procedure also is done electively. The more standard tracheotomy is done at the second or third tracheal ring. The tracheostomy tube is fixed in place by string ties knotted firmly at the side of the neck with a one-finger slack between the patient's neck and tie. Tracheostomies are difficult to keep in place in patients with very thick necks and when very high airway pressures are generated during positive-pressure ventilation of noncompliant lungs. One tracheostomy tube (Fig. 8–5) is made of a pliable material in which a spiral metal core is incorporated; this device

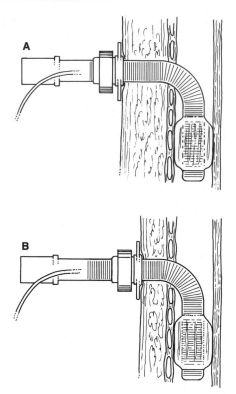

Figure 8–5. The Rusch Trach-O-Flex tracheostomy tube has a movable flange that permits adjustment for swelling (*A*) or neck size (*B*) at the level of the stoma.

also has a movable flange that can accommodate an edematous or thick, muscular neck wall (Rusch Trach-O-Flex). Additionally, the flange, which is available separately, can be put on a malleable endotracheal tube that is then placed through the stoma. This allows the tube and cuff position to be adjusted as needed by tightening the flange so that the tube is not propelled out of the stoma by the airway pressure. Substituting an ET tube through a tracheotomy is also helpful when cuff pressure complications such as a dilated trachea mandate moving the level of the cuff.

Special Purpose Tracheostomy Tubes. Fenestrated tracheostomy tubes are sometimes used to decrease airflow resistance while maintaining the stoma during weaning. Precut tubes often need the opening lengthened to assure that the fenestration lies within the lumen and not against the posterior tracheal wall. Normal secretion clearance and cough are impeded by the presence of the tube; therefore, many clinicians prefer the tracheostomy button.

Tracheostomy Buttons

Indications. Tracheostomy buttons (TBs) are cannulas that extend only from the skin to the anterior surface of the trachea (Fig. 8–6; see also Fig. 8–1). They (1) maintain the stoma when the ability to clear secretions or ventilate is in question and recannulization may be necessary, (2) provide an airway in intermittent conditions such as obstructive sleep apnea, and (3) allow occasional suctioning in chronic lung conditions. Although TBs cannot be cuffed, intermittent positive-pressure ventilation and manual deep breaths from a resuscitation bag can be delivered through a 15-mm adapter available for the Olympic button, if necessary. TBs have the advantage, during weaning and routine use, of creating little or no additional resistance to airflow or sputum clearance, because the tubes do not protrude into the airway. Speech, normal humidification, and normal cough flow all are possible when the buttons are capped.

Complications and Precautions. No complications from TBs have been reported, although irritation is sometimes seen at the stoma associated with the spacing rings. The buttons are easily coughed out if they have not been carefully sized for diameter; the retaining petals or flange is not large. The length of the button is either fixed (Kistner Plastic Tracheostomy) or adjustable (Olympic Trach-Button). Selection or adjustment to the correct length is essential to providing a resistance-free airway.

"Speaking" Tracheostomy Tubes or Adapters

Indications. Speech is possible for almost all patients with tracheostomy tubes when the cuff is deflated and the tube opening is

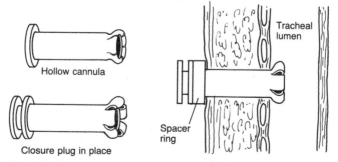

Figure 8–6. A tracheostomy button in place. Note that the cannula does not compromise the tracheal lumen, facilitating low-resistance breathing and sputum clearance.

temporarily occluded. However, the resistance created by exhaling past the tube makes this very difficult for weak patients and sometimes impossible for those with severe COPD. Positive-pressure ventilation also must be interrupted to allow speech in this manner. These problems are eliminated by the Pitt Speaking Tracheostomy Tube (Fig. 8–7), which has a port above the cuff through which a flow of air may be directed. A thumb valve controls the flow and diverts gas from a standard air or oxygen flowmeter into the supply tube. Practice and careful adjustment of airflow (usually 4 to 6 L/min) are necessary to prevent air-swallowing and gastric dilatation.

For patients who can have their ventilator tidal volumes satisfactorily adjusted to account for a blow-by leak, the Pitt Speaking Tracheostomy Tube is useful. The leak occurs because *the cuff must be deflated* when this device is in use; otherwise a ball-valve effect will occur, with potentially lethal consequences. A one-way valve assembly allows inspiration through the valve but closes on expiration, so that the exhaled air is directed through the larynx.

The Passy-Muir Valve can also be used in spontaneously breath-

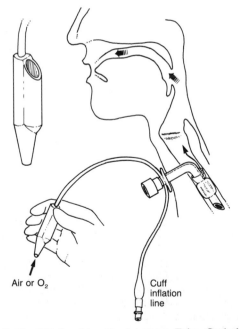

Figure 8–7. The Pitt Speaking Tracheostomy Tube. Occluding the port of the thumb control valve directs compressed air or oxygen into the trachea above the cuff. A flow of 4 to 6 L/min is suggested.

Air or O₂

Cuff inflation line

ing tracheostomized patients, as can the Olympic Trach-Talk. The work of breathing is increased with either device during spontaneous ventilation and may be intolerable for some patients. Fenestrated tracheostomy tubes also permit speech, particularly when they are corked and their cuffs are deflated.

MANAGEMENT OF TRANSLARYNGEAL AND TRACHEOSTOMY TUBES

Suctioning

Indications. Virtually all patients with transtracheal tubes in place require suctioning for both airway clearance (Chapter 9) and maintenance of tube patency. Complete humidification of the inspired gas with heated aerosols or water vapor at 100 per cent relative humidity at body temperature prevents inspissation of secretions in the tube and normalizes the air for the lower airways. The inner cannula on tracheostomy tubes no longer is necessary because of new, less adherent materials and improved humidification systems. However, if blood is seen in the tube, intraluminal clots may form, and the tube should be flushed with 5 to 10 ml of normal saline, followed by suctioning.

Secretion Clearance. Turning the head to the right, using curved-tip catheters, or using both methods is said to direct the catheter to the left main bronchus, but right main bronchus catheterization is the rule in blind suctioning. In general, suctioning cannot be counted on to clear secretions from any portion of the airway distal to the trachea. The methods of airway clearance described in Chapter 9 can be used to bring secretions to the level of the trachea.

Catheter Design. Catheter design and size influence the area reached by suctioning, the flow rate of gas or secretions from the lung, and the potential for mucosal trauma. In open-suction systems, the catheter should not be any larger than one-half the diameter of the ET or the tracheostomy tube, because air must be able to flow freely from the atmosphere to the catheter tip. This prevents potential evacuation of lung gases, atelectasis, and ultimately hypoxemia when suction is applied and secretions do not immediately fill the catheter.

In contrast, closed-suction systems are specifically designed to prevent the entry of ambient-pressure air into the lungs. To prevent the loss of positive end-expiratory pressure (PEEP) and interruption of ventilation during suctioning, the catheter is introduced through either a tightly fitting slit in the swivel adapter, or a special setup with a sleeved catheter and irrigation port (Ballard Trach Care) is placed between the ventilator circuit and the ET tube. The advantages of the latter device are the cost savings associated with repeated use of the same catheter over a 24-hour period and the reduction of opportunity for contamination. Disadvantages common to both closed-system methods are loss of lung volume, thereby defeating the PEEP preservation concept, and sometimes pressure limitation of the ventilator because of the increased airway resistance. The loss of lung volume occurs if suction is applied during the expiratory phase of the ventilator cycle; therefore, it is important to activate the suction only during the inspiratory phase when the ventilator can supply at least part of the volume that will flow out of the catheter (see above).

Placement of the catheter eyes also is a design feature of some concern. A catheter with an end hole surrounded by a beaded tip and a ring of side holes (Argyle Aero-Flo) has been designed to prevent invagination and trauma of the tracheal mucosa. Mucosal invagination also can be prevented by maneuvering a standard catheter in a constant sweeping motion whenever negative pressure is applied. Intermittent application of suction is also suggested, but this is likely to lower suction efficiency and does not decrease mucosal trauma.

Negative Pressure. The amount of negative pressure applied to the catheter also influences mucosal entrapment and lung gas evacuation. Pressures of 100 to 150 mmHg are usually suggested for adults, but may need to be increased if secretions are thick. A low negative pressure may seem optimal in reducing suction trauma, but it will significantly reduce the flow rate through the catheter, especially if resistance is already high owing to small-diameter catheter and to long, narrow connecting tubing interposed between the suction source and the catheter. Flow rate may become so slow at low aspirating pressures that suction efficiency is compromised.

Frequency. Frequency of suctioning is determined by the presence of secretions either observed in the ET tube or tracheostomy tube or heard in the central airways during auscultation. Many patients can cough secretions into or even out of the tube if the tube is disconnected from the ventilator. Airway trauma is prevented by suctioning only the depth of the tube in these patients. There is no rationale for routine suctioning every one or two hours. Suctioning cannot prevent the accumulation of secretions over the next hour and may actually encourage their formation by repeated irritation of the airway.

Cough stimulation is sometimes offered as a reason for routine suctioning. However, cough is mainly a central airway clearance mechanism, and if there are no central secretions present, neither cough nor suctioning is needed. The deep breath associated with a normal cough may be of value in overall lung care, but a deep breath is not usually elicited with an irritative cough and can be more reliably delivered by the methods described in Chapter 10. Peripheral crackles also are not an indication for suctioning, as they represent interstitial processes not associated with secretions or secretions well beyond the reach of the catheter, such as pulmonary edema.

Technique. Suctioning is begun with preoxygenation because a fall in the arterial oxygen tension (PaO_2) is so routinely observed during the procedure. The goal of preoxygenation is to convert a large proportion of the resident lung gas to 100 per cent O_2 to offset the amount used in metabolic consumption while ventilation is interrupted as well as to offset the volume lost through the suction catheter. An O_2-enriched resuscitation or anesthesia bag is used for preoxygenation; alternatively, the ventilator oxygen setting may be increased to an inspired O_2 fraction (FiO_2) of 1.00. Apneic patients are particularly prone to suction-induced hypoxemia because they do not inhale even room-air gas during the procedure. The entire suctioning procedure should not exceed 15 seconds and the time negative pressure is applied should be even shorter, as fall in PaO_2 is also related to suction duration. The catheter should be inserted rapidly *without suction* until it impacts; it is withdrawn slightly and then is removed with a constant, smooth twisting motion with suction applied. Ventilation with O_2-enriched gas should follow immediately. The procedure can then be repeated until the central airways are clear on auscultation.

Saline Instillation. Saline instillation prior to suctioning is probably of no value except to mechanically clean the artificial airway. There is little reason to believe that instilled solutions will remain in contact with secretions long enough to affect their consistency let alone to believe that they will actually find their way to secretions, particularly when one considers that lung volume is 3 to 6 L and the instilled volume is only 5 to 10 ml.

Cuff Pressures

Intracuff and Tracheal Wall Pressure. Because they prevent the escape of the ventilating gas, inflatable cuffs are a necessary adjunct to positive pressure ventilation. Secondary benefits of the inflated cuff are protection against major aspiration of gastric contents, blood, or other drainage and centering of the tube in the trachea. On the other hand, cuffs can cause considerable trauma if the pressure within the cuff is transmitted to the tracheal wall. Modern cuffs are designed so that they have a large resting volume. As the cuff is inflated, it conforms to the shape of the trachea, often filling the space and sealing the airway before the cuff material itself is stretched. Very little pressure is generated within the cuff unless the cuff is filled past this minimal occlusive volume, which usually requires less than 10 ml. The corresponding pressure should not exceed 25 cm H_2O at end-exhalation and is often much less. Some clinicians adjust intracuff pressure to 15 cm H_2O even if not required for adequate ventilation; this adds to the cuff's ability to prevent aspiration. Overfilling the cuff ("one more milliliter for good measure") will cause a rapid rise in intracuff and cuff-to-tracheal-wall pressure.

Depending on the amount of pressure transmitted to the tracheal wall, capillary, venous, or even arterial flow may be compromised in the area in contact with the cuff. When ventilation with PEEP is required, the intracuff pressure during exhalation must at least equal the PEEP to maintain the desired airway pressure. In addition, intracuff pressure will cycle higher with each inspiratory phase of the ventilator. Therefore, it may be impossible to maintain cuff pressure at low levels, particularly in patients with low lung compliance. Reducing tidal volume and flow rates may help, as these maneuvers reduce airway pressure.

Monitoring Intracuff Pressure and Volume. Intracuff pressure should be monitored to prevent overfilling the cuff and to alert the clinician to high-risk conditions. A four-way stopcock and blood pressure manometer or a commercially available aneroid manometer setup is easily attached to the cuff filling line for this purpose. Intracuff volume must also be monitored to detect gradual distention of the trachea at the cuff site. This is not always detected by increasing cuff pressures because the large resting volume of the cuff permits considerable expansion of the trachea before the cuff material itself is stretched, which results in a rise in intracuff pressure. Cuff volume is monitored by aspirating and measuring the volume of air in the cuff after it has been filled to the no-blow-by leak level.

The Pressure Easy Cuff Pressure Controller (CPC) is a convenient device for providing continuous monitoring of intracuff pressures within a range of 18 to 27 cm H_2O. The reservoir system of this device also adjusts the intracuff volume to maintain pressures within this range, but cannot adjust for incorrectly sized or grossly overfilled or underfilled cuffs. A pressure feedback line option is available to override the pressure-limiting characteristics of the CPC when PEEP levels are high and should be used if blow-by leak occurs during ventilation.

Cuff-Associated Complications

Innominate Artery Erosion. Pulsating of the tracheostomy tube or the ET tube is a serious premonitory sign of innominate artery erosion and hemorrhage. The area should be inspected through the fiberoptic bronchoscope and the tube repositioned so that the cuff or tube tip does not abut the artery. The Rusch armored tubes and movable flange will facilitate repositioning the cuff if a tracheostomy is in place. If hemorrhage occurs, overinflating the cuff of an ET airway may compress the artery enough to prevent exsanguination, suffocation, or both. If a tracheostomy is in place, a finger may be inserted in the stoma anterior to the tube and upward pressure applied to compress the artery between the finger and the sternum. Bright red blood of any amount in the tracheal aspirate must not be ignored: Very few patients survive to reach the operating room when frank hemorrhage begins.

Tracheoesophageal Fistula. Food or tube feedings aspirated from the trachea may indicate a tracheoesophageal fistula (TEF), particularly if the patient is not also receiving oral feedings. However, as mentioned above, cuffs do not give total protection against aspiration and, in addition, there is evidence for a decrease in the protective glottic closure reflex following tracheostomy, so food or feedings aspirated from the trachea may have come past the cuff via the larynx. Careful observation during meals and after tube feedings for coughing, in addition to examination with the fiberoptic bronchoscope, may help define the problem. Methylene blue dye is often used to color tube feedings. However, its appearance in the tracheal aspirate is not absolute proof of a TEF, as regurgitated material may leak through the glottis and past the cuff rather than through a fistula. Another indication of a TEF is gastric dilatation or constant eructation. These symptoms may occur if positive-pressure ventilation pushes air from the trachea into the esophagus through the TEF. This complication occurs more frequently when both a cuffed artificial airway and a standard nasogastric tube are present. Fine-gauge feeding tubes may help prevent the pressure necrosis that is thought to precede fistula formation.

Stoma Care

Bleeding during the immediate post-tracheostomy period is usually venous oozing, but arterial hemorrhage is a frequent cause of the 1 to 2 per cent mortality associated with the procedure. Suffocation by aspiration of blood is more likely than exsanguination. Close observation in the ICU is warranted for the first 24 hours after tracheostomy. Betadine-soaked tracheostomy dressings should be used around the stoma for the first two weeks. Prior ET intubation results in pressure-damaged laryngeal tissue that is easily colonized by bacteria, which enter through and also colonize the stoma. Two weeks of Betadine soaks is said to prevent colonization while giving the larynx time to heal, thereby decreasing the likelihood of infection and subsequent subglottic stenosis. Dressings should not be used after two weeks, in order to enhance inspection and cleaning of the area. Eventual colonization of the stoma is inevitable but should not be treated by antibiotic ointments unless infection is actually present.

Nutrition

Oral feeding, as indicated above, may be hampered by diminution of glottic closure reflexes. A soft rather than a liquid diet is often more manageable as the food texture provides cues to elicit the swallowing reflex. Although not without risk, letting the cuff down or using a fenestrated tube in spontaneously breathing patients may allow sufficient airflow through the larynx to cue the usual biofeedback mechanisms that prompt glottic closure and suspension of respiration when food is being swallowed. Examination and coaching of swallowing by a speech therapist are sometimes necessary when reinstituting a normal diet.

Activity

Placement of an artificial airway should not limit activity. Any necessary limitation depends entirely on the underlying condition and not on the presence of an artificial airway. Patients whose condition is stable benefit in muscle tone and strength and psychological status by being allowed, or assisted in, as normal a range of activity as possible. All intubated patients should get out of bed, at least to a chair, assuming hemodynamic and orthopedic contraindications are not present. Ventilator attachments are easily adjusted to the seated patient; assisted ventilation during walking or time away from the ventilator and ICU can be provided by a resuscitation bag with oxygen enrichment. Many patients can "ventilate" themselves with a self-inflating bag.

RECOMMENDED READING

1. Adams AL, et al.: Tongue extrusion as an aid to blind nasal intubation. *Crit Care Med,* 10:335–336, 1982.
2. Cane RD, et al.: Customizing fenestrated tracheostomy tubes: a bedside technique. *Crit Care Med,* 10:880–881, 1982.
3. Chapman GA, et al.: Evaluation of the safety and efficiency of a new suction catheter design. *Respir Care,* 31:889–895, 1986.
4. Chulay M, et al.: Efficacy of hyperinflation and hyperoxygenation suctioning intervention. *Heart Lung,* 17:15–22, 1988.
5. Czarnik RE, et al.: Differential effects of continuous versus intermittent suction on tracheal tissue. *Heart Lung,* 20:144–151, 1991.
6. Elpern EH, et al.: The technique of nasotracheal suctioning: How to prevent mucosal injury, hypoxemia, and atelectasis. *J Crit Illness,* 5:993–999, 1990.
7. Kleiber C, et al.: Acute histologic changes in the tracheobronchial tree associated with different suction catheter insertion techniques. *Heart Lung,* 17:10–14, 1988.
8. Long J, and West G: The Olympic Trach-Button as an interim airway following tracheostomy tube removal. *Respir Care,* 26:1269–1272, 1981.
9. Rogge JA, et al.: Effectiveness of oxygen concentrations of less than 100% before and after endotracheal suction in patients with chronic obstructive pulmonary disease. *Heart Lung,* 18:64–71, 1989.
10. Rudy EB, et al.: Endotracheal suctioning in adults with head injury. *Heart Lung,* 20:667–674, 1991.
11. Sasaki CT, et al.: The effect of tracheostomy on the laryngeal closure reflex. *Laryngoscope,* 87:1428–1433, 1977.
12. Sasaki CT, et al.: Tracheostomy-related subglottic stenosis: bacteriologic pathogenesis. *Laryngoscope,* 89:857–865, 876–877, 1979.
13. Stauffer JL, and Silvestri RC: Complications of endotracheal intubation, tracheostomy, and artificial airways. *Respir Care,* 27:417–434, 1982.

14. Stone KS, et al.: Effect of lung hyperinflation and endotracheal suctioning on heart rate and rhythm in patients after coronary artery bypass graft surgery. *Heart Lung,* 20:443–450, 1991.

15. Taft AA, et al.: A comparison of two methods of preoxygenation during endotracheal suctioning. *Respir Care,* 36:1195–1201, 1991.

16. Walsh JM, et al.: Unsuspected hemodynamic alterations during endotracheal suctioning. *Chest,* 95:162–165, 1989.

9

THERAPY TO IMPROVE AIRWAY CLEARANCE

PHYSIOLOGICAL RATIONALE FOR IMPROVING AIRWAY CLEARANCE

COMPONENTS OF NORMAL AIRWAY CLEARANCE

Mucociliary Membrane

As described in Chapter 1, the upper and lower airways are lined with ciliated epithelium. The mucociliary membrane is composed of two layers: a layer of cilia that beat in a serous fluid and a layer of mucus that rides on top and is propelled toward the pharynx by the cilia. Normal amounts of mucus are transported through the larynx and swallowed without notice. Excess amounts of mucus or other material in the airway stimulate the cough reflex, and the mucus is either expectorated or swallowed. Expectorated respiratory secretions are called sputum.

Cough

Cough is a normal defense mechanism that is activated in the presence of noxious gases, excess mucus, and foreign material such as food or fluids aspirated into the airways. A cough is a series of complex interactions. It involves inspiration to near total lung capacity (TLC); closure of the glottis and contraction of the abdominal muscles, resulting in an increased intrathoracic pressure and dynamic compression of the larger airways; and finally, rapid opening of the glottis to allow an explosive release of the pressurized air. The high flow rates and dynamic compression increase the velocity of the expired air; this in turn supplies the kinetic energy that ultimately shears mucus and foreign matter from the airway walls. Inability to take a deep breath, weak abdominal muscles or an unwillingness to contract them because of pain, and small airway collapse on expiration significantly reduce cough efficiency. An open glottis also reduces efficiency but to a lesser extent (see Chapter 8). Cough is an efficient airway clearance mechanism only when the depth of the tracheobronchial mucus is greater than normal. Therefore, requesting or encouraging cough in patients who do not have retained secretions is not particularly useful and is possibly irritating to airway mucosa. It also is painful in many postoperative situations (see Chapter 10).

Humidification

Warming and humidification of inspired air by the upper airway provide a gas that is nearly saturated in the lower airways and is completely saturated upon reaching the alveoli. When the upper airway is bypassed with an artificial airway, the inspired air is not adequately humidified. As the ambient air warms in the lower airways, the trachea and bronchi must supply all the moisture. As a result, the epithelium rapidly becomes desiccated, friable, easily injured, and penetrable by bacteria. Mucociliary transport is also less effective, possibly as a result of changes in mucus consistency, ciliary function, or both.

COMPROMISED AIRWAY CLEARANCE

Signs and Symptoms

Retained secretions are the hallmark of compromised airway clearance. Auscultation of gurgles or rhonchi and frequent cough, usually with expectoration, are the most prominent signs. Wheezing, atelectasis, and dyspnea are frequently found.

Causes of Secretion Retention

Mucus Hypersecretion. Mucus hypersecretion is the most frequent cause of retained secretions. Asthma, bronchiectasis [including that caused by cystic fibrosis (CF)], and chronic obstructive pulmonary disease (COPD) are the disease processes usually associated with excessive and abnormal airway secretions. Although pulmonary edema fluid sometimes fills the airways, airway clearance therapy is seldom used to treat pulmonary edema because diuretic therapy is more effective. Other alveolar space diseases, such as pneumonia, are not usually a cause of retained airway secretions unless cough is ineffective or an abscess forms.

Ciliary Dysfunction. Ciliary stasis results in an accumulation of mucus that compromises the airway lumen. Iatrogenic causes of ciliary dysfunction include smoking, high inspired oxygen fractions (FIO_2), and medications such as anesthetics, narcotics, and sedatives. The *ciliary dyskinesia syndrome* is a rare condition that is associated with repeated respiratory infections related to decreased or absent ciliary function.

Ineffective or Absent Cough. When reflex cough is absent or impaired following spinal cord trauma or neuromuscular disease, airway clearance is less effective despite normal production and consistency of mucus and normal ciliary action. It is not clear whether the inability to generate the expiratory flow rates necessary for clearance or the associated overall reduction in physical mobility further contributes to secretion retention, atelectasis, and infection in patients who cannot cough. Cough is also impaired in many persons with COPD, especially those with significant decreases in expiratory flow rates. Impaired cough in combination with mucus hypersecretion puts many patients with COPD at especially high risk for secretion retention problems.

Altered or Abnormal Mucus. Mucus that is either too "stiff" or too "loose" results in less than optimal transport velocities. Systemic dehydration also reduces tracheal transport velocity approximately 25 per cent in animals and probably in humans. Whether the decreased rate is caused by ciliary dysfunction or increased mucus viscosity or whether a decreased rate results in retained secretions is unknown. However, some combination of or all of these factors may explain the secretion retention seen in hypersecretory diseases, particularly when secretion viscosity is increased owing to purulence. Even when nonpurulent, the mucus in patients with CF has a slower transport rate than normal canine mucus of a similar viscoelasticity.

Bronchoconstriction and Airway Collapse. Narrowed airway caliber potentiates secretion retention by changing the depth of the mucus layer. Airway collapse is also thought to trap secretions distal to the collapsed segment and possibly to maintain atelectasis in areas served by the plugged airway that might otherwise be opened by deep breathing (see Chapter 10). Cough efficiency is also compromised, as constriction and collapse reduce expiratory flow rates.

Consequences of Retained Secretions

Retained secretions increase airway resistance. If excess secretions result in complete obstruction of some of the airways, a decrease in lung compliance also occurs. Both these conditions, either separately or in combination, cause an increase in the work of breathing that in turn causes the sensation of inappropriate respiratory effort; this is recognized by most persons as dyspnea. Partial or complete obstruction of the airways by secretions causes well perfused parts of the lung to be underventilated. This causes a fall in the arterial oxygen tension (PaO_2). The arterial carbon dioxide tension ($PaCO_2$) does not generally increase simply on the basis of regional ventilation and perfusion mismatching. However, alveolar hypoventilation may occur if the work of breathing is high, particularly if respiratory drive is abnormal, respiratory muscle fatigue is present, or both. Retained secretions have also been implicated in an increased incidence of pneumonia in certain patients, although the evidence for this is unclear.

THERAPY TO IMPROVE AIRWAY CLEARANCE

SPUTUM LIQUEFACTION

Systemic Hydration

Maintaining adequate systemic hydration is essential in keeping mucociliary clearance within normal limits. However, it is not known whether an increased fluid intake will thin normal airway secretions or change the composition of dried, inspissated mucus; the latter seems particularly unlikely. To prevent any decrease in mucociliary transport, most clinicians recommend a large fluid intake (1½ to 2 liters per day) for patients with COPD. In these and other individuals, inhalation of moisture-laden gases is also used to produce changes in mucus and to facilitate its clearance. Although these therapies may be less important than systemic hydration, they may be helpful, and a description of them follows.

Humidification Therapy

General Considerations
Humidification occurs when water is added to a gas mixture. Temperature is the most important factor in determining the capacity of a gas for holding water vapor. The actual content of water in relation to its capacity is the relative humidity of the mixture.

Methods and Purpose
Upper Airways. Oxygen delivered by nasal cannula is often humidified by bubbling the gas through water. This has little effect other than placebo and adds unnecessary expense. In unusually dry environments and with O_2 flows greater than 5 L/min, some patients may benefit from humidifying the oxygen, although there is no objective documentation of this.

Lower Airways. Gas reaching the lower airways must be completely saturated with water vapor at body temperature to prevent desiccation of the tracheal mucous membrane. This can be achieved by heating the carrier gas to 37° C. At this temperature it holds 44 mg of water per liter of gas. The corresponding water vapor pressure (PH_2O) is 47 mmHg. The Bennett Cascade humidifier is schematically depicted in Figure 9–1. This efficient, large-volume, heated humidifier and devices like it are frequently used as adjuncts to mechanical ventilation. Large-bore tubing carries the heated, humidified gas to the patient's artificial airway or, rarely, to the patient's mask.

The primary goal of these humidification devices is remedial; they are replacing water that ordinarily would be added by the upper airway were it not bypassed by a translaryngeal or tracheostomy tube. Condensation occurs if the gas temperature is just above body temperature when it reaches the airways so that water is deposited on the mucus lining the respiratory tract. Exposure to a saturated environment for 3 hours or longer modestly increases the volume and decreases the viscosity of sputum in vitro. Whether this occurs or is desirable in vivo is unknown.

Water vapors, heated in particular, have a soothing effect on the airways, and they may also decrease adherence of secretions to airway walls and facilitate clearance by cough. Perhaps for these reasons, both inpatients and outpatients often report improved or

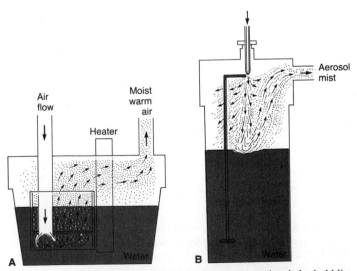

Figure 9–1. *A*, Heated humidifiers produce warm moist air by bubbling the gas mixture through a heated water bath. *B*, Gas-powered or jet nebulizers produce particles of water that are incorporated in the carrier gas. The amount and size of the particles determine the water content of the gas.

easier clearance following the use of both sophisticated steam-producing devices and simple substitutes such as tea kettles, hot showers, or baby-bottle warmers. Some patients, however, feel smothered by warm, moist air.

Complications and Precautions. Condensed water vapor must be emptied from tubings at relatively frequent intervals. Care should be taken in discarding the condensate, which is inoculated with the patient's bacterial flora, in order to prevent contamination of the environment. However, devices that increase humidity without generating particles have not been implicated in nosocomial infections (see Chapter 20). The temperature of the humidified gas must be monitored near the connection to the patient's airway to detect and prevent overheating or underheating.

THERAPEUTIC COUGH

General Considerations

Patients with excess airway secretions must cough to achieve airway clearance. Postural drainage, percussion, and vibration without cough are not efficient clearance therapies. Furthermore, young adult patients with CF achieve clearance with directed coughs alone that is comparable to chest physical therapy treatments that include cough.

Cough Positioning

Individuals who cough vigorously tend to assume a flexed position by bending forward at the waist. Supine patients are disadvantaged because their vital capacity (VC) is reduced in this position and they are not flexed. Supine patients therefore should be assisted to a Fowler's position with the knees up or, alternatively, should be turned to the side, again with the knees drawn up. These positions are particularly important for patients with abdominal incisions. They are much more effective in reducing pain than is pressing on the incision with a pillow, although this may also be helpful.

Huff Coughing

Huff coughing is a series of coughs performed with the glottis held open by saying the word *huff*. In COPD patients with significant airway collapse, this cough pattern is associated with higher flow rates than the normal glottis-closed pattern. Although cough is generally considered effective only in clearing the central airways, coughing to a low lung-volume may move dynamic compression more peripherally. Theoretically, this could increase cough velocity and promote clearance from smaller airways.

Quad Coughing

Clinicians can assist patients without functional abdominal muscles to cough by pushing upward and inward on the abdomen towards the diaphragm while the patient makes whatever expiratory effort is possible. The chest may be compressed at the same time. Hyperinflation via a bag-mask or bag-tube connection prior to the "cough" may enhance the expiratory flow rate by increasing VC and elastic recoil.

Cough Stimulation

A massaging pressure applied to the trachea with the index and middle fingers in the sternal notch will elicit a reflex cough. This maneuver, also known as tracheal tickle, is useful in obtunded patients. Clinicians can easily demonstrate this reflex on themselves. The tracheal tickle is not appropriate in confused patients; they often misinterpret the clinician's intent and think they are being strangled.

Predicting Cough Efficacy

Cough efficacy is evaluated by sputum expectoration, the patient's report of swallowed sputum, or clearing of gurgles on auscultation. The prediction of cough ability and efficacy prior to extubation is an important factor in the decision to extubate. Traditional values used to predict cough ability following extubation overlap with weaning criteria. These have included VC and maximum inspiratory force (MIF). Unfortunately, MIF does not reflect the maximum expiratory force (MEF), a measure of strength directly involved with cough. The best prediction of cough ability is "cough" peak flow measured prior to extubation by attaching a standard peak-flow meter to the tracheal tube and asking the patient to cough. Cough peak flow is consistently higher after extubation, presumably because the glottis can now close. Moderate to good postextubation cough ability is associated with pre-extubation values for cough peak flow > 100 L/min, MEF > 60 cm H_2O, and VC > 25 ml/kg.

CHEST PHYSICAL THERAPY

General Considerations

Chest physical therapy (CPT) is the general title for a group of airway clearance therapies consisting of postural drainage, percussion, and vibration. Although cough is not usually included in this list, no clinician should consider a treatment thorough unless it is accompanied by cough or suctioning if the patient's ability to cough is inadequate. Some clinicians also include abdominal diaphragmatic breathing, pursed-lip breathing, and inspiratory muscle training under the heading of CPT. These topics are discussed in Chapter 17.

Anatomical and Physiological Rationale

It has been demonstrated repeatedly that gravity increases mucociliary transport rates in the trachea. Put more simply, fluids run downhill. By extension, this is the rationale for postural drainage of the rest of the lung. Based on normal anatomy, drainage positions have been described for all segments of the lung. Whether these modest adjustments in body position and angle of tilt are useful in individual patients or those with abnormal lungs is open to question. On the other hand, both normal and diseased lungs are subject to other, more general influences of gravity that also influence secretion clearance. As illustrated in Figure 9–2, alveoli and airways are largest where the pleural pressure is most negative. This occurs where the lung tissue is least influenced by gravitational pull. Thus, pleural pressure is most negative in the apex of the lung in upright positions and in the uppermost portions of the upper lung when lying on one's side.

Pulmonary blood flow is also influenced by gravity (see Chapter 2), so blood volume is greatest in the dependent portions of the lung. The increased volume of blood adds to the tendency toward smaller alveoli and airways and airway closure at the bottom of the lung. Gross position changes obviously change these relationships within the lung. Such changes may open previously closed airways and permit drainage of pooled secretions even if the position is not entirely correct for the segment(s) of interest. These mechanisms also provide an explanation for the success of drainage

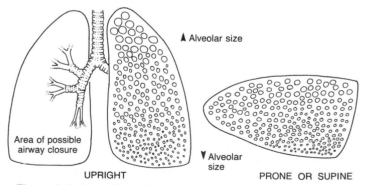

Figure 9–2. The effect of body position on the size of alveoli and airways. Note that alveoli and airways are larger in nondependent regions of the lung and smaller in dependent regions.

in horizontal side-lying or prone positions when head-down postures are contraindicated.

Indications

Acute. The presence of retained excessive or abnormal secretions in patients with weak coughs or in patients who become exhausted by coughing is an indication for CPT. Suctioning must be instituted if cough is significantly compromised. Additional or supporting indications include a decreased PaO_2 and roentgenographic evidence of atelectasis caused by airway plugging, that is, the lack of an air bronchogram. These findings are common in a wide variety of conditions. However, patients with COPD, respiratory or general neuromuscular dysfunction, altered consciousness, and intubation are those most likely to benefit from CPT.

Prophylactic. Some clinicians order prophylactic CPT to prevent the accumulation of secretions in all patients receiving mechanical ventilation or requiring prolonged bed rest. Others use CPT in patients who have pain that prevents cough, who have increased work of breathing, or who chronically aspirate. However, there is no evidence supporting prophylactic CPT in these groups. The therapeutic rationale is questionable particularly in the absence of retained secretions. Frequent position changes are mandatory in these conditions but achievement of this goal does not require a special treatment protocol.

Prophylactic therapy in hypersecretory COPD is advocated by many clinicians, but convincing evidence of reduced infections, fewer hospital days, or other objective measures of efficacy is lacking. Most COPD patients do not require daily therapy, but patients should be taught humidification and clearance therapies to use whenever they feel they are unable to cough and to clear their airways with their usual efficiency, particularly if the sputum becomes purulent. An occasional patient with voluminous sputum production is symptomatically better after instituting twice-daily postural drainage sessions on a regular, prophylactic basis. In contrast, younger patients with CF are almost universally treated at least twice daily with percussion, vibration, and postural drainage. Older CF patients may achieve the same mucus clearance with coughing sessions alone. Bronchiectasis is another condition that often benefits from daily prophylactic drainage therapy. In the postoperative period, prophylactic clearance therapy should be reserved for those patients known to have mucus hypersecretion.

Contraindications and Precautions

Increased intracranial pressure (ICP) is a contraindication to CPT, although the ability to monitor ICP allows cautious modifications of therapy, such as horizontal rather than head-down drainage. Other contraindications include active or recent lung hemorrhage; rib fractures, which prevent percussion and vibration but not drainage; lung abscess, if suction equipment is not available; and finally, uncontrolled hypoxemia that is aggravated by position changes. Patients to be treated with extra caution are those with extreme dyspnea, dysrhythmias, low cardiac output, hyperreactive airways, and a low PaO_2.

Techniques

Postural Drainage. Figure 9–3 shows the positions suggested for generalized drainage of the lung. Some or all of the positions indicated are used during CPT treatments in preference to the traditional 15 to 18 segmental positions, for the reasons given previously. In addition, exhaustion of the patient and the therapist frequently complicates the treatment regimen when compulsive attempts are made to drain all segments of the lung. Exact segmental drainage positions are still used when treatment of a localized bronchiectasis or abscess is indicated. Some clinicians advocate drainage of the unaffected lung following treatment of a localized area to remove any secretions that may have drained into the opposite lung. Unfortunately this means placing the affected lung down, which almost invariably increases ventilation-perfusion ($\dot{V}A/\dot{Q}$) mismatching and decreases the PaO_2. Without careful monitoring by oximetry or blood gases, this practice is questionable and may be dangerous.

Percussion. Percussion is an intuitive action that has a rational basis. Mucus is a gel that can become fluid when shaken or vibrated. Percussion on the surface of the chest sends waves of varying amplitude and frequency through the chest. These forces may change the nature of the sputum itself or physically dislodge the mucus by decreasing its adherence to airway walls. By whatever mechanism, percussion is known to increase tracheal transport velocity.

Percussion is performed by striking the chest wall over the area being drained. The hands are held in a cupped fashion (Fig. 9–4). This position traps air in the hand and cushions the blow, making it possible to strike firmly without injury. The striking action is from the wrists with the shoulders and elbows relaxed. Percussion is not risk free. The only deaths reported in conjunction with CPT were due to massive hemorrhage that occurred during percussion over lung abscesses that had previously bled. Clots may have been dislodged by the percussion. Fractured ribs have been reported in newborns. Care must also be taken in osteoporotic patients.

Vibration. Vibration is a fine, shaking pressure applied to the chest wall only during exhalation. It is said to facilitate exhalation of

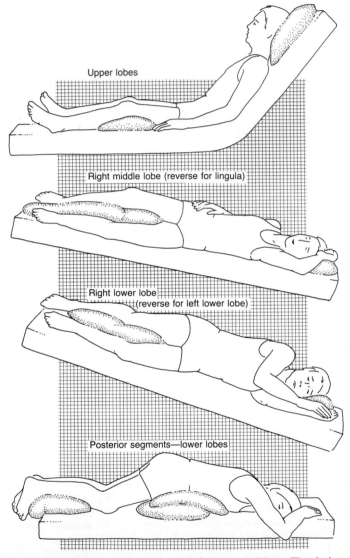

Figure 9–3. Frequently used postural drainage positions. The drainage angle is adjusted by raising the foot of the bed 12 inches for the middle lobes and 18 inches for the lower lobes or by using pillows under the hips.

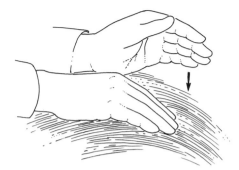

Figure 9–4. The position of the hands for percussion.

trapped air in addition to being another technique of shaking mucus loose and perhaps inducing cough. As always, the strength of the therapist must be adjusted to the patient's condition.

Physiological Changes During CPT

Several short-term physiological changes occur during CPT. Arterial PO_2 decreases in almost all patients owing to increased $\dot{V}A/\dot{Q}$ mismatch and shunt; however, arterial content generally does not change, and cardiac output increases in the majority of patients. The overall result is that O_2 transport often increases during CPT.

Evaluation of CPT

Some clinicians expect at least 30 ml of sputum per treatment. Yet most studies of the efficacy of airway clearance therapies report positive changes in flow rates and gas exchange despite small differences in sputum volume. At the very least, however, sputum expectoration should be increased and the chest should be clearing on auscultation. Symptomatic improvement is also an expected outcome of CPT. Additional benefits may include improved PaO_2, resolution of atelectasis, decreased work of breathing and dyspnea, and increased expiratory flow rates.

SUGGESTED THERAPEUTIC REGIMENS

General Considerations

Assisting or encouraging patients to cough effectively should always be attempted prior to instituting other more elaborate therapies. Too often this simple step is bypassed in favor of more

Table 9-1. AIRWAY CLEARANCE THERAPIES: ACUTE CONDITIONS

INDICATIONS	SUGGESTED TECHNIQUES
COPD, CF with secretion retention and exhaustion, poor cough, decreased PaO$_2$	CPT, huff coughing and suctioning, 3–4 times per day
Lung abscess *without* bleeding	CPT, coughing 2–3 times per day
Lung abscess, recent or current bleeding	Omit percussion; position with caution (see text)
Pneumonia with poor cough, underlying lung disease, weak, intubated, ventilated	CPT, coughing 2–3 times per day
Atelectasis with retained secretions (no air bronchogram)	CPT, coughing 3–4 times per day, deep breathing hourly
Atelectasis without retained secretions (air bronchogram present)	Deep breathing, positioning with atelectatic area uppermost
Coma with secretion retention and possible impairment of cough reflex	Stimulate coughing, add CPT and suctioning p.r.n., 2–3 times per day
Paralysis, weakness of respiratory or abdominal muscles, with secretion retention	CPT, quad coughing, assisted deep breathing, 3–4 times per day

KEY: COPD = chronic obstructive pulmonary disease, CF = cystic fibrosis, CPT = chest physical therapy.

Table 9-2. AIRWAY CLEARANCE THERAPIES: PROPHYLAXIS (TO PREVENT ACCUMULATION OF SECRETIONS)

INDICATIONS	SUGGESTED TECHNIQUES
COPD, CF with thoracic or abdominal incisions	CPT, coughing, deep breathing preoperatively and postoperatively 2–3 times per day until out of bed
COPD, effective cough	Encourage coughing; add CPT 2 times per day if sputum purulent
CF	
Young children	CPT, coughing 1–2 times per day
Teenagers, adults	Coughing only; compare efficacy with CPT plus coughing
Bronchiectasis	CPT, coughing daily in A.M.; increase frequency if sputum purulent
Coma (intubated or ventilated patient)	
Normal lungs	Frequent position changes, deep breathing, suction p.r.n.
Abnormal lungs	Same as for normal lungs plus CPT, 2 times per day
Prolonged bed rest	
Normal lungs	Frequent position changes, deep breathing
Abnormal lungs	Same as for normal lungs plus CPT with cough, 2 times per day

KEY: COPD = chronic obstructive pulmonary disease, CF = cystic fibrosis, CPT = chest physical therapy.

glamorous but not necessarily more effective therapy. Weak patients with limited reserves may benefit from CPT that brings secretions to the central airways. They can then direct all their energies to coughing out the secretions. If cough fails or is significantly compromised, the central airways can be cleared by nasotracheal suctioning via a nasopharyngeal airway (see Chapter 8). Tracheal suctioning, even in intubated patients, clears only the larger airways. CPT techniques are therefore often used in patients with artificial airways. However, CPT is not indicated in intubated patients who can cough vigorously and move about freely.

Type and Sequence of Therapy

The suggested sequence of a secretion clearance treatment is bronchodilator administration, moisture inhalation for 10 to 20 minutes, and finally assisted coughing. Chest physical therapy plus coughing or suctioning, if necessary, is substituted for cough alone if cough is ineffectual. This is very important, because *clearance* of excessive secretions is very dependent on cough and is much less efficient with CPT alone.

Tables 9–1 and 9–2 summarize the indications and therapies used to improve airway clearance. These therapies should be continued until the patient is mobile and can cough and until secretion production is reduced. Objective measures of efficacy include re-expansion of atelectatic lung and improved gas exchange. Bronchoscopy should be reserved for those with massive atelectasis who are unable to tolerate vigorous therapy or who have failed a 24- to 48-hour trial of therapy administered every four hours.

RECOMMENDED READING

1. AARC Clinical Practice Guide: Humidification during mechanical ventilation. *Respir Care,* 37:887–890, 1992.
2. AARC Clinical Practice Guideline: Nasotracheal suctioning. *Respir Care,* 37:898–901, 1992.
3. Brochard L, et al.: Constant-flow insufflation prevents arterial oxygen desaturation during endotracheal suctioning. *Am Rev Respir Dis,* 144:395–400, 1991.
4. Campbell EJ, et al. Subjective effects of humidification of oxygen for delivery by nasal cannula: A prospective study. *Chest,* 93:289–293, 1988.
5. Gaskell DV, and Webber BA: The Brompton Hospital guide to chest physiotherapy. Oxford, England, Blackwell Scientific Publications, 1973.
6. Kacmarek RM, and Pierson DJ: Assessment and management of airway protection, obstruction, and secretion clearance. *In* Pierson DJ, and Kacmarek RM (eds.): *Foundations of Respiratory Care.* New York, Churchill Livingstone, 1992, pp. 561–570.
7. Kigin C: Chest physical therapy. *In* Pierson DJ, and Kacmarek RM (eds.): *Foundations of Respiratory Care.* New York, Churchill Livingstone, 1992, pp. 777–792.
8. Martin TR: Defense mechanisms and immune reactions in the lungs. *In* Kelley WN (ed.): *Textbook of Internal Medicine,* 2nd ed. Philadelphia, J. B. Lippincott Co., 1992, pp. 1694–1700.

9. Mazzocco MC, et al.: Chest percussion and postural drainage in patients with bronchiectasis. *Chest,* 88:360–368, 1985.
10. Murray JF: The ketchup bottle method. *N Engl J Med,* 300:1155–1157, 1979.
11. Pierson DJ, and Hess DR: Respiratory care of the patient who is unresponsive, immobilized, or paralyzed. *In* Pierson DJ, and Kacmarek RM (eds.): *Foundations of Respiratory Care.* New York, Churchill Livingstone, 1992, pp. 1063–1074.
12. Tyler ML: Complications of positioning and chest physiotherapy. *Respir Care,* 27:458–466, 1982.
13. Wanner A, and Rao A: Clinical indications for and effects of bland, mucolytic, and antimicrobial aerosols. *Am Rev Respir Dis,* 122 (pt 2):79–87, 1980.

10

AIDS TO LUNG INFLATION

HYPERINFLATION THERAPY

DEFINITION

Hyperinflation therapy, or lung expansion therapy, includes any form of treatment that encourages or assists nonintubated patients in taking larger than usual inspirations, so that their tidal volume (V_T) is increased and approaches a normal inspiratory capacity (IC), which is equal to the V_T plus the inspiratory reserve volume. The augmented V_T can result from simple coaching to breathe deeply or from using one of several mechanical aids described below. Hyperinflation therapy does not ordinarily include positive end-expiratory pressure (PEEP), although the goals of both therapies are similar in that they are both designed to decrease atelectasis, the collapse of terminal airways and alveoli, and thereby to increase lung volume. Strictly applied, the term "hyperinflation therapy" describes promotion of dynamic changes in V_T during inspiration, whereas the goal of PEEP is to increase the static lung volume at end-expiration, or functional residual capacity (FRC). Furthermore, hyperinflation therapy is applied intermittently or for short periods and used to treat mild hypoxemia in patients who are not terribly sick, while PEEP is applied continuously and is used for conditions such as the neonatal and adult respiratory distress syndromes (NRDS, ARDS), which are characterized by pulmonary edema, diffuse atelectasis, refractory hypoxemia, and a very low FRC (see Chapter 14).

PHYSIOLOGICAL RATIONALE FOR HYPERINFLATION THERAPY

Atelectasis

Atelectasis, particularly in the postoperative period, is the most frequently cited indication for use of hyperinflation therapy. Atelectasis refers to a collapse of lung tissue that can occur at any structural level of the lung; it often is described as segmental or lobar. However, a more general classification, which recognizes the presence of atelectasis when it is not roentgenographically apparent, uses the terms microatelectasis and macroatelectasis.

Microatelectasis. Failure to fully expand the lung at normal intervals (approximately 10 times per hour) causes a diffuse collapse of air spaces, especially at the lung bases, that is called microatelectasis. This condition is related to decreased activity of the surfactant that normally reduces intra-alveolar surface tension. Although microatelectasis is a diffuse condition, the clearness of the chest roentgenogram (if the lungs are otherwise normal) indicates that only individual or very small groups of alveoli collapse. The condition is recognized by a widened alveolar to arterial oxygen difference, $P(A - a)O_2$. Microatelectasis is common among patients who cannot breathe deeply because of respiratory muscle dysfunction, obesity and chest wall disorders, recent surgery on the upper abdomen or thorax, restrictive lung diseases such as idiopathic pulmonary fibrosis, and coma due to drug overdosage. Microatelectasis can also be caused by breathing 100 per cent O_2. In this setting, once nitrogen is washed out of poorly ventilated alveoli, O_2 may be absorbed more rapidly than it is replenished, with alveolar collapse the result. Diffuse alveolar collapse also occurs in pulmonary edema.

Macroatelectasis. Macroatelectasis is roentgenographically evident as a diffuse or local infiltrate usually associated with volume loss. As noted above, diffuse atelectasis is often associated with pulmonary edema, whereas local atelectasis results from secretion retention or regional areas of altered lung mechanics. Areas of altered mechanics may result from anatomical compression of the lung during upper abdominal or thoracic surgery; an example is left lower lobe atelectasis following cardiac surgery. Air bronchograms are often seen in areas of atelectasis caused by local mechanical conditions, whereas secretion retention or plugging, by definition, results in airless bronchi. These roentgenographic findings are discussed in Chapter 6.

Immediate Effects of Lung Hyperinflation

Increased Lung Compliance. Microatelectasis is quickly resolved by taking deep breaths to total lung capacity (TLC). As alveoli reopen or grow larger, lung compliance increases as surfactant activity is restored.

Decreased Work of Breathing. When additional air spaces are recruited and compliance increases, the work required to breathe decreases. Work of breathing (WOB) amounts to only about 2 per cent of total O_2 consumption in persons with normal lungs. However, patients with restrictive lung diseases frequently have a high WOB and may feel less dyspneic when the WOB is decreased. Patients with COPD also often have increased WOB, although atelectasis is less likely to occur in this population.

Increased Arterial Oxygenation. Opening or enlarging the alveoli increases the tethering effect of the lung parenchyma on small airways. With the small airways open, shunt resolves, ventilation-perfusion ($\dot{V}A/\dot{Q}$) matching improves, or both occur. This typically leads to an improvement in the arterial O_2 tension (PaO_2) of 10 to 15 mmHg after as few as five sighs or yawns in the postoperative period. The PaO_2 falls over the next hour or so, but not all the way to the pre-sigh values. Subsequent yawns again produce about the same rise in PaO_2 but to a higher overall level. These stepwise increases continue for several hours. Because FRC increases in the upright position in most patients, the simple expedient of keeping the backrest elevated or assisting patients out of bed may significantly enhance the effect of hyperinflation therapy on PaO_2.

Increased Secretion Removal. It has been speculated that as lung volume increases and small airways remain open, once-trapped secretions can move centrally up the mucociliary transport system and eventually be coughed out. When retained secretions are the cause or result of atelectasis, positioning patients with their atelectatic segments uppermost results in an increase in the local transpulmonary pressure between the alveoli and the pleural space; the pressure increases both alveolar size and airway caliber (see Chapter 9 and Fig. 9–2). Adding hyperinflation therapy while the patient is in this position may enhance drainage of secretions by further increasing airway caliber. Collateral ventilation also is enhanced and may result in regassing the area distal to the obstructing secretions.

Long-Term Effects of Hyperinflation Therapy

General Effects. Other than the effects on PaO_2 just mentioned, which last only hours, the long-term effects of hyperinflation therapy have not been studied. However, if hyperinflation therapy effectively prevents or treats atelectasis, the duration of the patient's stay in the hospital may be decreased, and there should be a lower incidence of other associated conditions such as pneumonia. In contrast, an undesirable long-term effect, increased air trapping, has been observed in patients with COPD who used intermittent positive-pressure breathing (IPPB) as part of a home-care regimen.

Ventilatory Muscle Training. During the 1980s much attention focused on the role of the ventilatory muscles, both in the development of and potentially in therapy for chronic ventilatory insufficiency. Resting the ventilatory muscles by means of part-time ventilatory assistance can be very efficacious when done correctly in appropriately selected patients (see Chapter 17). Considerable enthusiasm has also been generated for exercises aimed specifically at strengthening the ventilatory muscles (especially those of inspiration) and improving their endurance. A regimen of daily inspiratory muscle exercise by means of graded inspiratory resistance, when continued for a period of weeks or months, was initially touted as effective in reducing dyspnea and increasing patients' abilities to walk and carry out other activities of daily living. Wider clinical experience with this therapy, however, has been discouraging; getting patients to continue the exercises indefinitely is difficult, and more recent studies have called the initially promising results into question.

LIMITATIONS OF HYPERINFLATION THERAPY

Duration of Effects

The temporary nature of the physiological effects of hyperinflation therapy is its major limitation. If decreased surfactant activity is the cause of alveolar collapse and subsequent microatelectasis, hyperinflation therapy will reverse these conditions only if spontaneous deep breathing returns or if some of the alveoli remain at their new size and surface tension remains normal. On the other hand, if coughing is stimulated by deep breathing and mucous plugs are coughed out during the course of the treatment, the benefit derived may be longer lasting or even permanent.

Carbon Dioxide Retention

Hyperinflation therapy should not be used to treat CO_2 retention. In contrast to the effect on PaO_2, CO_2 elimination is not substantially affected by reopening alveoli (see Chapter 2). An increased $PaCO_2$ may be temporarily lowered if the deep breaths are repeated so rapidly that total alveolar ventilation is increased; however, it will be at the cost of a significant increase in WOB, which most patients will not be able to maintain unless IPPB is used. As soon as therapy is stopped the $PaCO_2$ will rise again, unless there has been a change in the underlying condition. It is easy to get a false sense of security from measurement of blood gases obtained during IPPB therapy.

ASSOCIATED THERAPIES

Turning and Coughing

Turning. Traditional care for the postoperative patient is to have the patient turn, cough, and deep breathe every two hours. Turning results in a redistribution of the FRC, such that lung volume is greatest in the portion of the lung that is uppermost (see Increased Secretion Removal and Chapter 9). This phenomenon can be used to advantage in the treatment of localized atelectasis by positioning patients so that the atelectatic area is superior relative to the rest of the lung. Because the more normal lung is dependent in this position, the PaO_2 almost always increases owing to improved matching of $\dot{V}A/\dot{Q}$, reduction of shunt, or both. Whether turning or positioning is important in preventing atelectasis is speculative because it has not been studied, but it is a theoretically reasonable maneuver that is also useful in preventing vascular stasis.

Coughing. Coughing is frequently overemphasized in the treatment and prevention of atelectasis. Opening atelectatic lung requires large lung volumes, an inspiratory maneuver. Taking a deep breath is part of a normal cough but is incidental to its main purpose, airway clearance, which is an expiratory maneuver. Therefore cough is required only when secretions are present. Although mucociliary stasis does occur during anesthesia, nonsmoking patients with otherwise normal airways (and even smokers without chronic bronchitis) do not produce or retain enough mucus during the operative period to hinder its clearance by ciliary transport in the postanesthesia period. However, patients with mucus hypersecretion prior to surgery, or with any other condition that significantly reduces mobility, *are* at increased risk of secretion retention. They should be assisted to cough effectively when secretions are auscultated in the central airways. Preoperative secretion clearance measures are essential in this population (see Chapter 9).

Analgesia

Patients with thoracic (particularly lateral) and abdominal incisions obviously will have significant pain with coughing and cannot be expected to cough effectively unless given adequate analgesia. The postoperative routine for patients with retained secretions, in addition to turning, coughing, and deep breathing, should include appropriate analgesia with narcotic or other agents. Epidural anesthesia can be of great assistance in patients with poor lung inflation due to postoperative pain.

TYPES OF HYPERINFLATION THERAPY

Voluntary Deep Breathing

Definition. The easiest, most natural, and least expensive method of achieving lung hyperinflation is to breathe to TLC. Unfortunately, patients often need to be reminded or encouraged to take deep breaths, and costs escalate rapidly when a nurse or a respiratory care practitioner must go to the bedside. Thus, on the theory that the patient will continue to perform the maneuver correctly once taught to do so, an enormous collection of devices has been developed to provide positive feedback and to coach the patient in obtaining a maximum, sustained inhalation without the constant presence of health care personnel.

Technique or Pattern of Breathing. Deep breathing is most effective when inspiration is slow, when the maximum inflation is held for several seconds, and when the deep breaths are repeated. Slow inspiratory rates allow time for lung areas with narrowed airways and decreased compliance to fill, resulting in better overall distribution of the inhaled volume. The slow inspiration and end-inspiratory pause at TLC theoretically promote alveolar stabilization by allowing time for replenishing surfactant, for redistributing air in the lung, and for reopening of alveoli. Mechanical aids to hyperinflation, described below, should be judged according to their success in facilitating this pattern of breathing.

How many deep breaths need to be taken has not been well studied in the clinical setting; however, at least three deep breaths are used in laboratory studies in which it is necessary to control for lung compliance. Five yawns, as mentioned earlier, have been shown to be physiologically effective, at least as measured by an increase in PaO_2. Ten deep breaths has become the clinical tradition, perhaps because that is the observed frequency of sighs normally occuring in one hour.

Frequency and Duration of Therapy. No studies have been done regarding the frequency of deep breathing and the subsequent incidence or resolution of atelectasis. However, lung hyperinflations are usually prescribed at hourly intervals during the waking hours and at least every four hours at night in the early postoperative period. Treatments are probably unnecessary when patients are getting out of bed regularly or are able to freely move about in bed. Further study is needed to determine if this regimen is both prophylactically and therapeutically satisfactory.

Complications. No complications have been described as a result of voluntary or encouraged deep breathing. Barotrauma is associated, however, with large lung volumes and is a potential complication of hyperinflation therapy no matter how it is administered.

Rebreathing Devices

Description. Rebreathing devices are tubes or cannisters designed to stimulate ventilation by adding the patient's exhaled CO_2 to the inspired air. Minute ventilation will increase, but rate is favored more than volume. Additionally, the devices do nothing to control inspiratory flow rate or allow for a pause at maximum inflation; as a result the chances of effectively reversing alveolar collapse are small with these devices.

Complications. Potential complications include hypoxemia if the patient's V_T is less than the dead space of the device. This is particularly likely in children, but can be overcome by bleeding oxygen into the tube or cannister.

Blow Bottles, Gloves, or Balloons

Description. Blow bottles (Fig. 10–1) are devices in which fluid is moved from one container to another by means of air pressure. Balloons and their frequent substitute, examination gloves, also require air pressure; all three emphasize the wrong maneuver, exhalation. Positive feedback is provided only during exhalation, while any hyperinflation and presumed benefit occur only if a deep breath is taken in preparation to transferring the fluid or blowing up the balloon or glove. Furthermore, these maneuvers can be done with frequent small breaths and the fluid may even be moved by means of a Valsalva maneuver rather than a deep breath.

Complications. Increased airway and alveolar closure are possible if exhalation is always begun at FRC. Temporary reductions in cardiac output may occur, particularly in hypovolemic patients, if positive intrathoracic pressure is sustained.

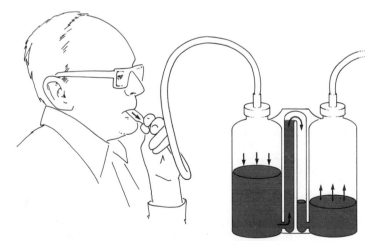

Figure 10–1. Blow bottles assist lung hyperinflation *only* if the patient takes a deep breath prior to blowing the fluid from one bottle to the next.

Intermittent Positive-Pressure Breathing

Description

IPPB devices assist lung hyperinflation by applying positive pressure to the airways. Whether hyperexpansion is actually achieved depends on the amount of pressure applied and the compliance of the chest wall and lungs. Lungs with low compliance require high distending pressures and will not be expanded at the traditional 10 to 15 cm H_2O pressure used during standard IPPB treatments. If inspired volumes are monitored during IPPB treatments, pressures can be adjusted appropriately to achieve large VT breaths, assuming that the pressure capabilities of the IPPB machine are not exceeded. Inflation hold settings are not available on simple IPPB devices; however, patients can be instructed to pause at TLC during the treatment.

Clinical Indications

Patients with significant ventilatory muscle weakness, chest wall deformity, or both may not be able to take large VT breaths on their own and are likely to require IPPB rather than voluntary deep breathing or incentive spirometry (see Incentive Spirometry, later). Inspiratory capacity should be measured with and without properly adjusted IPPB assistance to determine the necessity for IPPB over voluntary methods in individual patients.

Contraindications

IPPB should not be used on semicomatose, restless, or confused patients: They will be unable to cooperate sufficiently to receive a satisfactory hyperinflation treatment. The esophagus opens at a pressure of about 15 to 20 cm H_2O; esophageal and subsequent gastric insufflation, dilation, and vomiting are likely in noncooperating patients.

Complications

Nosocomial Infection. Nosocomial tracheobronchitis and pneumonia have been observed in some patients receiving IPPB therapy, as discussed in Chapter 20. The source of contamination was found to be the nebulizer, which adds moisture or medication to the inhaled gas. Proper cleaning techniques are available and this should no longer be a problem. In fact, it is doubtful if moisture needs to be added if the IPPB treatment is given in the same manner as deep breathing or incentive spirometry, that is, 10 breaths per hour.

Barotrauma. Barotrauma is possible with all maneuvers that distend the lungs, and IPPB is no exception. The term "barotrauma" actually is a misnomer, since high volume, not high pressure, is the most likely direct cause of pneumothorax and pneumomediastinum. Hence, IPPB is problematical only if the pressure used results in a high lung volume. Lung conditions that may add to the incidence of pneumothorax in patients include necrotizing pneumonia, localized narrowing of airways, and areas of low compliance that lead to uneven gas distribution and overinflation of small groups of alveoli.

Increased Airways Resistance. Increased airways resistance occasionally occurs after IPPB therapy in patients with airway hyperreactivity. One of the proposed mechanisms of the increased airways resistance is stimulation of stretch receptors in the lung. This complication has not been documented in other forms of hyperinflation therapy.

Other Potential Complications. Other possible complications include excessive oxygenation when O_2 is the pressure source driving the IPPB device; alveolar hyperventilation and respiratory alkalosis due to overenthusiastic use or incorrect administration; gastric distention, particularly in uncooperative patients; impaction of secretions, if they are loosened and move distally to smaller airways during the treatment; and impaired venous return, which rarely is of clinical significance in the spontaneously breathing patient.

Incentive Spirometry

Description

Incentive spirometry (IS) is a method of encouraging voluntary deep breathing by providing visual feedback to patients of the inspiratory volume they have achieved. Incentive spirometry has gained great popularity, particularly in the postoperative setting, where it is used to prevent or treat postoperative atelectasis. The efficacy of this or any other deep breathing therapy in this setting needs further study.

Types of Incentive Spirometers

Incentive spirometers were introduced in 1969. They fall into two general categories, depending on whether the feedback, or incentive, is generated by flow or volume.

Flow-Oriented Incentive Spirometers. Flow-oriented incentive spirometers (Fig. 10–2) usually consist of one or more plastic chambers that house a freely movable, colored Ping-Pong ball. When patients inhale at sufficiently high inspiratory flow rates the ball or balls rise, providing visual incentive. The devices work because flow equals volume per unit time; they are constructed so that the balls will not rise without a rather brisk flow rate. Patients must be instructed, however, that the goal is to keep the balls elevated for as long as possible in order to assure a maximum sustained inhalation. If not so instructed they will soon learn that the balls can be snapped to the top of the chamber by a rapid, very brief, and therefore low-volume breath. On the other hand, a very slow inspiration will not budge the balls but may achieve a TLC breath. The decided advantage of flow-oriented IS has been its cost per unit.

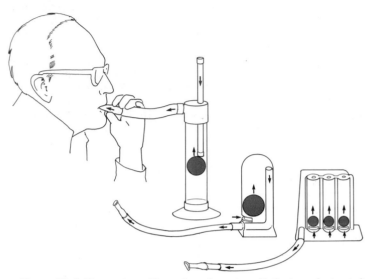

Figure 10–2. Flow-oriented incentive spirometers. Patients are instructed to inhale briskly to elevate the ball(s) and to keep them floating as long as possible. The volume inhaled is unknown.

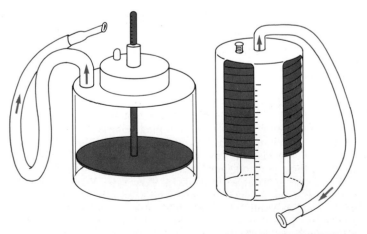

Figure 10–3. Volume-oriented incentive spirometers. The inspired volume is known and the goal is obtained by inhaling until the bellows reach a predetermined level.

Volume-Oriented Incentive Spirometers. The original Bartlett-Edwards incentive spirometer is pictured along with a new-generation volume-oriented IS device in Figure 10–3. Volume-oriented devices usually have bellows that are raised to a preset volume by the inhaled breath. An achievement light and counter are incorporated when the bellows are not visible to provide positive reinforcement and accountability for self-directed therapy. Often a small leak is included and arranged so that the light will not go on unless the bellows are held at the desired volume for a short time to ensure a period of inflation hold at TLC. Because the feedback mechanism is directly tied to the desired goal of a larger V_T breath, volume-oriented IS has a theoretical advantage over flow-oriented IS. Costs also are comparable between them.

Determining the Desired Volume

Incentive spirometry should encourage patients to breathe to the level of a normal inspiratory capacity (IC). Knowing the IC the patients could generate before surgery is helpful in setting the volume, which, allowing for pain, is realistically about one half to three quarters of their preoperative IC. Alternatively, the best of three directed postoperative inspirations can be the goal if the volume achieved is at least one half of their predicted IC. It is important, however, not to set the desired value too high, as negative feedback is quite possible if the patient repeatedly fails to achieve the desired goal.

INTEGRATED APPROACH TO ASSESSMENT AND MANAGEMENT OF ATELECTASIS

Acute lobar or segmental atelectasis in a postoperative or acutely ill patient, usually initially detected by chest radiograph, is a frequent cause for respiratory care consultation. At one time, semi-emergency fiberoptic bronchoscopy was routinely performed in patients with lobar collapse, but this has been shown to be unnecessary in the majority of patients if an appropriate regimen of lung inflation and chest physiotherapy is promptly initiated. Figure 10–4 illustrates in algorithmic form a reasonable clinical approach to atelectasis in hospitalized patients. This approach incorporates elements of several forms of therapy, and it is not certain that all of them (e.g., chest percussion) are necessary. However, in the absence of studies to clarify this issue, the practical approach shown in the figure should prove effective with few adverse effects and minimal patient discomfort.

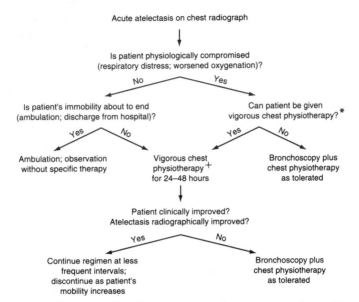

Acute atelectasis on chest radiograph

Is patient physiologically compromised
(respiratory distress; worsened oxygenation)?

No — Yes

Is patient's immobility about to end
(ambulation; discharge from hospital)?

Can patient be given
vigorous chest physiotherapy?*

Yes — No

Yes — No

Ambulation; observation
without specific therapy

Vigorous chest
physiotherapy†
for 24–48 hours

Bronchoscopy plus
chest physiotherapy
as tolerated

Patient clinically improved?
Atelectasis radiographically improved?

Yes — No

Continue regimen at less
frequent intervals;
discontinue as patient's
mobility increases

Bronchoscopy plus
chest physiotherapy
as tolerated

Figure 10–4. Algorithm for assessment and management of acute lobar or segmental atelectasis. (Reproduced with permission from Wilkins RL, and Pierson DJ: Assessment and management of acute atelectasis. *In* Pierson DJ, and Kacmarek RM (eds.): *Foundations of Respiratory Care.* New York, Churchill Livingstone, 1992, pp. 851–857.)

*Patient not immobilized by traction or spinal injury; no intracranial hypertension or other contraindication to head-down position if required; no rib fractures or other injuries causing sufficient pain to prevent effective chest physiotherapy; sufficient personnel available to administer treatment.

†Sample regimen: bronchodilator aerosol administered by metered-dose inhaler, followed by vigorous deep breathing and sustained maximum inhalation, along with encouraged coughing; this followed by postural drainage of affected lobe accompanied by chest percussion; entire sequence repeated every four hours.

RECOMMENDED READING

1. American Association for Respiratory Care. AARC Clinical Practice Guideline: Incentive Spirometry. *Respir Care*, 36:1402–1405, 1991.
2. Bartlett RH: Respiratory therapy to prevent pulmonary complications of surgery. *Respir Care*, 29:667–676, 1984.
3. Celli BR, et al.: A controlled trial of intermittent positive pressure breathing, incentive spirometry, and deep breathing exercises in preventing pulmonary complications after abdominal surgery. *Am Rev Respir Dis*, 130:12–15, 1984.
4. Harver A, et al.: Targeted inspiratory muscle training improves respiratory muscle function and reduces dyspnea in patients with chronic obstructive pulmonary disease. *Ann Intern Med*, 111:117–124, 1989.
5. Johnson NT, and Pierson DJ: The spectrum of pulmonary atelectasis: Pathophysiology, diagnosis, and therapy. *Respir Care*, 31:1107–1120, 1986.

6. Marini JJ, et al.: Acute lobar atelectasis: A prospective comparison of fiberoptic bronchoscopy and respiratory therapy. *Am Rev Respir Dis*, 119:971–978, 1979.
7. O'Donohue WJ, Jr: Postoperative pulmonary complications: When are preventive and therapeutic measures necessary? *Postgrad Med*, 91:167–175, 1992.
8. Realy AM: Hyperinflation therapy. *In* Scanlon CL, et al. (eds.): *Egan's Fundamentals of Respiratory Care*, 5th ed. St. Louis, C.V. Mosby, 1990, pp. 633–654.
9. Ricksten S, et al.: Effects of periodic positive airway pressure by mask on postoperative pulmonary function. *Chest*, 89:774–781, 1986.
10. Stiller K, et al.: Acute lobar atelectasis: A comparison of two chest physiotherapy regimens. *Chest*, 98:1336–1340, 1990.
11. Wilkins RL: Lung expansion therapy. *In* Pierson DJ, and Kacmarek RM (eds.): *Foundations of Respiratory Care*. New York, Churchill Livingstone, 1992, pp. 843–849.
12. Wilkins RL, and Pierson DJ: Assessment and management of acute atelectasis. *In* Pierson DJ, and Kacmarek RM (eds.): *Foundations of Respiratory Care*. New York, Churchill Livingstone, 1992, pp. 851–857.

11

RESPIRATORY CARE DRUGS

DRUG THERAPY

GENERAL PRINCIPLES OF DRUG ADMINISTRATION

Despite sound intentions, prescribed drugs often fail to produce anticipated therapeutic effects. In some cases this results from poor patient compliance; in others it stems from limited knowledge of drug metabolism, routes of administration, or adverse effects.

Drug Metabolism

Drug metabolism is determined primarily by genetic factors, age, body size, and route of excretion. Very young and very old people in general do not metabolize drugs as rapidly as others do. Since most recommended drug dosages are intended for an average male adult weighing 70 kg at an ideal body weight, patients who differ from this description should have dosages adjusted accordingly. Drugs excreted by the kidneys, such as the aminoglycoside antibiotics, can rapidly reach toxic levels when renal function is impaired. Doses of theophylline and other drugs metabolized by the liver must be reduced when hepatic function is abnormal. Cigarette smoking increases the breakdown of theophylline by the liver and may increase the requirements for theophylline in young asthmatic patients. In contrast, the effects of age and liver dysfunction often counter this result in older patients with chronic obstructive pulmonary disease (COPD).

Route of Administration

The intensity, duration, and nature of a drug's effect depend on the route by which it is given. Intravenous administration provides the quickest drug effect but is potentially dangerous and limited to hospitals. The inhaled route provides almost immediate absorption and onset of action for agents acting directly on the airways, offering the potential for full therapeutic effect at the lowest possible dose with the fewest side effects. However, this route is subject to error in administration and requires patient capability and cooperation. Intramuscular drugs are absorbed relatively rapidly but are often painful for the patient, as is the subcutaneous route. The oral route is ideal for most drugs taken chronically. Patient compliance is a problem, however, and absorption may vary in terms of rapidity and completeness. An increasing number of drugs can now be given topically through the skin, although at present none of the main respiratory care drugs are in this category.

Adverse Effects

Rashes and the asthmatic reactions seen after administration of penicillin are examples of drug allergy, an antigen-antibody reaction to part or all of a drug molecule or to some other component of the product given a patient. This allergic response requires prior exposure to the offending agent and is relatively uncommon. More common are direct and undesirable side effects, such as tachycardia after epinephrine, that result from the drug's usual pharmacological action. Dose-related toxicity is experienced at greater than usual drug dosage—e.g., convulsions at high blood levels of theophylline. Tachyphylaxis, in which previously effective amounts of an agent become less so and require higher doses, is occasionally observed with ephedrine but is not a clinically important problem with inhaled bronchodilators. Common drug interactions include the heightened tachycardia, cardiac dysrhythmias, and nervousness seen in patients who use both sympathomimetics and theophylline.

DRUGS USED IN RESPIRATORY CARE

Sympathomimetics

Description and Actions. Sympathomimetic agents, or adrenergic agonists, include epinephrine and norepinephrine, the natural hormonal transmitters of the sympathetic nervous system, and drugs of related chemical structure with similar effects. Those like epinephrine and isoproterenol, which are related to catechol, are known as catecholamines, although some sympathomimetics (terbutaline, metaproterenol, albuterol, and others) are not catecholamines. These drugs differ in the extent to which individual preparations stimulate different adrenergic receptors in the lung and elsewhere. Adrenergic receptors have been classified into alpha, beta-1, and beta-2; stimulation of each type produces different effects, as summarized in Table 11–1. In general, the more beta-2 stimulation a drug produces in proportion to its alpha and beta-1 effects, the more it approaches the ideal bronchodilator—that which relieves bronchospasm without adverse effects elsewhere in the body. No pure beta-2 agent exists, although

Table 11–1. EFFECTS OF ADRENERGIC RECEPTOR STIMULATION

EFFECT	ALPHA	BETA-1	BETA-2
Bronchoconstriction	↑	—	↓ ↓
Cough	—	—	↓
Heart rate	↓	↑ ↑	—
Ectopy	↑	↑	—
Blood pressure	↑	— or ↑	— or ↓
Tremor	—	—	↑
CNS stimulation	?	?	↑

several drugs available today are much more beta-2 selective than those available a few years ago.

Available Preparations. Table 11–2 compares the main sympathomimetic drugs available today. Epinephrine, the only agent available in aerosol form without prescription, is also the least selective beta-2 and potentially the most dangerous: It is short-acting and produces about equal stimulation of alpha, beta-1, and beta-2 receptors. Isoproterenol, also short-acting, is beta selective but stimulates beta-1 and beta-2 receptors equally. Of the so-called beta-2 selective drugs, which are also longer-acting than epinephrine and isoproterenol, isoetharine and metaproterenol are less so than are albuterol (salbutamol), terbutaline, and pirbuterol. Salmeterol, an ultra long-acting beta-2 selective agent, is currently available in Europe but not in the United States. Ephedrine, which like epinephrine is available in numerous preparations without prescription, is not used in aerosol form and stimulates all three kinds of adrenergic receptors.

Indications and Administration. The differences in rapidity of onset, maximum bronchodilator effect, and duration in the various sympathomimetics used in aerosol form are shown in Table 11–3. These differences are clinically useful and aid in selecting the appropriate drug for a given patient with asthma or COPD. Their relative beta-2 selectivity makes albuterol, terbutaline, pirbuterol, and bitolterol preferable to those agents listed above them in Table 11–3 for patients who have concomitant hypertension or heart disease, who are middle-aged or older, or who complain of nervousness or palpitations after taking bronchodilators.

Since all sympathomimetic bronchodilators work by the same mechanism regardless of their route of administration, it does not make sense to give two or more agents by the same or different routes in the same patient at the same time. This will only compound side effects without adding therapeutic benefit. Since the site of action is in the lung, the magnitude of pharmacological effect is related to how much drug is delivered to the bronchial tree. For equivalent bronchodilator response, nearly ten times the total dose must be given by mouth as by inhalation. On the other

Table 11-2. SYMPATHOMIMETIC BRONCHODILATORS

DRUG	RELATIVE BETA-2 SELECTIVITY	METERED-DOSE INHALER	AEROSOL SOLUTION	PARENTERAL PREPARATION	ORAL TABLET/ELIXIR	BRAND NAMES
Epinephrine	−	+	+	+	−	Medihaler-Epi Primatine (others)
Isoproterenol	−	+	+	+	−	Isuprel Medi-haler-Iso Duo-Medihaler (others)
Ephedrine	−	−	−	−	+	Numerous combination products
Isoetharine	+	+	+	−	−	Bronkosol Bronkometer
Metaproterenol	+	+	+	−	+	Alupent Metaprel
Albuterol	+ +	+	+	+ *	+	Ventolin Proventil
Terbutaline	+ +	−	+ *	+	+	Brethine Bricanyl
Pirbuterol	+ +	+	−	−	−	Maxair
Bitolterol	+ +	+	−	−	−	Tornalate
Salmeterol	+ +	+ †	−	−	−	−

*Not available in the United States.
†Also available in a dry-powder inhaler.

Table 11–3. SYMPATHOMIMETICS AVAILABLE AS METERED-DOSE AEROSOL INHALERS

DRUG	ONSET OF EFFECT (min)	PEAK EFFECT (min)	DURATION OF EFFECT (hr)	DOSE PER ACTIVATION (mg)	RELATIVE SAFETY FOR PATIENTS OVER 40 OR WITH HYPERTENSION OR HEART DISEASE
Epinephrine	1–2	15	1–1	0.06–0.130	–
Isoproterenol	1–2	15	1–2	0.06–0.125	+
Isoetharine	2–3	15	2–4	0.24	+ +
Metaproterenol	2–5	15–30	3–5	0.65	+ +
Albuterol	5–15	60–90	4–6	0.10	+ + +
Terbutaline	5–15	60–90	4–6	0.20	+ + +
Pirbuterol	5–15	60–90	4–6	0.20	+ + +
Bitolterol	5–15	60–90	4–6	0.37	+ + +

hand, adverse effects are more proportional to the total quantity of drug entering the body, so that one can expect significantly more side effects when an agent is given orally than when it is given by inhalation. For this reason the aerosol route, whether by metered-dose inhaler (Table 11–3) or nebulized solution (Table 11–4), is preferable to injection (Table 11–5) or tablet (Table 11–6). When sympathomimetics are delivered by aerosol, the actual dose deposited in the lower respiratory tract is unknown but comprises a small fraction (probably 5 to 10 per cent) of that leaving the nebulizer. The quantity of drug recommended for use with a hand or powered nebulizer is greater than that delivered via a metered-dose inhaler (MDI); for this reason patients "refractory" to the latter often respond to the same drug administered by the former route. However, numerous studies have shown MDI and nebulizer administration to be clinically equivalent if sufficient doses are given via MDI, and this device should be the one initially used in view of its lower cost and less requirement for personnel time.

Adverse Effects. Tachycardia, nervousness, palpitations, and generalized central nervous system excitation are the most common adverse effects of sympathomimetics. These result from direct pharmacological actions of these drugs on alpha and beta-1 receptors. Allergy to these agents is exceedingly rare. Other effects are tachyphylaxis, especially with ephedrine, and clinical tolerance, which may reflect poor administration technique, psychological dependence, or worsening of the underlying disease process in addition to reduced pharmacological effectiveness. Overuse of MDI sympathomimetics is less a problem today than in the past, primarily because of the increased safety and specificity of currently available agents. Tremor from beta-2 selective agents is due to direct stimulation of skeletal muscle beta-2 receptors by the drug.

Table 11–4. SYMPATHOMIMETICS AVAILABLE IN SOLUTION FOR AEROSOL ADMINISTRATION

DRUG	CONCENTRATION (%)	ADULT STARTING DOSE	DURATION OF EFFECT (hr)
Isoproterenol	0.5	2.5 mg (0.5 ml)*	1–2
Isoetharine	1	5 mg (0.5 ml)*	2–3
Metaproterenol	5	10 mg (0.2 ml)*	3–5
Albuterol	0.5‡	2.5 mg* (0.5 ml)	4–6
Terbutaline†	1	0.25 mg (0.25 ml)*	4–6

*In 2–2.5-ml total delivered volume.
†Not approved for use by this route in the United States.
‡Also available in 3-ml unit doses (0.083% solution)

Table 11–5. SYMPATHOMIMETICS AVAILABLE FOR PARENTERAL ADMINISTRATION

DRUG	PREPARATION	ROUTE	DURATION OF EFFECT (hr)	INDICATION	RELATIVE SAFETY†
Epinephrine	0.1% aqueous solution	Subcutaneous	1–1½	Acute bronchospasm	—
Epinephrine	0.2% suspension in oil	Intramuscular	4–6	Acute bronchospasm	+
Terbutaline	Aqueous solution	Subcutaneous	4–7	Acute bronchospasm	+ +
Albuterol	Aqueous solution*	Intramuscular, intravenous	4–6	Status asthmaticus	+ +

*Not available in the United States.
†Relative safety for patients over 40 or with hypertension or heart disease.

Table 11-6. SYMPATHOMIMETICS AVAILABLE IN TABLET FORM

DRUG	DOSE (mg)	DURATION OF EFFECT (hr)
Ephedrine	25–50	2–4
Metaproterenol	10–20	3–5
Albuterol	2–4	4–6
Terbutaline	2.5–5	4–7*

*Also available in sustained-action formulation lasting 6 to 12 hr (4 mg).

Monitoring. Since no quantitative measure of serum levels is available for sympathomimetics, monitoring for efficacy and toxicity must be done clinically. Bronchodilator response can be quantified by using serial measurements of peak flow rate determined by a hand-held flow meter or by using the forced expiratory volume in one second (FEV_1), obtained by spirometry. These techniques have proved useful both in adjustment of chronic dosage and in management of acute asthma attacks.

Theophyllines

Description and Actions. The methylxanthines, of which theophylline is the major representative, are phosphodiesterase inhibitors that decrease the breakdown of cyclic AMP, raising its availability and promoting bronchodilation. Sympathomimetics also raise cyclic AMP levels, but the two classes of drugs may do this by separate mechanisms and thus be synergistic, not competing. Theophylline and its relatives cause bronchial smooth muscle relaxation and strengthen respiratory muscle contraction. They also stimulate the cardiovascular system and cause diuresis. Central nervous system stimulation is another prominent effect of these drugs: They lower the seizure threshold, cause convulsions at high blood levels even in normal individuals, and act centrally to stimulate respiration.

Theophylline is metabolized mainly by the liver. Hepatic clearance is increased with cigarette smoking and some other processes that stimulate enzyme systems, is variably affected by acute infectious illnesses, and is decreased by liver disease and heart failure. Certain drugs, such as some erythromycins and cimetidine, also slow metabolism of theophylline by the liver.

Available Preparations. Several theophylline-like drugs are available and all act by being converted to theophylline in the body. These include aminophylline, which can be given intravenously, orally, or rectally; and anhydrous theophylline, which is usually administered only by mouth. Oxtriphylline, or choline theophyllinate, is another commonly prescribed oral agent. Both aminophylline and theophylline are available in sustained-release, long-acting preparations as well as in the original shorter-acting tablets and elixirs. Theophylline, along with ephedrine, is available over the counter in numerous combinations with antihistamines and other drugs.

Indications and Administration. Theophyllines are used to treat bronchospasm in patients with asthma and COPD. The drugs' bronchodilator effect is directly dependent on serum level. These drugs may be given intravenously or orally.

Intravenous Therapy. Intravenous therapy with aminophylline has two phases, a loading dose and continuous maintenance infusion. The loading dose is determined by weight regardless of hepatic or renal function: infusion of 6 milligrams per kilogram (mg/kg) over 20 to 40 minutes will produce a serum concentration of about 10 to 15 micrograms per milliter (μg/ml). If the patient has been, or may have been, taking a theophylline preparation prior to admission, but does not have signs of gastrointestinal, cardiovascular, or neurological toxicity, then giving half the usual loading dose (3 mg/kg) will raise the serum level about 5 μg/ml and should be relatively safe. Patients who have been taking theophylline in whom higher than therapeutic levels may exist should not be given a loading dose.

After loading, a maintenance infusion should be begun. The originally recommended dose of 0.9 mg/kg/hr has proven too high for many patients and is safe to give only to children and healthy young cigarette smokers. Otherwise healthy adult nonsmokers under age 40 should be begun on 0.6 mg/kg/hr. Older adult asthmatic patients and COPD patients without signs of cor pulmonale or liver impairment should be started on 0.4 mg/kg/hr, and if liver disease or heart failure is suspected or present, the appropriate initial infusion rate is 0.2 mg/kg/hr. Serum level should be checked within 12 hours after the loading dose is given and subsequent doses adjusted accordingly. Intravenous aminophylline should never be given without documentation of the resulting serum theophylline concentration within the first 24 hours. Subsequent determinations should be guided by therapeutic response and the patient's clinical course; dose requirements often vary considerably during the course of an acute hospitalization.

Oral Therapy. Oral therapy follows intravenous therapy, with the same total daily dose. If parenteral aminophylline is being replaced by oral theophylline, a conversion ratio of approximately 1.2 to 1.0 (aminophylline/theophylline) can be used. Thus, a patient receiving 1200 mg of intravenous aminophylline over 24 hours may be switched to 1000 mg of oral theophylline per day. This could be given in divided doses every 8 to 12 hours using a sustained-action preparation.

Adverse Effects and Monitoring. Patients vary widely and unpredictably in the serum concentration resulting from a given dosage of theophyllines. Thus, although dosing schedules are provided as general outlines, serum levels are mandatory. The optimal therapeutic concentration is 10 to 20 µg/ml. No effect may be likely at levels less than 5 µg/ml, and the 5 to 10 µg/ml range may be suboptimal. Gastrointestinal, cardiac, and neurological side effects commonly occur at levels above 20 µg/ml but may occur at lower levels in some patients. Serum theophylline levels of inpatients should be checked either on an every-other-day basis or when drug dosages are changed. Levels in outpatients are checked when the clinical response is not optimal, when clinical toxicity is suspected, when starting or stopping a drug such as cimetidine that affects theophylline metabolism, or to assure maximal therapeutic effect prior to a trial of corticosteroids.

Anticholinergics

Description, Actions, and Available Preparations. Atropine and other anticholinergic drugs inhibit the action of acetylcholine on autonomic nerve endings innervated by postganglionic cholinergic nerves. This opposes the actions of the vagus nerve and is especially useful in preventing or reversing bronchospasm of reflex or irritant origin.

Indications and Administration. Atropine is an effective bronchodilator for many patients, particularly those whose bronchoconstriction is strongly influenced by irritant receptors, but drying of respiratory secretions and tachycardia make it a suboptimal agent, particularly for regular or prolonged use. The quaternary ammonium compound ipratropium bromide (Atrovent) is a more effective bronchodilator than atropine and lacks virtually all of its adverse effects. Ipratropium is available in both solution and MDI in Europe but only the MDI is marketed in the United States. Although clinically useful in only a minority of patients with asthma, ipratropium is at least as effective in COPD as the beta-2 agonists, and is a first-line drug for this condition. Two puffs (0.018 mg ipratropium/puff) every 4 to 6 hours provide acceptable bronchodilatation for most patients; this dose may be doubled if needed, but unlike the situation with beta-2 agonists, little additional benefit is obtained by further increasing the delivered dose. Peak bronchodilator effect may not occur for 60 minutes or more.

Adverse Effects. Atropine and its relatives can cause tachycardia, urinary retention, blurred vision, decreased bowel motility, and drying of respiratory secretions. These effects are pronounced after parenteral administration but usually do not occur after direct application to the respiratory tract. Ipratropium is essentially free of adverse effects in most clinical applications.

Monitoring. Since blood levels of atropine and other anticholinergics are not routinely available, responses are generally followed clinically, as with the sympathomimetics.

Corticosteroids

Description and Actions. The corticosteroids are a potent group of natural and synthetic hormones that are used in conditions characterized by inappropriately severe immune or inflammatory reactions. Their known effects include decreased exudation and migration of inflammatory cells, protection of cell membranes against damage by a variety of agents, and decreased release of vasoactive amines and other mediators. Corticosteroids also decrease fluid leakage from blood vessels and edema formation and increase responsiveness to sympathomimetic agents.

Available Preparations. Although numerous steroid preparations are available, the following are usually used in respiratory disorders:
Parenteral Preparations. Hydrocortisone (Solu-Cortef, Cortef, others), methylprednisolone (Solu-Medrol, others), and dexamethasone (Decadron) are most commonly used. Relative doses are 20 mg for hydrocortisone, 4 mg for methylprednisolone, and 0.75 mg for dexamethasone.
Oral Preparations. Prednisone (Deltasone, others) and prednisolone (Delta-Cortef, others) are the main preparations and have about equal potency.
Inhaled Preparations. Beclomethasone dipropionate (Vanceril, Beclovent), flunisolide (Aerobid), and triamcinolone (Azmacort) are the most widely used agents in North America.

Indications and Administration. Because of their potential toxicity, systemic corticosteroids should generally be used only after other agents have been tried in optimal doses with unacceptable results. Inhalation of steroids has become the primary therapy for asthma in outpatients, but is not effective in acute exacerbations or in status asthmaticus. The following are guidelines for administration of corticosteroids in different clinical situations.
Status Asthmaticus. Intractable asthma should be treated with intravenous hydrocortisone (100 to 1000 mg/24 hr) or intravenous methylprednisolone (80 to 1000 mg/24 hr) every four to six hours. Treatment should be continued until the attack subsides and then tapered over several days.
Acute Asthma Attacks. Attacks of lesser severity usually respond to oral prednisone or prednisolone (20 to 40 mg/24 hr) either every morning (q.A.M.) or twice daily for two to four days, depending on the severity of attack. Treatment should be tapered over four to six days after improvement occurs. Each asthmatic patient tends to respond similarly during repeated episodes, so therapy can be tailored to past responses.

Chronic Asthma Maintenance. Most asthmatic patients can be controlled with inhaled corticosteroids (e.g., triamcinolone [Azmacort]), two to four puffs three to four times a day. When oral steroids are used, the lowest A.M. dose of prednisone or prednisolone should be used that maintains remission, with an attempt made to switch stable patients to an every-other-day (q.o.d.) dose or inhaled preparations whenever possible. Beclomethasone dipropionate, four puffs (200 µg) four times daily (q.i.d.), is equivalent to about 8 mg of prednisone and can help lower the oral dose even when complete substitution is unsuccessful.

COPD with Acute Exacerbation. In patients requiring hospitalization, give intravenous methylprednisolone, 2 mg/kg/24 hr (0.5 mg/kg every six hours), for 72 hr. Whether treatment should be tapered over several days or abruptly stopped is unproven.

Stable COPD. In patients requiring a diagnostic or therapeutic trial, theophylline, sympathomimetic, and perhaps anticholinergic therapy should first be optimized. After baseline spirometry, a treatment regimen of prednisone or prednisolone, 20 to 40 mg q.A.M. for two to three weeks, can be instituted. If repeat spirometry shows that the FEV_1 has improved by 20 to 30 per cent or more, medication should be reduced to the lowest daily or q.o.d. dose that maintains effects. If the steroids do not produce improvement, their use should be tapered and discontinued over a one- to two-week period. Inhaled steroids have not been shown to be effective in COPD.

Adverse Effects. *Acute Effects.* Acute effects include mild euphoria and a sense of well-being. Short-term therapy (from hours to a few days) can produce restlessness, insomnia, and frank psychosis. Peptic ulceration and upper gastrointestinal bleeding can also occur.

Long-Term Effects at Greater Than Physiological Replacement Doses. These include fluid retention; potassium loss and metabolic alkalosis; increased susceptibility to infections, especially tuberculosis and fungal infections; hyperglycemia and glycosuria; osteoporosis and vertebral compression fractures, especially in postmenopausal women; myopathy involving the proximal shoulder muscles and hip girdle; cataracts; weight gain in adults and growth arrest in children; and cushingoid features such as moon facies. Behavioral changes may also occur, including attempts at suicide. Inhalation of steroids is not infrequently associated with development of oral candidiasis (thrush), especially at high doses. This can be decreased or prevented with the use of spacer devices for inhalation.

Withdrawal. Prolonged corticosteroid therapy at or above normal physiological needs causes pituitary-adrenal suppression that is manifested as adrenal insufficiency during withdrawal. Symptoms include depression, weakness, fatigue, anorexia, and weight loss. Hypotension and hypoglycemia are common findings. After steroids have been used in high doses for more than two to four months, six to nine months may be required for full adrenal recovery.

Monitoring. Since blood levels of corticosteroids are not routinely available, therapy is monitored by objective measurement of the physiological abnormality being treated, such as the FEV_1, as well as by clinical effect, such as reduction in the frequency of asthma attacks. An overall goal should be to discontinue systemic therapy as soon as possible, or at least to use the lowest possible dose.

Cromolyn

Description, Actions, and Available Preparations. Disodium cromoglycate, or cromolyn sodium (Intal), is a topical agent administered by inhalation for the prophylaxis of asthma. Cromolyn is not a bronchodilator. It seems to stabilize mast cell lysosomal membranes so that release of histamine and other vasoactive amines does not occur on exposure of the mast cells to stimuli that otherwise would trigger an asthma attack.

Indications and Administration. Although cromolyn may be valuable in preventing asthma attacks, including those induced by exercise, it has no place in the management of an attack or in status asthmaticus. It also usually is ineffective in COPD. Cromolyn is ineffective if taken by mouth and therefore is administered by inhalation. Cromolyn usually is prescribed q.i.d. Several weeks' therapy may be required to see an effect.

Adverse Effects. Cromolyn generally causes no side effects, other than occasional irritant effects of the powder in the upper airway.

Mucolytic Agents and Expectorants

Description, Actions, and Available Preparations. A wide variety of compounds are said to facilitate sputum expectoration. The main mechanisms include dilution with water administered systemically or topically; bronchial gland stimulation via vagal stimulation with guaifenesin (glyceryl guaiacolate), via the blood with a supersaturated solution of potassium iodide (SSKI) or iodinated glycerol (Organidin), or through topical application of hypotonic or hypertonic saline and other irritants; mucoprotein or DNA breakdown with acetylcysteine (Mucomyst); and the surfactant effect achieved with sodium bicarbonate.

Indications and Administration. Although many of these agents may increase sputum expectoration, it is not clear whether they do so by helping patients bring up what is already there or by increasing sputum production through their irritative actions. Their use is generally limited to persons with cystic fibrosis and other conditions that cause thick, inspissated secretions and to those individuals who have difficulty raising secretions spontaneously. Even in these patients, the value of the agents is unclear. Agents relying on vagal stimulation or dispersion through the bloodstream are given by mouth; those producing mucosal wetting or irritation are often aerosolized.

Adverse Effects. Hypotonic or hypertonic aerosols can cause bronchospasm, as can Mucomyst. Patients may become sensitized to iodides, Mucomyst, and other agents, which may also become less effective with repeated administration.

Antitussives

Description and Actions. Antitussive agents are intended to stop patients from coughing. The most important peripherally acting antitussives are mucosal anesthetics such as cocaine, lidocaine, and tetracaine, and the oral agent benzonatate. Central antitussives include the narcotics, of which codeine is most important, and a number of non-narcotic drugs such as caramiphen and dextromethorphan. Most of these drugs are metabolized by the liver.

Available Preparations. Cocaine, tetracaine, and lidocaine are used to suppress cough during bronchoscopy and other procedures. Lidocaine is also used in intubated patients with cough. In outpatients, the most important antitussive agent is codeine. Codeine is preferable to morphine and most other narcotics as an antitussive because it has less addiction potential, produces less sedation, causes less respiratory depression, and is less likely to lead to tolerance. Codeine is effective by itself (adult dose: 5 to 20 mg q four to six hr) and is also available in numerous combinations with other agents. Hydrocodone is another commonly used narcotic antitussive available in numerous preparations. Of the many non-narcotic cough suppressants the most widely prescribed effective agents are benzonatate (Tessalon), caramiphen (Tuss-Ornade), and dextromethorphan (many available preparations).

Indications and Administration. Cough is an airway protection and clearance mechanism that can be either effective, relieving the stimulus by expelling secretions, or ineffective, when no sputum is present or the patient is unable to raise it. Since retention of secretions in the airways is harmful, suppressing a productive cough is usually ill advised. Therapy should instead be directed at reducing sputum production by treating its underlying cause. Patients too weak or obtunded to cough effectively are likewise not appropriate candidates for antitussives. When nonproductive cough is a troublesome symptom in itself, however, and interferes with sleep or causes headache, muscle soreness, or social inconvenience, suppressing it is appropriate. In general, antitussives should be used for short-term rather than chronic cough suppression; most chronic coughs have a specific identifiable cause that can be treated with specific therapy, such as bronchodilators, treatment of sinus disease, avoidance of smoking, and so on. Patients who have trouble raising sputum may need mucokinetic rather than antitussive therapy.

Adverse Effects. The most important adverse effect of antitussive therapy is secretion retention, with consequent worsening of airflow obstruction and risk of infection. Proper patient selection is crucial, and the actual number of justifiable indications for these agents is relatively small. Respiratory depression is a major threat with any narcotic as well as with other depressant drugs.

Respiratory Stimulants

Acute Stimulants. Respiratory drives vary with metabolic rate. Just as hypothermia, hypothyroidism, and sedating drugs depress these drives, any process or agent that produces hypermetabolism tends to increase them and, so far as the patient is capable, to augment ventilation. Thus, fever, hyperthyroidism, and general stimulant drugs such as amphetamines all stimulate ventilation. A few other drugs, including doxapram (Dopram), also stimulate the ventilatory regulatory center more or less selectively. However, except for occasional use in accelerating postanesthetic awakening, such acute stimulants have little clinical use. Although they increase the frequency and depth of spontaneous ventilation, they do so at the expense of increased work of breathing. Furthermore, controlled studies have demonstrated that these drugs do not alter the course of acute ventilatory failure. If used to avoid intubation or for other purposes, respiratory stimulants must be given by continuous intravenous infusion and their effects monitored in a critical care unit.

Chronic Stimulants. Progesterone can be given orally over prolonged periods (Provera, 20 mg 3 times daily) to stimulate ventilation in patients with COPD or the obesity-hypoventilation syndrome whose mechanical limitations are not insurmountable but whose normal drive to breathe is lacking. Two weeks may be required to see an effect.

Paralyzing Agents

Description and Actions. These drugs are used to decrease voluntary muscle activity during mechanical ventilation. Both nondepolarizing and depolarizing agents are available. They are given by repeated intravenous bolus and produce paralysis but not sedation.

Available Preparations. The three paralyzing drugs most commonly used are pancuronium bromide (Pavulon) and tubocurarine (curare), which are nondepolarizing agents, and succinylcholine (Anectine), which is a depolarizing agent. Pancuronium produces flaccid paralysis within two to three minutes after intravenous injection. The paralysis lasts 40 to 60 minutes. Pancuronium is the drug of first choice for use during ventilator care (dose = 0.8 mg/ kg). Curare has similar effects of slightly shorter duration. Succinylcholine acts rapidly and causes muscle fasciculations, which may be severe; its effect disappears within five to ten minutes.

Indications and Administration. Paralyzing agents are important in anesthesia and are indicated in severe tetanus to control muscle spasms. They may be useful in prolonged or repetitive seizure activity, although they do not affect brain electrical activity and do not actually stop the seizure. Short-acting paralyzing agents are helpful during difficult endotracheal intubation. These drugs are occasionally necessary during mechanical ventilation in cases of uncontrollable agitation; this indication occurs very infrequently with respiratory care by experienced personnel. Finally, in some cases of refractory, life-threatening hypoxemia in the adult respiratory distress syndrome (ARDS), paralysis may improve oxygenation by decreasing peripheral oxygen utilization. When necessary, paralysis should be managed by an anesthesiologist or other physician experienced in such care, and paralyzing agents must always be used in conjunction with sedation with a benzodiazepine, a narcotic, or both.

Adverse Effects. A paralyzed patient is rendered incapable of breathing spontaneously and will die if disconnected from the ventilator. When paralyzed, patients are more difficult to monitor and neurological status is hard to assess. Since patients remain wide awake, use of these drugs without concomitant adequate sedation may lead to serious adverse effects.

RECOMMENDED READING

1. Braga PC, and Allegra L (eds.): *Drugs in Bronchial Mucology*. New York, Raven Press, 1989.
2. Cherniack RM (ed.): *Drugs for the Respiratory System*. New York, Grune & Stratton, 1986.
3. Chernow B (ed.): *Essentials of Critical Care Pharmacology*. Baltimore, Williams & Wilkins, 1989.
4. Consensus Conference on Aerosol Delivery. *Respir Care*, 36:916–1044, 1991.
5. Gilman AG, et al. (eds.): *Goodman and Gilman's The Pharmacological Basis of Therapeutics*, 8th ed., New York, Pergamon Press, 1990.

6. Hess D: How should bronchodilators be administered to patients on ventilators? *Respir Care*, 36:377–394, 1991.
7. Pierson DJ: Drugs used in respiratory care. *In* Pierson DJ, and Kacmarek RM, (eds.): *Foundations of Respiratory Care.* New York, Churchill Livingstone, 1992, pp. 175–194.
8. US Pharmacopeial Convention, Inc.: USP DI. *Drug Information for the Health Care Professional,* 10th ed. Rockville, Md, USPC, 1990.
9. Witek TJ Jr, and Schachter EN (eds.): Advances in respiratory care pharmacology. *Probl Respir Care*, 1:1–153, 1988.
10. Ziment I: Drugs used in respiratory therapy. *In* Burton GG, et al. (eds.): *Respiratory Care: A Guide to Clinical Practice*, 3rd ed. Philadelphia, J. B. Lippincott, 1991, pp. 411–448.

12

AEROSOL THERAPY

GENERAL CONSIDERATIONS

An aerosol is a suspension of liquid droplets or solid particles in a gaseous medium. In aerosol therapy, a pharmacological agent constitutes the dispersed substance, and the gas is inhaled by a patient for the purpose of diagnosing or treating lung disease. Several of the most important drugs in respiratory care can have a higher therapeutic index (ratio of desired effects to side effects) when delivered as aerosols than when administered orally or parenterally. Included are the beta-adrenergic agonists, anticholinergics, and corticosteroids used in the treatment of asthma and chronic obstructive pulmonary disease (COPD). This chapter first describes the important physical characteristics of aerosols and the equipment used to generate and deliver them in the clinical setting, and then summarizes the main aspects of aerosol therapy, including indications, techniques, and precautions. Humidity therapy and the use of bland aerosols are described in Chapter 9.

PHYSICAL CHARACTERISTICS OF AEROSOLS

Penetration and Deposition

Penetration applies to the depth within the respiratory tract that particles of a given size are capable of reaching, whereas *deposition* refers to those mechanisms that enhance the settling of aerosol particles within the airway. Of numerous factors affecting deposition, the most important are inertia, sedimentation, and brownian diffusion (Table 12–1).

Retention and Clearance

Retention is the amount of a substance present in the respiratory tract at a specific point in time. *Clearance* is the removal of a deposited aerosol that does not become absorbed by the airway mucous membrane. The rate at which particles are cleared depends on where within the lung they are deposited: Particles deposited on ciliated epithelium are cleared relatively rapidly (less so, however, in the presence of chronic bronchitis or COPD), while those

Table 12–1. FACTORS AFFECTING PARTICLE DEPOSITION IN THE RESPIRATORY TRACT

FACTOR	DEPOSITION BY INERTIA	DEPOSITION BY SEDIMENTATION	DEPOSITION BY DIFFUSION
Particle size	Large (>5 μ)	Medium (1–5 μ)	Small (<1 μ)
Site of deposition	Upper respiratory tract; large airways	Smaller airways	Terminal airways; alveoli
Geometrical factors	Large angles of airway bifurcation	Horizontal airway surfaces	Small sizes of individual air spaces; nearness of surfaces
Aerodynamic factors	High airflow rates	Low airflow rates	Very low to zero airflow
Maneuvers that increase deposition	Rapid inspiration	Breath-holding	Breath-holding

that reach the alveoli and other nonciliated areas must first be phagocytosed by macrophages and may be cleared very slowly.

Factors Affecting Particle Deposition

The effectiveness of a therapeutic aerosol depends on the dose deposited at the appropriate site in the respiratory tract, which in turn is determined by *particle size, ventilatory pattern*, and *airway anatomy and geometry*, among other factors (Table 12–1). Clinically useful aerosol particles are in the range of about 1 to 10 micrometers (μ) in size; those smaller than 0.5 to 1.0 μ are likely to be exhaled, while particles larger than 10 μ are generally deposited in the upper respiratory tract and delivery apparatus.

The best size range for airway delivery (as with bronchodilators) is 2 to 5 μ in mass median aerodynamic diameter (MMAD), which indicates that 50 per cent of the aerosol's particles have a diameter larger and 50 per cent have a diameter smaller than this value. Drugs acting on the lung parenchyma rather than the airways, such as ribavirin and pentamidine, are most effective at an MMAD of 1 to 3 μ.

Aspects of *ventilatory pattern* that affect penetration and deposition of therapeutic aerosols include inspiratory flow rate, breath-holding, and tidal volume. The optimal inspiratory flow rate for airway deposition of liquid aerosols, as from a metered-dose inhaler (MDI), is 0.5 L/sec, whereas higher flow rates (>1.0 L/sec) are required for generation and dispersal of dry-powder aerosols. Breath-holding at end-inspiration, ideally for 10 seconds, enhances deposition due to particle settling. Tidal volume mainly affects the amount of aerosol delivered to the lung parenchyma.

Anatomical and pathological factors are mainly those affecting airway diameter. The narrower the airways (e.g., in small children or in acute asthma) the less aerosol is deposited distally. In addition, the presence of an endotracheal or tracheostomy tube markedly reduces the quantity of drug deposited in the lower respiratory tract. These facts do not mean that other delivery routes should be used, but rather that larger doses of inhaled medication will be required.

EQUIPMENT

In respiratory care, aerosols are generated by nebulizers, which are classified as large-volume or small-volume aerosol generators; MDIs, used either alone or with auxiliary devices such as spacers; and dry-powder inhalers (DPIs).

Large-Volume Aerosol Generators

These generators include ultrasonic, hydrodynamic, and jet nebulizers. *Ultrasonic nebulizers* (Fig. 12–1) create an aerosol by applying electrical energy to a piezoelectric transducer, which converts the electrical energy to high-frequency sound waves. The latter are focused either directly or indirectly on the solution to be nebulized, forming a spray of aerosol particles. These nebulizers are highly efficient, producing particles mainly in the range of 1 to 10 μ, and generate large volumes of aerosol (1 to 6 ml/min of nebulized solution). They are used mainly for delivery of saline to facilitate sputum production and expectoration and are seldom used for delivery of medication. *Hydrodynamic (Babbington) nebulizers* and *large-volume jet nebulizers* (LVN; see Fig. 9–1B) also produce very large volumes of nebulized solution and are likewise used mainly for sputum induction or secretion liquefaction or, in the case of jet nebulizers, for continuous humidification during mechanical ventilation.

Small-Volume Aerosol Generators

These generators are designed exclusively for administration of medication. All *small-volume nebulizers* (SVNs), regardless of manufacturer or external appearance, operate by the same mechanism as described in Chapter 9 and illustrated in Figure 9–1B, but have a smaller solution capacity (usually 10 to 15 ml). A typical example is diagrammed in Figure 12–2. Usually 2 to 6 ml of medication solution is added, with 2.5 to 3.5 ml recommended for bronchodilator use. Larger volumes take too long to nebulize, while proportionally more medication is lost if a smaller volume is employed. All SVNs leave a specific volume of solution in the unit after nebulization is complete, and this "dead volume" is generally 0.5 to 1.0 ml, depending on the manufacturer. This represents the amount of solution that adheres to the walls, cap, and system connections (e.g., corrugated tubing, mouthpiece, mask). Dead

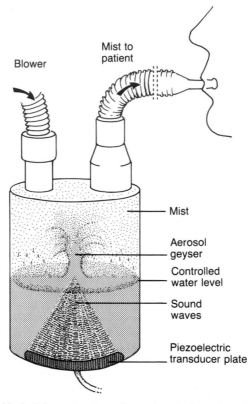

Figure 12–1. Schematic of an ultrasonic nebulizer. Sound waves produced by an electrically powered piezoelectric transducer physically disrupt the water into an aerosol geyser. The largest droplets rain out while those of respirable size are delivered to the patient.

volume can be minimized by periodically tapping the sides of the nebulizer during use until the unit is dry.

More drug is delivered via SVN when administered only during inspiration rather than throughout the respiratory cycle. With hand-held administration this requires the patient to occlude a finger port or other mechanism in the driving gas line with each inspiration. Such a degree of continuous patient compliance is often unattainable, and in such circumstances higher doses (or, rather, addition of more drug to the nebulizer) may be required.

Metered-Dose Inhalers

Figure 12–3 illustrates the general design of an MDI, a self-contained unit consisting of a pressurized canister containing drug

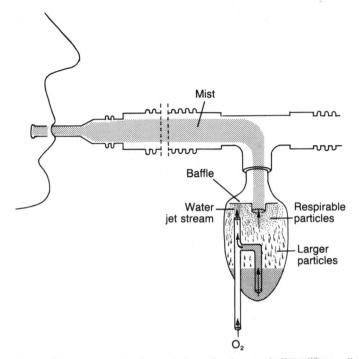

Figure 12–2. Schematic of a typical small volume nebulizer. The medication solution is drawn into the stream of oxygen (or air) and blown against a baffle, generating the aerosol. Larger particles "rain out" and are re-nebulized until all the solution has been consumed.

and propellant, a valve, and a mouthpiece. With each actuation of the device the prescribed quantity of drug is released in a volume of propellant gas that is usually 60 to 90 ml. Most of the *particles* are in the 2- to 5-μ range, but most of the *drug* is released in larger particles that impact in the mouthpiece or in the patient's oropharynx. Even with ideal technique only 9 to 12 per cent of the delivered drug actually reaches the patient's lower airway; with suboptimal usage the amount can be far lower. For maximal lower-airway deposition the patient's inspiratory flow rate should be about 0.5 L/sec, followed by a breath-hold (see subsequent section).

Because the chlorofluorocarbon (CFC) propellants used in all MDIs are soon to be banned world wide because of their potential effect on the atmosphere, these most widely used devices for aerosol therapy are likely to be phased out or markedly altered in their design in the future.

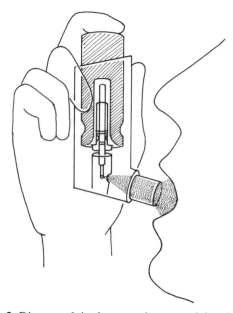

Figure 12–3. Diagram of the features of a metered-dose inhaler. After shaking the canister, the patient holds it upright and presses down, activating the metering valve and discharging a preset volume of propellant and medication. Most clinicians consider the open-mouth technique to be ideal, although effective therapy can also be given with the lips sealed around the mouthpiece.

Spacers

Spacers, also called auxiliary or accessory devices, are extensions to an MDI designed to eliminate the need for hand-eye coordination and also to reduce the amount of drug delivered by impaction to the patient's upper airway. Lung deposition using a spacer is comparable to that resulting from proper use of an MDI alone. Figure 12–4 shows three of the most commonly used spacer devices.

Clinically, MDIs with spacers are at least as effective in delivering aerosolized bronchodilator as MDIs used alone or SVNs, and outperform MDIs used with suboptimal technique. MDIs used with spacers have been shown in numerous studies to be as effective as SVNs both in the emergency department and during hospitalization for asthma or COPD.

Dry-Powder Inhalers

DPIs are becoming more widely used as replacements for CFC-powered MDIs. DPIs are breath actuated and require a higher inspiratory flow rate to generate and disperse the aerosol: 1 to 2 L/sec is considered optimal. They vary somewhat in design; Figure 12–5 illustrates two current types of DPI.

AEROSOL THERAPY

INDICATIONS AND GOALS

The overall purposes of aerosol therapy are to facilitate bronchial hygiene, to condition inspired gas, and to deliver medication. In *bronchial hygiene*, aerosols have the goals of hydrating dried retained secretions, improving the efficacy of cough, and restoring and maintaining normal function of the mucociliary clearance system (see Chapter 9). Cool, bland aerosol therapy is commonly used in both children and adults with *upper airway inflammation.* This applies to primary disorders such as croup and epiglottitis and also to the consequences of therapy such as laryngeal edema following extubation. There are few objective data substantiating this use, but most clinicians (and patients) feel it reduces discomfort. *Humidification of inspired gases*, especially during mechanical ventilation, is another major goal of aerosol therapy, as discussed in Chapter 9.

Delivery of medication to the lower airways and lung parenchyma is the fourth main goal of aerosol therapy. Drugs most commonly delivered by aerosol include beta-adrenergic agonists and anticholinergic bronchodilators (e.g., albuterol and ipratropium, respectively), corticosteroids (e.g., beclomethasone, triamcinolone), nonsteroidal anti-inflammatory agents for the airways (e.g., cromolyn sodium), antiviral agents (e.g., ribavirin), and pentamidine (for treatment or prevention of *Pneumocystis carinii* pneumonia). Aminoglycoside antibiotics (e.g., gentamicin, tobramycin) are also sometimes given by aerosol, or by direct instillation into the trachea in intubated patients.

PRACTICAL ASPECTS

Technique

The advantages and disadvantages of the use of SVN, MDI, and DPI for the delivery of aerosolized bronchodilators and other medications are compared in Table 12–2. Tables 12–3 through 12–8 list the recommended techniques for clinical aerosol administration using the devices described in this chapter, including their use

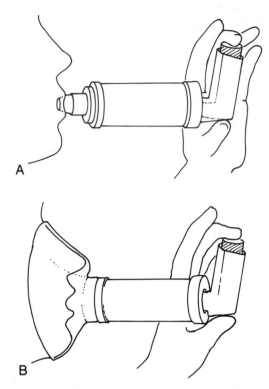

Figure 12–4. Examples of spacer devices for use with an MDI. *A,* Aerochamber with mouthpiece. *B,* Aerochamber with face mask.

in patients who are intubated and undergoing mechanical ventilation (Tables 12–4 and 12–7).

Dosing Strategies

Delivery Device. For years clinicians and patients alike believed that nebulizers were inherently more effective than MDIs in relieving airflow obstruction in asthma and COPD. This was largely because the doses recommended for the two delivery methods were markedly different—typically fivefold to tenfold larger for SVN than for MDI. Used correctly and with therapeutically equivalent doses of the same drug, many studies have now demonstrated that there is no inherent difference in effectiveness between the SVN and the MDI.

Beta-Agonist Bronchodilators. Numerous studies have shown that the regimen of two puffs every four to six hours that has been

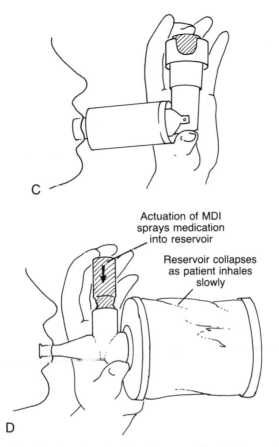

Actuation of MDI
sprays medication
into reservoir

Reservoir collapses
as patient inhales
slowly

Figure 12–4 *Continued C,* Combined metered-dose inhaler and spacer (Azmacort). *D,* InspirEase. With the last device, the metered-dose inhaler is discharged into the reservoir, away from the patient; the reservoir then collapses as the patient inhales. With several types of commercial spacer devices, a whistle or other indicator is activated if the patient inhales too rapidly.

recommended for decades in the United States is insufficient to produce maximal bronchodilation, and that currently available beta-agonists can generally be used at these higher doses, at least short term, without significant side effects. This has been found to be the case for both asthma and COPD, and in patients whose condition is stable, during acute exacerbations, and when patients are intubated and mechanically ventilated. Many authorities recommend that a dose-response relationship be determined for each patient, using objective outcome measures such as peak expiratory flow rate (PEFR) or forced expiratory flow in the first second

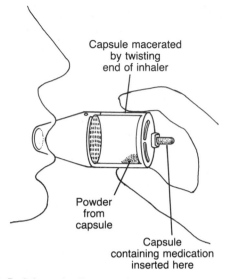

Capsule macerated
by twisting
end of inhaler

Powder
from
capsule

Capsule
containing medication
inserted here

Figure 12–5. Schematic diagram of one type of dry powder inhaler (Rotahaler). Inspiratory flowrate must be sufficient (e.g., > 1.0 L/sec) to generate the aerosol by dispersing the powdered medication.

(FEV$_1$) for spontaneously breathing patients, and peak inspiratory pressure or auto-PEEP for ventilated patients. When this is done, considerably higher doses are usually required. The patient's status should be carefully monitored for adverse effects, but these have generally not been observed when careful dose-response titration has been employed. The reader should consult the sources listed in Recommended Reading at the end of this chapter for more complete explanation and actual dosing schedules.

COMPLICATIONS AND PRECAUTIONS

Aerosol therapy is generally safe when administered according to the principles described in the preceding sections. However, the clinician should be aware of several potential hazards, which include precipitation of bronchospasm and cough, swelling of dried retained secretions, fluid overload, drug reactions, and nosocomial infection. In addition, recently there has been concern about adverse environmental effects to caregivers and others in the vicinity and also to the global environment.

Bronchospasm and Cough

Bland aerosol therapy irritates the airway mucosa, and in some patients this irritation can be severe enough to produce clinical

Table 12–2. ADVANTAGES AND DISADVANTAGES OF SMALL-VOLUME NEBULIZERS (SVN), METERED-DOSE INHALERS (MDI), AND DRY-POWDER INHALERS (DPI)

ADVANTAGES	DISADVANTAGES
SVN	
Less patient coordination required	Expensive
	Wasteful
High doses possible (even continuous)	Contamination possible if not carefully cleaned
No chlorofluorocarbon release	Not all medications available
	Pressurized gas source required
	More time required
MDI	
Convenient	Patient coordination required
Inexpensive	Patient activation required
	Results in pharyngeal deposition
	Has potential for abuse
	Difficult to deliver high doses
	Not all medications available
	Dependent on ozone-depleting chlorofluorocarbons
MDI with Auxiliary Device	
Less patient coordination required	More complex process for patient who can use MDI alone
	More expensive than MDI alone
	Less portable than MDI alone
DPI	
Less patient coordination required	Requires high inspiratory flow
	Most units are single dose
Breath-holding not required	Can result in pharyngeal deposition
No chlorofluorocarbon release	Cannot be used with intubated patients
Breath activated	Not all medications available
	Difficult to deliver high doses

From Kacmarek RM, and Hess D: The interface between patient and aerosol generator. *Respir Care* 36:952–976, 1991. With permission.

bronchospasm, manifested by wheezing, cough, and reduction in PEFR or FEV_1. This complication is most commonly seen with the use of ultrasonic or hydrodynamic humidifiers, which can potentially deposit large quantities of fluid on the airway surface. Administration of bronchodilator prior to use of these devices may reduce or eliminate this complication. All treatments with ultrasonic or hydrodynamic humidifiers should be monitored by the clinician, using periodic auscultation for adventitious breath sounds as well as overall observation of the patient.

Swelling of Dried Retained Secretions

Hydration of secretions can increase their volume substantially, with the potential for airway obstruction if the patient is unable to cough and expectorate adequately. This problem would be of greatest concern during the use of ultrasonic or hydrodynamic nebulizers. During and after therapy with these devices, patients

Table 12–3. TECHNIQUE FOR USE OF A SMALL-VOLUME NEBULIZER (SVN)

Place drug in nebulizer.

Dilute with physiological saline (0.9%) to 4 ml total volume.

Incorporate a finger port into the driving gas system to provide intermittent nebulization during inspiration only.

Set driving gas flow at 6–8 L/min.

Connect patient to SVN via a mouthpiece or mask (in some patients a nose clip may be necessary).

Instruct patient to inspire through open mouth if using a mask or to close lips around mouthpiece.

Grasp nebulizer chamber firmly in hand to maintain temperature during treatment.

Have patient inhale slowly (0.5 L/sec) at normal tidal volume.

Have patient occasionally inspire to total lung capacity and incorporate a 4–10-sec breath-hold.

Tap sides of nebulizer to minimize dead volume.

Continue treatment until no aerosol is produced.

Monitor patient for presence of side effects (e.g., tachycardia or tremor) and beneficial effects (e.g., improved breath sounds, peak flow, and FEV_1).

From Kacmarek RM, and Hess D: The interface between patient and aerosol generator. *Respir Care* 36:952–976, 1991. With permission.

should be carefully monitored for respiratory distress. Airway suctioning should be performed if spontaneous removal of secretions appears to be inadequate.

Fluid Overload

Total body fluid overload, with associated electrolyte disturbances, could theoretically occur from prolonged use of ultrasonic or hydrodynamic nebulizers. This is potentially a problem in infants and children, in whom the volume of delivered fluid would be proportionally greater than in adults, and for this reason the use of these nebulizers should generally be avoided in such patients. Because the fluid output of jet nebulizers is much less, these devices should not be associated with a risk of this complication.

Drug Reactions

Any adverse reaction to a drug may occur with aerosol administration (see Chapter 11). However, because considerably less drug is required for therapeutic effectiveness with aerosol than with other administration routes, such reactions should be infrequent.

Table 12–4. TECHNIQUE FOR USE OF A SMALL-VOLUME NEBULIZER (SVN) DURING MECHANICAL VENTILATION

Place drug in nebulizer.

Dilute with physiological saline (0.9%) to 4 ml total volume.

Insert nebulizer into inspiratory limb of ventilatory circuit at least 18 inches from Y.

Use intermittent nebulizer flow from ventilator if available.

If continuous flow is used, set at 6–8 L/min.

Set ventilator rate at 4–8/min or higher if not contraindicated.

Set tidal volume at 12 ml/kg or more unless contraindicated. If pressure support rate drops, add back-up synchronized intermittent mandatory ventilation rate.

With children, adjust ventilator flow to ensure that total flow is unchanged during pressure-limited ventilation.

With children (and some adults), readjust tidal volume during continuous-flow nebulization to maintain constant tidal volume and peak airway pressure.

Tap sides of nebulizer to minimize dead volume.

Continue treatment until no aerosol is produced.

Remove equipment from ventilator circuit.

Return ventilator to pretreatment settings.

Monitor patient for presence of side effects (e.g., tachycardia or tremor) and beneficial effects (e.g., improved breath sounds, peak flow, and FEV_1).

From Kacmarek RM, and Hess D: The interface between patient and aerosol generator. *Respir Care* 36:952–976, 1991. With permission.

Table 12–5. TECHNIQUE FOR USE OF A METERED-DOSE INHALER (MDI) WITHOUT SPACER

Warm MDI to body temperature.

Assemble apparatus.

Shake canister vigorously.

Hold canister upright.

Open mouth.

Place aerosol at mouth opening.

Begin to inspire slowly at inspiratory flows <0.5 L/min.

Actuate MDI.

Continue to inspire to total lung capacity.

Hold breath for 4–10 sec.

Wait 3–10 min between actuations.

Rinse mouth and pharynx if inhaling steroids.

Monitor patient for presence of side effects (e.g., tachycardia or tremor) and beneficial effects (e.g., improved breath sounds, peak flow, and FEV_1).

From Kacmarek RM, and Hess D: The interface between patient and aerosol generator. *Respir Care* 36:952–976, 1991. With permission.

Table 12–6. TECHNIQUE FOR USE OF A METERED-DOSE INHALER (MDI) WITH SPACER

Warm MDI to body temperature.

Shake canister vigorously.

Hold canister upright.

Actuate MDI.

Place mouthpiece in mouth.

Close lips about mouthpiece.

Inspire slowly (≤ 0.5 L/sec) from spacer.

Continue to inspire to total lung capacity.

Hold breath 4–10 sec.

Repeat inspiration with breath-hold if indicated by spacer manufacturer.

Wait 3–10 min between subsequent actuations.

Monitor patient for presence of side effects (e.g., tachycardia or tremor) and beneficial effects (e.g., improved breath sounds, peak flow, and FEV_1).

From Kacmarek RM, and Hess D: The interface between patient and aerosol generator. *Respir Care* 36:952–976, 1991. With permission.

Nosocomial Infection

Aerosol administration to patients has the potential for airway contamination with bacteria or other infectious agents. Because the warm, wet environment provided by all aerosol generators constitutes an ideal growth medium for bacteria, clinicians should

Table 12–7. TECHNIQUE FOR USE OF A METERED-DOSE INHALER (MDI) DURING MECHANICAL VENTILATION

Place MDI adapter into circuit.

Adjust ventilator to deliver volume-limited breaths or use a manual ventilator.

Warm MDI to body temperature.

Shake MDI vigorously.

Place MDI in circuit.

Actuate MDI immediately after the beginning of a mechanical breath; if spacer is used, actuate 1–2 sec before mechanical breath or near end-exhalation, depending on the rate.

Apply a 2–3-sec inflation hold, if not contraindicated.

Wait 1 min between actuations.

Return ventilator to pretreatment settings.

Monitor patient for presence of side effects (e.g., tachycardia or tremor) and beneficial effects (e.g., improved breath sounds, peak flow, and FEV_1).

From Kacmarek RM, and Hess D: The interface between patient and aerosol generator. *Respir Care* 36:952–976, 1991. With permission.

Table 12–8. TECHNIQUE FOR USE OF A DRY-POWDER INHALER (DPI)

Assemble apparatus.

Open capsule (technique specific for each device).

Exhale normally to functional residual capacity.

Place inhaler mouthpiece in mouth.

Seal lips around mouthpiece.

Inhale rapidly (>60 L/min) through device; breath-hold unnecessary.

Repeat process until capsule is empty.

Rinse mouth after inhalation if medication is a steroid.

Monitor patient for presence of side effects (e.g., tachycardia or tremor) and beneficial effects (e.g., improved breath sounds, peak flow, and FEV_1).

From Kacmarek RM, and Hess D: The interface between patient and aerosol generator. *Respir Care* 36:952–976, 1991. With permission.

exercise meticulous care in setting up and refilling them, and appropriate infection control measures should be followed at all times.

All aerosol equipment used on patients should be sterile before use and should be changed every 24 hours. This applies to small-volume as well as to large-volume devices. Unlike aerosol generators, humidification systems do not generate particles and thus provide no mechanism for transporting bacteria from the device to the patient. When humidification systems produce large volumes of condensate in the delivery tubing, as sometimes occurs during mechanical ventilation, these should be changed periodically; most clinicians recommend that this be done every 48 hours, although recent studies suggest that less frequent changes are acceptable.

Escape of Aerosols into the Environment

Clinical aerosol administration poses potential hazards to persons other than the patient to whom the treatment is given. The clinician administering the aerosol could be affected, as could others (patients, visitors, and other staff) in the vicinity. The greatest risk is from the spread of tuberculosis through coughing during the treatment; the existence and magnitude of other risks, as from environmental inhalation of pentamidine and ribavirin, are controversial.

Measures recommended to reduce the risk of transmission of tuberculosis during aerosol therapy include:

1. Prompt recognition and treatment (prophylactic or therapeutic) of tuberculosis in HIV-positive patients and others at increased risk for tuberculosis.

2. Performance of sputum induction and administration of aero-

solized pentamidine or ribavirin in facilities that meet the CDC guidelines for prevention of tuberculosis (see Recommended Reading), including at least six air exchanges per hour or use of special filters in the room in which the treatment is administered.

3. Strict adherence by the clinician to protective procedures established by the hospital or other health care facility when dealing with patients at high risk for tuberculosis.

Although the medical use of CFCs amounts to only 0.4 to 0.5 per cent of worldwide production of these compounds, they are believed to be a major cause of atmospheric damage and are scheduled to be banned everywhere by the year 2000. The pharmaceutical industry is working to develop and market alternative propellants and delivery devices, and increased use of DPIs and other non-CFC delivery devices can be expected.

RECOMMENDED READING

1. American Association for Respiratory Care. AARC Clinical Practice Guideline: Selection of aerosol delivery device. *Respir Care*, 37:891–897, 1992.
2. Chaisson RE, and McAvinue S: Control of tuberculosis during aerosol therapy administration. *Respir Care*, 36:1027–1035, 1991.
3. Consensus Conference on Aerosol Delivery. *Respir Care*, 36:914–1044, 1991.
4. Hess D: How should bronchodilators be administered to patients on ventilators? *Respir Care*, 36:377–394, 1991.
5. Kacmarek RM: Humidity and aerosol therapy. *In* Pierson DJ, and Kacmarek RM (eds.): *Foundations of Respiratory Care.* New York, Churchill Livingstone, 1992, pp. 793–824.
6. Kacmarek RM, and Hess D: The interface between patient and aerosol generator. *Respir Care*, 36:952–976, 1991.
7. Morrow PE: Conference on the scientific basis of respiratory therapy: Aerosol therapy. Aerosol characteristics and deposition. *Am Rev Respir Dis*, 110:88–99, 1974.
8. Newman SP: Aerosol deposition considerations in inhalation therapy. *Chest*, 88(suppl 2):152s–160s, 1985.
9. Newman SP, and Clarke SW: The proper use of metered dose inhalers. *Chest*, 86:342–344, 1984.
10. Svedmyr N: Clinical advantages of the aerosol route of drug administration. *Respir Care*, 36:922–930, 1991.
11. U.S. Department of Health & Human Services. Guidelines for preventing the transmission of tuberculosis in health-care settings with special focus on HIV-related issues. *MMWR*, 39(RR-17):20–22, 1990.

13

THERAPY TO IMPROVE VENTILATION

FAILURE OF VENTILATION

OVERVIEW

Definition

As discussed in Chapter 7, respiratory failure due to failure of ventilation is present when the arterial carbon dioxide tension ($PaCO_2$) significantly exceeds the normal limit of approximately 40 mmHg. This condition is called hypercapnia. A $PaCO_2$ of 50 mmHg or greater meets most textbook definitions of ventilatory failure.

Acute and Chronic Ventilatory Failure

The distinction between acute and chronic ventilatory failure relates not to the degree of hypercapnia in the two conditions, which may be the same, but to the acuteness of the rise in $PaCO_2$ and its effect on the pH. Assuming that no other acid-base derangements are present, a rapid rise in $PaCO_2$ of 10 to 15 mmHg will cause the pH to fall from 7.40 to 7.30 regardless of the original $PaCO_2$ level. A pH of 7.30 or lower caused by a rise in $PaCO_2$ is the hallmark of acute ventilatory failure, which may also be called acute respiratory acidosis. Acute respiratory acidosis of this sort is life-threatening and requires therapeutic intervention. However, chronic respiratory acidosis due to sustained hypercapnia results in compensatory metabolic alkalosis. The pH is normalized by this process, so immediate therapy is not required.

These points are illustrated in the arterial blood gas values of the four patients described in Table 13–1. Patient A has acute ventilatory failure and patient B has chronic ventilatory failure, despite their identical $PaCO_2$ values. Of these two, only patient A, whose respiratory acidosis is acute, requires prompt treatment. Patient C initially has normal blood gases, whereas patient D initially has chronic ventilatory failure and respiratory acidosis. Both patients require therapy to improve ventilation when they decompensate because their respiratory acidosis is acute. Note also

Table 13–1. ARTERIAL BLOOD GAS VALUES FOR ACUTE AND CHRONIC VENTILATORY FAILURE

	PATIENT A	PATIENT B	PATIENT C Baseline (chronic)	Acute	PATIENT D Baseline (chronic)	Acute
pHa	7.25	7.38	7.40	7.25	7.38	7.25
PaCO$_2$	55	55	40	60	60	80
PaO$_2$	75	75	90	70	70	50
HCO$_3^-$	24	32	24	25	36	37

KEY: pHa = arterial pH, PaCO$_2$ = arterial carbon dioxide tension, PaO$_2$ = arterial oxygen tension, HCO$_3^-$ = bicarbonate ion.

that patient D suffers from concurrent failure of oxygenation (arterial oxygen tension [PaO$_2$] = 50 mmHg) due to hypoventilation. Therapy to improve oxygenation is discussed in Chapter 14.

Pathophysiology of Ventilatory Failure

The alveolar ventilation equation (PaCO$_2$ = $\dot{V}CO_2/\dot{V}A$), introduced in Chapter 2, states that the PaCO$_2$ is directly proportional to the body's CO$_2$ production ($\dot{V}CO_2$) and inversely proportional to the gas exchanged in the lung, the alveolar ventilation ($\dot{V}A$). Alveolar ventilation is equal to the amount of gas inspired in a given minute, the minute ventilation ($\dot{V}E$), minus the amount of inspired gas that does not participate in gas exchange, the dead space ventilation ($\dot{V}D$). Thus, $\dot{V}A = \dot{V}E - \dot{V}D$. Hypercapnia occurs (1) when $\dot{V}CO_2$ increases and $\dot{V}A$ does not; (2) when $\dot{V}A$ decreases; and (3) when $\dot{V}E$ remains constant and $\dot{V}D$ increases more than $\dot{V}A$.

Causes of Ventilatory Failure

Obstructive Pulmonary Diseases. These disorders reduce $\dot{V}A$. They also may increase $\dot{V}D$ a small amount and augment $\dot{V}CO_2$ if the work of breathing is high. Examples include upper airway obstruction due to aspirated foreign bodies or oropharyngeal muscle relaxation during sleep and lower airway obstruction due to asthma, chronic obstructive pulmonary disease (COPD), or cystic fibrosis.

Restrictive Pulmonary Diseases. These disorders also reduce $\dot{V}A$ and increase $\dot{V}D$, $\dot{V}CO_2$, or both slightly. They include obesity and other abnormalities of the thoracic cage; respiratory muscle dysfunction due to generalized neuromuscular disease, spinal cord injury, or bilateral diaphragmatic paralysis; pneumonia and fibrotic processes occupying lung tissue; and occupation of the pleural space by effusion or fibrothorax.

Pulmonary Vascular Diseases. Vascular diseases, in particular massive pulmonary thromboembolism, may occasionally increase $\dot{V}_D$ enough to cause acute ventilatory failure.

Disordered Ventilatory Regulation. Abnormal control of breathing, including that caused by depressant drug overdose and neurological illness, may limit $\dot{V}_A$.

THERAPY FOR ACUTE VENTILATORY FAILURE

GENERAL GOALS

Because acute ventilatory failure is an immediate threat to life, therapy must commence instantly. Three simultaneous processes are involved: patient assessment, which is discussed in Chapters 6 and 16; general supportive measures, discussed in the following section; and specific therapy for the underlying cause or causes of ventilatory failure.

IMPROVING VENTILATORY FUNCTION WITHOUT INTUBATION OR MECHANICAL VENTILATION

Decreasing Airflow Obstruction and Resistance

Aspirated food or other foreign material should be removed immediately from the upper airway. Proper humidification of inspired gases should be provided to patients with endotracheal tubes or tracheostomies to prevent mucus impaction. Airway clearance techniques, discussed in Chapter 9, are also helpful in patients with pneumonia or COPD. Bronchospasm should be treated with sympathomimetic agents, corticosteroids, and theophylline or ipratropium as indicated. Inhaled mixtures of helium and O_2 are theoretically useful in acute upper airway obstruction because helium is less dense than air, reduces turbulent flow, and should help the O_2 reach the alveoli. Helium is prohibitively expensive, however, and its efficacy in reducing airflow resistance diminishes rapidly as the fraction of inspired O_2 (FIO_2) is raised. Helium-oxygen mixtures are used clinically mainly for short-term administration to children with postextubation stridor, to avoid the need for reintubation.

Improving Respiratory Muscle Performance

Nutrition and respiratory muscle endurance training (see Chapter 17) may preserve and augment respiratory muscle performance over the long term. Nevertheless, they cannot forestall or substitute for mechanical ventilation in acute ventilatory failure.

Decreasing Ventilatory Demand

Carbon dioxide production may be reduced by lowering body temperature to normal with antipyretics and cooling blankets. Excessive muscular activity also should be reduced by sedatives, if necessary, and patients should not be given excessively high caloric loads early in their management.

Decreasing Dead Space Ventilation

Although less can be done to reduce $\dot{V}D$ than $\dot{V}CO_2$, therapy for the underlying pulmonary disorder may help normalize $\dot{V}D$. Anticoagulants are used to prevent pulmonary thromboembolism.

Improving Ventilatory Drives

The best way to improve ventilatory drives is to eliminate any limitation of them. Selective antagonists such as naloxone (Narcan) will reverse the depressant effects of narcotics not only in patients with overdoses of "street" drugs but also in patients who have received narcotics in the hospital. Barbiturates and other sedative-hypnotic drugs also depress ventilation but lack specific antagonists. These drugs should be administered with caution, especially in patients with chronic respiratory disease. The same caution should be extended to the benzodiazepines, although an antagonist to these drugs is now available.

Respiratory stimulants such as doxapram (Dopram) are occasionally recommended to avoid mechanical ventilation. However, these agents do nothing to reverse the underlying cause of ventilatory failure; they add to the patient's already excessive ventilatory burden; and they do not affect the ultimate clinical outcome.

Intravenous feedings containing only glucose induce a state of semistarvation that depresses ventilatory drives. This situation can be improved with adequate nutrition, albeit at the expense of increased $\dot{V}CO_2$.

ENDOTRACHEAL INTUBATION

General Considerations

Intubation of the airway is often necessary in patients with or without acute ventilatory failure. These patients also may require mechanical ventilation, but the indications for these therapeutic modalities are not the same. Ventilatory failure may be treatable by intubation alone in patients with upper airway obstruction, for example. The insertion of endotracheal tubes and their management are discussed in Chapter 8.

Indications for Intubation (see also Chapter 8)

Prevention or Reversal of Acute Upper Airway Obstruction. This is a major indication for endotracheal intubation. Patients with chronic or recurrent obstruction may benefit from permanent tracheostomies.

Protection Against Aspiration. Such protection may be required in comatose patients with impaired gag reflexes if they have ventilatory failure or if it is anticipated.

Tracheobronchial Toilet. Clearance can be facilitated by intubation in patients with voluminous secretions and impaired cough defenses, especially if their consciousness is impaired.

Providing a Closed System. Providing such a system for mechanical ventilation, for therapy to improve oxygenation, or for both is perhaps the most common reason for intubation. The indications for mechanical ventilation follow; therapy to improve oxygenation is discussed in Chapter 14.

MECHANICAL VENTILATION

Indications for Mechanical Ventilation

Acute Ventilatory Failure. Any patient who is apneic or has severe acute respiratory acidosis (elevated $PaCO_2$ with pH less than 7.25) should be intubated and mechanically ventilated. The indications for instituting mechanical support for ventilation vary somewhat in other situations, depending upon the clinical setting.

Failure of Oxygenation. This condition, discussed in Chapter 7, may require intubation and mechanical ventilation even in the absence of respiratory acidosis. Patients with the adult respiratory distress syndrome (ARDS) from any cause, or who have sustained severe trauma or have undergone recent major surgery, should be ventilated if their spontaneous tidal volume (V_T) is less than 5 ml/kg, since despite adequate CO_2 elimination these individuals are likely to develop worsening hypoxemia because of inadequate expansion of their lungs.

Head Trauma. Head trauma may cause apneic episodes or an acutely changing neurological status that necessitates mechanical ventilation. In addition, since hypocapnia causes cerebral vasoconstriction and thereby reduces post-traumatic brain swelling and intracranial pressure, such patients are often deliberately hyperventilated to a $PaCO_2$ of 25 to 30 mmHg for the first 24 to 48 hours. After 24 to 48 hours, the effect of hyperventilation is lessened because of the brain's re-establishment of normal pH through its buffering system. The $PaCO_2$ must be allowed to rise slowly (over a 24-hour period) to avoid rebound acidosis in the central nervous system.

Chronic Obstructive Pulmonary Disease. Acute ventilatory insufficiency in COPD is nearly always manageable without mechanical ventilation if patients are alert on admission. Since these patients pose special problems in ventilator weaning and muscle function, the goal of therapy must be to avoid mechanical ventilation. In experienced hands, mechanical ventilation becomes necessary in only about 5 to 10 per cent of patients, unless depressant drugs are injudiciously given or the patients must undergo general anesthesia. Patients with COPD whose consciousness is seriously disturbed, however, should be intubated and ventilated, as should those with uncontrollable agitation or mania that renders them uncooperative. If respiratory acidosis worsens substantially during the initial treatment and the pH falls significantly below 7.30, intubation and mechanical ventilation may be unavoidable. This does not apply to patients whose $PaCO_2$ values rise by 2 to 4 mmHg on institution of low-flow O_2 therapy even if their pH values dip below the 7.30 cutoff.

Respiratory Muscle Dysfunction and Disordered Ventilatory Regulation. Patients whose intrinsic lung function is adequate but in whom acute ventilatory failure results from muscle weakness or ventilatory center depression by drugs or disease should be intubated if they are unable to protect their airways. They should be ventilated if they manifest any of the following: progressive hypoventilation with pH falling to or below 7.30; vital capacity (VC) less than 10 to 15 ml/kg; VT less than 5 ml/kg; and maximum inspiratory force less than -20 to -25 cm H_2O.

Kinds of Mechanical Ventilation

Intermittent Negative Pressure Ventilation. This kind of mechanical ventilation attempts to duplicate the spontaneous breathing pattern mechanically. As described in Chapter 2, inspiration normally results from respiratory muscle contraction that creates a negative pleural pressure. This increases the transpulmonary pressure, the pressure gradient between the pleural space and the alveoli that accounts for lung distention. Alveolar pressure then becomes more negative as the alveoli expand, and gas flows into the alveoli from the mouth, where atmospheric pressure is zero (Fig. 13–1).

INSPIRATION

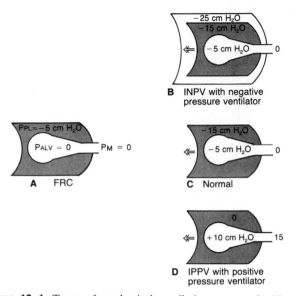

Figure 13–1. Types of mechanical ventilation compared with spontaneous ventilation. Diagrams *B* to *D* (at right) show airway and pleural pressure at end-inspiration, after a breath from functional residual capacity (FRC, *A*). P_{PL} = pleural pressure; P_{ALV} = alveolar pressure; P_M = mouth, or atmospheric, pressure; FRC = functional residual capacity; INPV = intermittent negative pressure ventilation; IPPV = intermittent positive pressure ventilation; arrows denote direction of motion of diaphragm.

This normal situation can be duplicated if negative pressure (suction) is applied intermittently to the outside of the body, producing chest wall expansion that in turn creates a negative pleural pressure (see Fig. 13–1*B*). This technique is used in negative pressure tank ventilators ("iron lungs"), portable cuirasses, and "poncho" wrap ventilators and is effective if the lungs and chest wall are normal. However, intermittent negative pressure ventilation cannot insure an adequate $\dot{V}_A$ in patients whose respiratory system compliance (C_{RS}) is reduced. It also is not applicable to patients with failure of oxygenation except that caused solely by alveolar hypoventilation.

Intermittent Positive Pressure Ventilation. Intermittent positive pressure ventilation (IPPV) creates a transpulmonary pressure gradient during inspiration, not by sucking on the chest wall to generate a negative pleural pressure but instead by blowing gas into the lungs and generating a positive alveolar pressure (see Fig. 13–1D). In its simplest form this is accomplished by mouth-to-mouth resuscitation, and positive pressure ventilation may be achieved quite effectively with a properly used manual resuscitation bag and mask. For periods longer than minutes to a few hours, however, mechanical ventilation with IPPV is required.

Positive pressure ventilators are described in terms of how they terminate the inspiratory phase of the ventilatory cycle. Pressure-cycled machines allow gas to flow into the patient until a preselected airway pressure is reached. Pressure, not V_T, is thus constant, and the delivered V_T can vary considerably, especially in patients with abnormal C_{RS}.

Most ventilators currently used for continuous support of critically ill patients are volume-cycled, which means that a preset V_T is delivered each time the ventilator cycles, even if a very high airway pressure must be generated. Time-cycled ventilators allow gas to flow into the patient until a preselected inspiratory duration is achieved. Since currently available time-cycled ventilators have high-pressure capabilities, they are used in patients with severe respiratory failure more or less interchangeably with volume-cycled machines.

All currently used ventilators have safety features designed to prevent delivery of dangerous pressures or volumes. With the high-pressure alarm set, a volume- or time-cycled ventilator may in fact be pressure-cycled if the dialed volume or inspiratory time is not reached before the set pressure cutoff occurs in a given breath.

Modes of Mechanical Ventilation With Positive Airway Pressure

Spontaneous Ventilation. Spontaneous ventilation (SV) may be achieved on ventilators that allow the machine rate to be set at zero so that patients breathe spontaneously through the ventilator circuit (Fig. 13–2). Individual systems vary in the resistance that must be overcome during spontaneous breathing, so SV may involve considerably more respiratory work than free breathing on a T-piece. The T-piece is a piece of tubing that connects the intubated patient with a source of humidified and, most commonly, oxygenated gas. Positive pressure may be added to the system in both inspiration and expiration, allowing the patient to receive continuous positive airway pressure (CPAP). Pressurizing the inspiratory phase only (pressure support ventilation [PSV]) may be used either to reduce the work of spontaneous breathing or as a mode of ventilatory support (see below).

Intermittent Mandatory Ventilation. Intermittent mandatory ventilation (IMV) allows the patient to breathe in what is essentially two modes at once (see Fig. 13–2). Spontaneous breaths, as in SV, are interrupted at preset intervals by machine-delivered breaths.

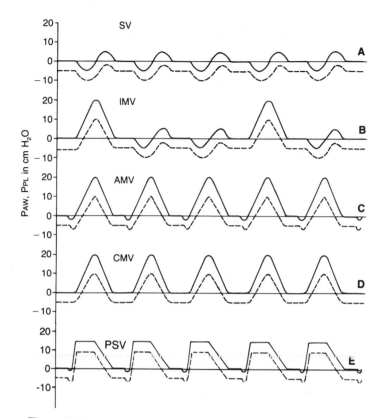

Figure 13–2. Modes of mechanical ventilation with positive pressure (*B* to *E*) compared with spontaneous ventilation (SV, *A*). IMV = intermittent mandatory ventilation; AMV = assisted mechanical ventilation (or assist-control mode); CMV = controlled mechanical ventilation; PSV = pressure support ventilation. Solid line = airway (PAW) or alveolar pressure; dashed line = pleural pressure.

The latter cannot be triggered by the patient on demand, and their rate is fixed at a set frequency. Some ventilators, however, allow synchronization of the machine breaths so that they follow spontaneous exhalation. Synchronous IMV offers the theoretical advantage of avoiding stacking a machine breath on top of a spontaneous breath, but studies have indicated that stacking is not a serious problem in clinical practice. Patients may or may not contribute the SV portion of IMV shown in Figure 13–2*B*, depending on the set mandatory rate, the patient's V̇E demand, and the patient's ventilatory drive and capability.

Controlled Mechanical Ventilation. Controlled mechanical ventilation (CMV) delivers a preset number of ventilator breaths to the patient; additional breaths cannot be triggered from the machine or initiated spontaneously as in IMV (see Fig. 13–2). When high machine rates are employed in the IMV mode, say 18 or even 25 breaths/min, patients take few if any spontaneous breaths and thus are effectively receiving CMV. Paralyzed patients who can make no spontaneous ventilatory efforts are managed on CMV. In others who can make spontaneous efforts to trigger the ventilator, CMV results in air hunger and subjective distress unless the machine rate is set high enough to over-drive the patient's urge to breathe; significant hyperventilation is usually the result.

Assisted Mechanical Ventilation. Assisted mechanical ventilation (AMV) should always be delivered with a CMV back-up rate; this combination often is called assist/control (see Fig. 13–2). In this mode all breaths are from the machine but the preset rate can be exceeded by a triggering effort from the patient. If the patient makes no inspiratory effort, the set rate determines ventilatory frequency, and the patient is effectively on CMV. The key difference between CMV and AMV with back-up is that with the latter, patients can initiate more frequent breaths if desired.

Pressure Support Ventilation. Pressure support, or inspiratory assist, adds a set level of positive pressure to the breathing circuit during the inspiratory phase of SV. It is thus similar to intermittent positive pressure breathing (IPPB), except that very high inspiratory flows can be generated—higher than with IMV or AMV in most settings (see Fig. 13–2). If the PSV level is set high enough, the same VT can be achieved as with IMV or AMV, and PSV can be used as a stand-alone ventilatory support mode so long as the patient's ventilatory drive is intact. With PSV the patient receives only breaths that are initiated spontaneously; if no breaths are taken by the patient, no inspiratory flow is delivered. Adding a low level of pressure support (e.g., 5 cm H_2O) can counteract the extra work of breathing added by the endotracheal tube and ventilator circuit during SV or low-rate IMV.

Pressure Control Ventilation. With some ventilators, inspiratory pressure support can also be delivered at a set cycling frequency; in this instance it is called pressure control ventilation (PCV). This mode has recently been applied in severe ARDS using an inspiratory phase longer than the expiratory phase of each respiratory cycle (pressure control with inverse ratio ventilation [PCIRV]), in an attempt to improve arterial oxygenation. While an improved PaO_2 has been achieved in some instances, PCIRV increases air trapping and auto-PEEP and thus also increases the likelihood of cardiac impairment and barotrauma. At present, PCIRV should be used primarily in investigational settings, and then only with great caution. PCV alone may be quite useful.

High-Frequency Ventilation. In this largely investigational mode, the ventilator's cycling rate is (1) increased to 60 to 100 breaths/min, (2) supplemented by a more rapidly cycling jet of gas flow delivered through low-compliance circuits with V_T at or below calculated anatomical V_D, or (3) oscillated at a very rapid rate (up to 6000 cycles/min or more). How high-frequency ventilation works is not completely understood, and this mode is not indicated as the preferred method of ventilatory support in any intensive care setting.

Choosing the Appropriate Ventilator Mode

Although much controversy exists regarding the best ventilator mode for a given patient, data documenting any clear-cut advantage of one mode over another are lacking in most instances. For the majority of patients being managed with short-term mechanical ventilation for respiratory failure either IMV or AMV with back-up will suffice, with little difference apparent between them so long as they are used judiciously. In some circumstances, however, there are at least theoretical reasons for choosing one mode over the others.

Controlled mechanical ventilation is the only feasible mode in patients who are totally apneic. Whether the ventilator is set up for CMV, AMV, or IMV in such patients, as long as they make no spontaneous efforts at ventilation they are in fact receiving CMV. Any patient who is awake and is capable of taking or at least initiating a breath should be permitted to do so by being on either AMV with back-up or IMV. Thus, patients who are initially apneic but will recover to breathe on their own—for example, drug overdose patients or postoperative patients—should be set up on either IMV or AMV, with the set machine rate sufficient to support them completely at first.

Assisted mechanical ventilation with back-up may be used in any patient with respiratory failure who needs ventilatory assistance, unless severe respiratory alkalosis refractory to machine adjustment and sedation occurs. In such patients IMV may be tried, although most dyspneic, agitated patients will continue to hyperventilate on IMV if they are capable of doing so. Assisted mechanical ventilation has the advantages of being able to respond to increased patient $\dot{V}CO_2$ by increasing $\dot{V}E$, and of being able to decrease $\dot{V}O_2$ and $\dot{V}CO_2$ in patients with a high degree of work of breathing on SV or IMV.

Intermittent mandatory ventilation may be useful for patients with airflow obstruction who trap air in their lungs at a high V_T. Intermittent mechanical ventilation at a low rate should clearly not be used in patients who are heavily sedated or paralyzed with pancuronium bromide or other agents. Patients whose neurological status fluctuates, as after severe head trauma, cerebrovascular accident, or drug overdose with varying levels of consciousness, should not be placed on IMV unless the machine rate is sufficient to provide all the ventilation needed. Finally, when mechanical ventilation is provided through a small (7-mm inner diameter or less in average-sized adult) endotracheal tube, the work required to overcome the tube's resistance may raise $\dot{V}O_2$ and $\dot{V}CO_2$ unacceptably if IMV is employed with a low machine rate, unless PSV is added at a level sufficient to overcome this additional work of breathing.

Initial Ventilator Set-up

It is seldom possible to predict a patient's oxygenation and ventilation needs so accurately in initially setting up the ventilator that no subsequent adjustments are necessary. Matching the machine to the patient's requirements, therefore, must be thought of as an evolving process rather than as a single task performed only once. The initial settings are chosen according to predictions based on what is known of the patient and the disease and are modified as arterial blood gas results reveal the patient's needs.

Inspired Oxygen Fraction. An FIO_2 of 1.00 should be used initially in most patients, particularly those whose initial oxygenation status is unknown. This is reduced by a fraction gauged according to the initial PaO_2 on an FIO_2 of 1.00. Choosing an optimal PaO_2 target value in consideration of the patient's primary disease process is discussed in the next chapter.

Tidal Volume. In healthy people, V_T normally is 5 to 7 ml/kg; periodic sighs of two to several times that volume are added to stimulate surfactant production and to prevent atelectasis. In the management of acute respiratory failure, a V_T of 10 to 12 ml/kg is generally used, without intermittent sigh breaths, although some clinicians prefer a lower V_T. Patients with very low C_{RS}, in whom these volumes cause an excessively high peak and mean airway pressures, should be given somewhat smaller volumes, as should patients with severe air trapping, which occurs in status asthmaticus and severe COPD.

Frequency. While a patient's exact $\dot{V}E$ requirement cannot be accurately predicted, the initial ventilator rate (f) should be chosen to approximate a reasonable clinical estimate based on the V_T used. Whether IMV or AMV is the mode of choice, the initial f should provide all the breaths the patient is judged to need. With IMV, the machine f is subsequently reduced in an empirical fashion, according to the patient's ability to contribute spontaneously as shown by arterial blood gas results. In the case of AMV, when the patient is triggering the ventilator and establishing his own f, the machine back-up f should be set within two to four breaths of this rate. In this way, serious hypoventilation will not occur if the patient stops triggering the ventilator. A back-up of ten breaths/ min in a patient breathing 24 times/min would be insufficient to prevent life-threatening respiratory acidosis if the patient's status changed and triggering stopped.

Inspiratory Flow Rate. Although currently manufactured ventilators have inspiratory peak flow rates that are adjustable from zero to 120 L/min, the most common initial rate setting is between 50 and 80 L/min. Differences in inspiratory flow rate seldom make a clinically important difference in the distribution of ventilation, but patients with air trapping and expiratory airflow obstruction should have fast inspiratory rates (70 to 100 L/min) in order to maximize expiratory time. In addition, patients who are alert usually prefer a faster inspiratory peak flow rate over a slower one. With such patients some bedside experimentation will usually produce a rate affording maximal comfort.

Fighting the Ventilator

Patient agitation and distress during mechanical ventilation develop in four main circumstances: (1) incorrect set-up of the ventilator for the patient's metabolic or psychological needs; (2) an acute change in clinical status; (3) an obstructed airway; and (4) malfunction of the ventilator. "Fighting the ventilator" must always be regarded as a potentially life-threatening problem and approached as an emergency.

Agitation and distress manifested on initiation of mechanical ventilation call for a careful check of the equipment and procedures followed by empirical adjustment of V_T, inspiratory flow, and triggering sensitivity. Calm reassurance, followed by moderate sedation if needed, will enable most patients to tolerate mechanical ventilation without distress, provided the settings chosen result in arterial blood gas values in the normal range.

The sudden onset of agitation and fighting the ventilator in a patient who previously tolerated it means either that the patient's condition has worsened abruptly or that a malfunction has developed in the ventilator or artificial airway. When this happens the following steps should be taken:

a. Disconnect the patient from the ventilator and provide manual ventilation with a self-inflating resuscitator.
b. Quickly check the patient's vital signs, chest motion and symmetry, and breath sounds.
c. Briefly survey the bedside monitoring equipment to make sure it is working.
d. Suction the airway and make sure the endotracheal or tracheostomy tube is patent.
e. Draw an arterial blood specimen for blood gas measurements and perform a more detailed general examination of the patient

to see if a process away from the chest is the main cause of respiratory distress.

This protocol will disclose the source of most instances of sudden patient distress during mechanical ventilation. Under no circumstances should the patient be sedated or paralyzed without a careful assessment for the cause of the agitation being made; distress in this situation should be viewed as an important clinical sign, not an irritation. (The proper use of paralyzing agents in respiratory care is discussed in Chapter 11.)

Complications of Mechanical Ventilation

General Complications. The general complications of acute ventilatory failure and its management include acid-base disturbances, O_2 toxicity, hemodynamic consequences of raised intrathoracic pressure, barotrauma, nosocomial infection, mechanical failure of ventilators and other apparatus, and a host of other developments to which all patients in the ICU setting are predisposed. These deserve special mention in this chapter.

Acute Respiratory Alkalosis in Patients With Chronic Hypercapnia. Patients with abnormal ventilatory drives, with or without chronic airflow limitation, may have long-standing, compensated respiratory acidosis. When such patients are mechanically ventilated they may become severely alkalemic and subsequently may lose their secondary metabolic alkalosis and be ventilator-bound as a result (Table 13–2).

In Table 13–2, the patient's baseline state is typical of that of many patients with severe but stable COPD. An acute rise in PCO_2 of 30 mmHg results in life-threatening acidemia, and the patient is placed on a mechanical ventilator. The initial settings are made for an "average" patient without consideration for this patient's chronic compensated respiratory acidosis, and the first postintubation arterial blood gas specimen shows severe alkalemia due to the now unopposed metabolic alkalosis chronically maintained by

Table 13–2. MECHANICAL VENTILATION IN SEVERE COPD

CONDITIONS	BASELINE STATE	ACUTE VENTILATORY FAILURE	ONE HOUR OF MECHANICAL VENTILATION	TWO DAYS AT SAME VENTILATOR SETTINGS
pHa	7.38	7.25	7.55	7.40
$PaCO_2$	55	85	40	40
HCO_3^-	32	36	34	24

KEY: pHa = arterial pH, $PaCO_2$ = arterial carbon dioxide tension, HCO_3^- = bicarbonate ion.

this patient to offset the hypercapnia. This degree of alkalemia is as threatening to the patient's life as was the initial acidemia. If no adjustments are made in ventilator settings to restore the "normal" PCO_2 for this patient (making the erroneous assumption that a PCO_2 of 40 is normal for all patients), over the next two or three days the patient's kidneys will excrete the "extra" bicarbonate and the previous compensation will be lost. Thus, when the acute episode is over and an attempt is made to wean the patient from the ventilator, he or she will be forced to do so in the face of ventilatory mechanics unchanged from what they were before the exacerbation, and will "fail." Care must be taken that such patients not be overventilated and that their acid-base balance be kept as close to their accustomed state as possible.

Barotrauma. Pneumothorax, pneumomediastinum, and subcutaneous emphysema occurring during mechanical ventilation are termed barotrauma. Despite this term, these complications are more directly related to maximum distending volume than to peak inspiratory airway pressure. Barotrauma is most likely to occur in patients ventilated with tidal volumes above 15 ml/kg. It also occurs in patients with severe ARDS treated with high levels of PEEP, although this may reflect the underlying disease process more than its therapy. Patients with COPD and status asthmaticus are particularly susceptible to barotrauma during mechanical ventilation, especially if PEEP is used, since lung volumes in these patients are high to begin with. Equipment for performing emergency tube thoracostomy should be kept at the bedside of patients identified as being at increased risk for development of pneumothorax during mechanical ventilation, since this complication can be rapidly fatal if not treated promptly.

RECOMMENDED READING

1. Benson MS, and Pierson DJ: Auto-PEEP during mechanical ventilation of adults. *Respir Care*, 33:557–565, 1988.
2. Branson RD: Enhanced capabilities of current ICU ventilators: Do they really benefit patients? *Respir Care*, 36:362–376, 1991.
3. Conference on Mechanical Ventilation. *Respir Care*, 32:403–478, 517–614, 1987.
4. Hudson LD, et al.: Does intermittent mandatory ventilation correct respiratory alkalosis in patients receiving assisted mechanical ventilation? *Am Rev Respir Dis*, 132:1071–1074, 1985.
5. Kacmarek RM: Methods of providing mechanical ventilatory support. *In* Pierson DJ, and Kacmarek RM (eds.): *Foundations of Respiratory Care*. New York, Churchill Livingstone, 1992, pp 953–972.
6. Kirby RR, et al. (eds.): *Clinical Application of Ventilatory Support*. New York, Churchill Livingstone, 1990.
7. MacIntyre NR: Respiratory function during pressure support ventilation. *Chest*, 89:677–683, 1986.
8. MacIntyre NR: New forms of mechanical ventilation in the adult. *Clin Chest Med*, 9:47–54, 1988.
9. Pierson DJ: Indications for mechanical ventilation in acute respiratory failure. *Respir Care*, 28:570–577, 1983.

10. Pierson DJ: Complications of mechanical ventilation. *Curr Pulmonol,* 11:19–46, 1990.
11. Pierson DJ: Respiratory therapy techniques. *In* Kelley WN (ed.): *Textbook of Internal Medicine*, 2nd ed. Philadelphia, J. B. Lippincott, 1992, pp. 1836–1842.
12. Slutsky AS: Nonconventional modes of ventilation. *Am Rev Respir Dis,* 138:175–183, 1988.
13. Tobin MJ: What should the clinician do when the patient "fights the ventilator"? *Respir Care*, 36:395–406, 1991.

14

THERAPY TO IMPROVE TISSUE OXYGENATION

CAUSES OF IMPAIRED TISSUE OXYGENATION

OVERVIEW

As noted in Chapter 7, any disruption in the steps of respiration can limit the utilization of O_2 by the tissues. The adequacy of O_2 for aerobic metabolism is best assessed by examining O_2 supply and demand.

DETERMINANTS OF OXYGEN DEMAND

The body's consumption of oxygen ($\dot{V}O_2$) is defined by the Fick equation as the product of cardiac output ($\dot{Q}T$) and peripheral O_2 extraction as expressed by the difference between the arterial O_2 content (CaO_2) and the mixed venous O_2 content ($C\bar{v}O_2$); thus $\dot{V}O_2 = \dot{Q}T \times (CaO_2 - C\bar{v}O_2)$ or $C(a-\bar{v})O_2$.

DETERMINANTS OF OXYGEN SUPPLY

The supply of O_2 to the tissues is determined by both the amount of O_2 transported to the periphery and the amount of O_2 extracted by the tissues. Oxygen transport is the product of $\dot{Q}T$ and CaO_2; CaO_2 is equal to the amount of O_2 carried by hemoglobin (1.34 ml O_2/gm hemoglobin × gm hemoglobin/100 ml blood × arterial O_2 saturation [SaO_2]) + the normally small amount dissolved in blood (0.003 ml O_2/100 ml blood) × arterial O_2 tension (PaO_2). Oxygen extraction is governed by $\dot{V}O_2$, the partial pressure of O_2 in capillaries adjacent to the tissues (this cannot be measured directly, but the O_2 tension in mixed venous blood ($P\bar{v}O_2$) provides an approximation), and the willingness of hemoglobin to release O_2 to the tissues (as expressed by the position of the O_2-hemoglobin

211

dissociation curve and the partial pressure of O_2 at which half the hemoglobin is saturated, the P50).

PATHOPHYSIOLOGY OF IMPAIRED TISSUE OXYGENATION

Abnormalities in any of the variables affecting O_2 supply may impair tissue oxygenation unless O_2 demand diminishes proportionately. These abnormalities often exist concurrently but may be categorized in the following fashion (see also Table 14–1).

Failure of Arterial Oxygenation

This condition involves inadequate oxygenation of arterial blood as reflected by a PaO_2 of 50 mmHg or less. Hypoxemia occurs with a normal (10 to 15 mmHg) or widened gradient between the alveolar and arterial PO_2 $[P(A-a)O_2]$. Hypoxemia with a normal $P(A-a)O_2$ is present with a low inspired O_2 tension, which occurs at high altitude or during a fire, and with the alveolar hypoventilation seen in drug overdosage and other conditions, in which the arterial carbon dioxide tension ($PaCO_2$) is greater than approximately 40 mmHg. Hypoxemia with a widened $P(A-a)O_2$ occurs clinically with ventilation-perfusion ($\dot{V}A/\dot{Q}$) mismatching, as in asthma and chronic obstructive pulmonary disease (COPD), and with shunt due to severe pneumonia or the adult respiratory distress syndrome (ARDS). A fall in $\dot{Q}T$ in the presence of fixed shunt worsens hypoxemia appreciably.

Failure of Oxygen Transport

Inadequate O_2 delivery to the peripheral tissues is reflected in a $P\bar{v}O_2$ of less than 40 mmHg and in lactic acidosis resulting from anaerobic metabolism. This can be caused (1) by a low CaO_2 due either to a low PaO_2 or SaO_2, as in the aforementioned hypoxemic states; (2) by a low hemoglobin concentration, as in anemia; or (3) by a displacement of O_2 from hemoglobin, as in carbon monoxide (CO) poisoning. The other major cause of poor O_2 transport is impaired $\dot{Q}T$. This is seen with dysrhythmias, left ventricular dysfunction, and the kinds of circulatory shock outlined in Chapter 7.

Failure of Tissue Oxygen Extraction

An inability of the cells to extract O_2 from arterial blood or to use it for aerobic metabolism results in lactic acidosis and a $P\bar{v}O_2$ that is normal or even elevated. Reductions in the P50 due to alkalemia and other factors may limit O_2 release from hemoglobin in certain situations. However, the only major clinical condition involving pure failure of O_2 uptake is cyanide (CN) poisoning, in which CN prevents the intracellular metabolism of O_2. Rarely,

Table 14–1. INADEQUATE TISSUE OXYGENATION: PATHOPHYSIOLOGY AND CLINICAL FEATURES

	PROCESS	CLINICAL EXAMPLES	$P_{A}O_2$	$P_{A}O_2$	CaO_2	O_2 TRANSPORT	TISSUE UPTAKE	↑ PaO_2 WITH ↑ FiO_2	APPROPRIATE THERAPY
I.	**Respiratory Failure**								
	Alveolar hypoventilation	Drug overdose	↓	↓	↓	↓	nl	↑↑	Increase $\dot{V}_A$
	$\dot{V}_A/\dot{Q}$ mismatching	COPD, asthma	nl	↓	↓	↓	nl	↑↑	Low FiO_2
	Shunt (generalized)	ARDS	nl	↓	↓	↓	nl	± to ↑	High FiO_2, PEEP
	Shunt (localized)	Lobar pneumonia; atelectasis	nl	↓	↓	↓	nl	± to ↑	Treat primary process (PEEP may increase shunt)
II.	**Failure of O_2 Transport**								
	Insufficient hemoglobin	Anemia	nl	nl	↓	↓	nl	↑↑	Increase hemoglobin (high FiO_2)
	Abnormal hemoglobin	Carbon monoxide poisoning	nl	nl	↓	↓	nl	↑↑	High FiO_2
	Low cardiac output	Shock; left ventricular failure	nl	nl	nl	↓	nl	↑↑	Increase cardiac output
III.	**Failure of Tissue O_2 Extraction**								
	Impaired tissue O_2 extraction	Cyanide poisoning	nl	nl	nl	nl	↓	↑↑	Nitrites; thiosulfate (high FiO_2)

KEY: nl = normal, O_2 = oxygen, COPD = chronic obstructive pulmonary disease, ARDS = adult respiratory distress syndrome, $\dot{V}_A$ = alveolar ventilation, FiO_2 = fraction of inspired oxygen, PEEP = positive end-expiratory pressure, $P_{A}O_2$ = alveolar oxygen tension, PaO_2 = arterial oxygen tension, CaO_2 = arterial oxygen content, $\dot{V}_A/\dot{Q}$ = ventilation/perfusion.

patients with severe cardiogenic shock or septic shock (e.g., with extremely high or low systemic vascular resistance) may manifest impaired peripheral oxygen extraction because of effective pretissue left-to-right shunting.

THERAPY TO IMPROVE TISSUE OXYGENATION

GENERAL GOALS

Some of the preceding pathophysiological processes require highly specific treatments; for example, CN poisoning will respond only to certain antidotes. Nevertheless, ordinarily, any patient with impaired tissue oxygenation should benefit from a general approach that attends to peripheral O_2 utilization. Clinicians frequently focus on arterial blood gases in assessing and following patients. This is appropriate in many cases, as the diagnosis of respiratory failure can be made only if the pH, $PaCO_2$, and PaO_2 are available, and supplemental O_2 is usually essential in improving tissue oxygenation. Yet the PaO_2 and the SaO_2, which is derived from it, are only two of the variables involved in O_2 transport. In certain situations the clinician should monitor the $\dot{Q}T$ and $P\bar{v}O_2$ in addition to the PaO_2.

OXYGEN AS A DRUG

Indications

To Correct Hypoxemia. The most obvious use of O_2 is in raising PaO_2 to reverse or diminish hypoxemia. In acute respiratory failure this is immediately lifesaving. In chronic respiratory failure, O_2 is given to reverse pulmonary hypertension and cor pulmonale, to increase exercise capability, and to improve quality of life, as discussed in Chapter 17.

Since PaO_2 is the most commonly monitored parameter of impaired oxygenation, the clinician must understand how high it should be raised and why. These goals are related to the O_2-hemoglobin dissociation curve. Figure 14–1 shows this curve, with two points emphasized by vertical and horizontal lines. Arterial O_2 content is mainly determined by SaO_2; thus, once hemoglobin is saturated, little additional CaO_2 is achieved by raising PaO_2. In Figure 14–1, point A, at PaO_2 = 40 mmHg, indicates that SaO_2 = 75 per cent and CaO_2 = 15 ml/dl. Raising PaO_2 to 60 mmHg,

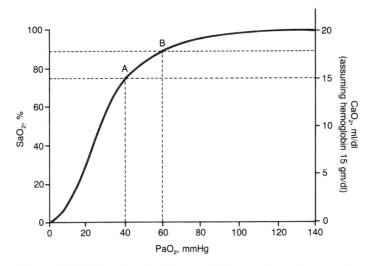

Figure 14–1. General goals of oxygen therapy as shown by two points on the hemoglobin-oxygen dissociation curve. Raising PaO_2 from 40 mmHg (Point A) to 60 mmHg (Point B) increases arterial O_2 saturation (SaO_2) from 75 to about 90 per cent and arterial O_2 content (CaO_2) from 15 to 18 ml/dl. This corrects hypoxemia of a life-threatening degree. Less additional benefit is achieved by further increasing PaO_2, as indicated by the flatter shape of the curve above 60 mmHg.

as at point B, increases SaO_2 to about 90 per cent and CaO_2 to approximately 18 ml/dl. Further raising PaO_2 to the normal level of 90 mmHg produces a smaller increase in SaO_2 and CaO_2, and additional increases above 90 mmHg gain little O_2-carrying capacity. To optimize CaO_2, a basic goal of therapy should be to raise PaO_2 to 60 to 90 mmHg.

Because achieving a PaO_2 higher than 90 mmHg may require potentially toxic levels of inspired O_2 fraction (FiO_2) (see p. 217 and Fig. 14–2) and raising PaO_2 beyond this value achieves little additional O_2-carrying capacity, doing so is rarely justified in the care of patients with acute respiratory failure. Maintaining a PaO_2 of 150 mmHg offers no clinically detectable advantage over a value of 60 to 90 mmHg in any but a few circumstances. One such situation is the need to improve oxygenation by dissolving more O_2 in blood, a temporary measure sometimes used in severe anemia. Another is the need to displace CO from hemoglobin, as will be discussed. The third circumstance is hyperventilation of a patient with head trauma and other neurological insults in an attempt to reduce cerebral blood flow and intracranial pressure; such patients may develop a very low cerebral tissue PO_2 due to

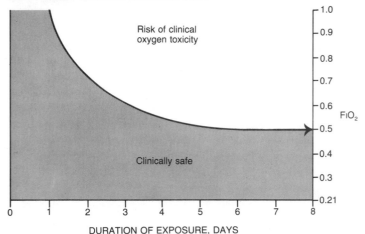

Figure 14–2. General relationship among FIO_2, the duration of exposure, and risk of clinically significant oxygen toxicity, consistent with clinical experience and the very limited data available from studies in acutely ill patients.

intense cerebral vasoconstriction and may benefit from a high PaO_2, although little objective evidence for this currently exists.

To Prevent Hypoxemia. Supplemental O_2 should be given prophylactically during bronchoscopy and other procedures that might compromise oxygenation, during sleep in individuals shown to have physiologically significant dysrhythmias and other complications of arterial desaturation, and during exercise in certain patients whose exertion is limited by hypoxemia.

To Treat Carbon Monoxide Poisoning. As described in Chapter 7, CO is displaced from hemoglobin in direct proportion to the PaO_2. In CO poisoning the treatment goals are both to supply O_2 to tissues and to remove the CO molecules. In this case, raising PaO_2 far beyond 90 mmHg—even beyond one atmosphere if a hyperbaric facility is immediately available—is appropriate and may be life-saving. Such therapy is needed only long enough to reduce the carboxyhemoglobin level to 5 to 10 per cent, a few hours at most.

To Facilitate Gas Absorption From Body Cavities and Tissues. O_2 therapy may be used to hasten anesthetic gas elimination after surgery and to treat air embolism.

Adverse Effects

Diminished Hypoxic Ventilatory Drive. Hypoxic ventilatory drive diminishes greatly when PaO_2 is raised above about 65 mmHg. In patients whose breathing is stimulated primarily by hypoxemia—such as COPD patients with acute hypoxemic respiratory failure—suddenly relieving this stimulus can produce severe hypoventilation. For this select group of patients, then, the goal of O_2 therapy should be to raise PaO_2 only out of the immediately life-threatening range (e.g., to 50 to 60 mmHg).

Absorption Atelectasis. Ventilation to individual alveoli is not the same throughout the lungs, and when nitrogen is rinsed out during 100 per cent O_2 breathing, the less well-ventilated alveoli tend to collapse as more O_2 is absorbed from them than is replaced. This effect is observed in normal individuals breathing very high FIO_2, as manifested by increased $P(A-a)O_2$. Localized atelectasis may be exaggerated distal to focal airway obstructions.

Acute Airway and Central Nervous System Effects. Ciliary dysfunction and impaired mucus clearance from the tracheobronchial tree occur within the first few hours of 100 per cent O_2 breathing by healthy individuals. Acute airway irritation develops after about 12 hours, with cough, substernal burning during inspiration, dyspnea, sore throat, and nasal stuffiness. Reversible tracheobronchitis and a mild restrictive ventilatory defect follow. These effects are irritative rather than destructive and resolve on discontinuation of O_2 breathing. Exposure to hyperbaric O_2 leads to muscle twitching, nausea, vertigo, paresthesias, mood changes, and diminished alertness, followed by generalized convulsions if exposure continues. These effects occur in about two hours at three atmospheres and in a few minutes at six atmospheres; they are usually not seen at pressures below two atmospheres. Like the acute airway changes, these neurological manifestations are reversible.

Parenchymal Pulmonary O_2 Toxicity. Exposure to high FIO_2 produces a syndrome resembling ARDS both clinically and pathologically. This process is accelerated in animals by hypermetabolic states such as hyperthermia and sepsis; by administration of corticosteroids, insulin, and catecholamines; and by x-ray irradiation. It is slowed by processes decreasing metabolic rate, by antioxidants, and by adrenergic blocking drugs. These observations have not been completely confirmed in humans.

Figure 14–2 illustrates the general relationship between pulmonary O_2 toxicity, FIO_2, and duration of exposure. The curve in the figure is consistent with available data in humans, but it must be pointed out that these data are incomplete. Documentation of human O_2 toxicity at FIO_2 less than 0.70 is scarce, whether in healthy or in severely ill individuals. An FIO_2 of 0.50 appears clinically safe for many weeks if required in the treatment of hypoxemia. Although the mechanism is not known, hypoxemia appears to protect the lung from O_2 toxicity to some extent. One problem in identifying a safe FIO_2 and in clarifying the pathophysiology of O_2 toxicity is that the conditions requiring the highest FIO_2 and the longest exposure are clinically and pathologically similar to O_2 toxicity itself. A good clinical rule is to administer sufficient O_2 to keep PaO_2 in the 60- to 90-mmHg range, remembering the exceptions mentioned earlier, utilizing positive end-expiratory pressure (PEEP) as described later in this chapter, and reversing the primary disease process as completely and rapidly as possible.

THERAPY WITH LOW FIO_2 OXYGEN

Indications

Oxygen administration may be thought of in two general categories, low FIO_2 and high FIO_2, based upon how much supplemental O_2 is required to raise PaO_2 out of the life-threatening range. As discussed in Chapter 7, hypoxemia resulting from hypoventilation or $\dot{V}A/\dot{Q}$ mismatching is reversed by a modest increase in FIO_2, whereas that attributable to shunt requires high FIO_2, with or without physical measures such as PEEP, to raise PaO_2 acceptably. Patients with COPD and asthma, both of which are characterized physiologically by generalized $\dot{V}A/\dot{Q}$ mismatching (with or without concomitant hypoventilation), constitute the major group for whom low FIO_2 oxygen therapy is appropriate. Two concepts are crucial to this form of O_2 administration: (1) only a modest increment in FIO_2 is needed, and (2) because of the sensitivity of some of these patients to an oversupply of O_2, it must be administered under carefully controlled circumstances.

Methods of Delivery

"Venturi" Masks. These devices rely upon air entrainment around a jet of O_2 (Bernoulli effect) for precise dilution of the latter to a controlled FIO_2 of 0.24, 0.28, 0.35, or 0.40, depending upon the O_2 flow rate and the jet orifice diameter. This precisely accurate FIO_2 is present in the mask but not necessarily in the patient's airways, for two reasons: First, hyperpneic individuals entrain room air around the mask, and second, it is difficult for many patients, especially if they are dyspneic or confused, to keep a mask in correct position. Thus, the statement that the FIO_2 is known when Venturi masks are used is misleading.

Nasal Prongs. With the use of plastic cannulas inserted into the patient's nostrils, pure O_2 can be administered at flow rates up to

5 or 6 L/min (higher flows dry airway mucosae and do not further increase FIO_2). The resulting FIO_2 ranges from about 0.24 to a maximum of 0.35 to 0.40 in most patients. Although the desired FIO_2 is not preset as it is with Venturi masks, the resulting tracheal FIO_2 is in the same range, and nasal prongs have the advantage of being more comfortable to wear and thus easier to keep in place. Nasal prongs are equally effective in raising tracheal FIO_2 whether the patient breathes nasally or orally, so long as the nasal passages are not completely obstructed. Humidification of oxygen delivered via nasal prongs or Venturi masks is unnecessary.

Monitoring

Because supplemental O_2 is given to correct hypoxemia and because the signs and symptoms of hypoxemia are of little value in seriously ill patients, the effects of O_2 therapy must always be assessed by arterial blood gas measurement. That the exact FIO_2 is unknown with either Venturi mask or nasal prongs is unimportant, as long as O_2 administration is constant and each change in therapy is followed by blood gas measurements. Blood gas should also be measured whenever there is a change in the patient's condition during O_2 therapy. Pulse oximetry is helpful in monitoring O_2 therapy in patients whose SaO_2 values remain below about 97 per cent, but should not be the sole monitor of O_2 therapy in acutely ill patients. Transcutaneous PO_2 monitors are not sufficiently reliable for routine use in acutely ill adult patients (see Chapter 16).

THERAPY WITH HIGH-FIO_2 OXYGEN

Indications

Hypoxemia primarily due to shunt responds less well to supplemental O_2 than it does in hypoventilation and $\dot{V}A/\dot{Q}$ mismatching, and delivery of FIO_2 of 0.50 or greater is usually required, at least initially. This is true whether the shunt is from a localized process or a more diffuse, generalized process in the lung. High-FIO_2 oxygen therapy is also indicated for CO poisoning and in profound anemia until the hemoglobin concentration can be restored.

Methods of Delivery

Masks. Currently available oxygen masks can deliver O_2 at any FIO_2 up to and including 1.00, but different equipment must be used, depending upon the patient's minute ventilation ($\dot{V}E$) and inspiratory flow rate. Standard hospital O_2 flowmeters used for nasal oxygen can deliver only about 15 L/min, so that even with tight-fitting partial rebreathing masks or nonrebreathing masks patients who are dyspneic and/or hyperpneic entrain room air during inspiration and lower the effective FIO_2 substantially. More than one flowmeter can be used to supply a single mask, but the most effective means of delivering high-FIO_2 therapy at high flow rates is to utilize any of several high-flow air-O_2 blenders (e.g., Downs flow generator). When used with appropriately fitted masks, such devices can deliver any set FIO_2 at up to 100 L/min or more.

Endotracheal Intubation With Spontaneous Breathing via a T-piece. In contrast to the situation with most masks, using a closed system with endotracheal intubation allows accurate delivery of any FIO_2 between 0.21 (room air) and 1.00. Because the protective apparatus of the upper airway is bypassed, gases administered through an endotracheal tube must be filtered and completely humidified. Room-air entrainment during inspiration still can occur if the patient's peak inspiratory flow exceeds the system's delivery rate, so that an extension tube should be added to the expiratory side of the T-piece. This extension tube should be long enough so that the stream of mist emanating from it is not interrupted during inspiration. Because continuous flow is provided during exhalation to wash away expired gas, this extension tube does not increase mechanical dead space significantly.

Monitoring

As with other forms of O_2 therapy, the adequacy of closed-system, high-FIO_2-supplement O_2 administration should be monitored by arterial blood gas measurement following each therapeutic adjustment or when a clinical change occurs (see Chapter 16).

POSITIVE END-EXPIRATORY PRESSURE

Rationale and Goals

PEEP is a mechanical means of increasing end-expiratory lung volumes during tidal breathing, either spontaneously or by ventilator. This approach is used in addition to supplemental O_2 therapy for acute, diffuse restrictive processes producing failure to oxygenate arterial blood. Figure 14–3 illustrates diagrammatically the rationale for the use of PEEP. In part A, the lung is normal, as is functional residual capacity (FRC), the volume at end-expiration. In the presence of an acute diffuse process whose effect on pulmonary function is restrictive, as in part C, hypoxemia is worsened by the increased numbers of collapsed or marginally ventilated alveoli at the lower FRC. If positive pressure at end-expiration enables the lung to assume its previous FRC, as in part D, the lung will be held at higher volumes throughout the ventilatory cycle. Oxygenation will be optimized if FRC is thereby

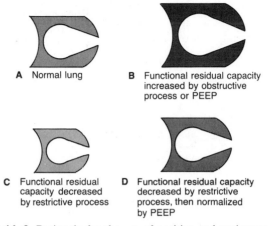

A Normal lung

B Functional residual capacity increased by obstructive process or PEEP

C Functional residual capacity decreased by restrictive process

D Functional residual capacity decreased by restrictive process, then normalized by PEEP

Figure 14–3. Rationale for the use of positive end-expiratory pressure (PEEP).

returned to normal. However, if this end-expiratory positive pressure is applied to the normal lung or to one already enlarged by diffuse obstructive disease, an abnormally high FRC will be produced as in part B, with deleterious effects on gas exchange and increased risk of barotrauma. Properly used, then, PEEP restores an abnormally low FRC to or toward normal. As discussed below, how vigorously this restoration should be pursued and how its effects should be monitored are matters of considerable disagreement.

Definitions

Continuous Positive Pressure Ventilation. By convention, the term continuous positive pressure ventilation (CPPV) is used when PEEP is delivered via a ventilator and airway pressure never drops to zero (atmospheric) (Fig. 14–4). This is accomplished by pressurizing both inspiratory and expiratory sides of the circuit. Even when the patient triggers ventilator breaths in the assist-control mode, end-expiratory pressure is not allowed to fall below the set value.

Expiratory Positive Airway Pressure. With expiratory positive airway pressure (EPAP), only the expiratory side of the circuit is pressurized, and the patient must lower pressure to or below atmospheric pressure in order to inspire. This results in lower mean pleural and intrathoracic pressure, but the patient must work

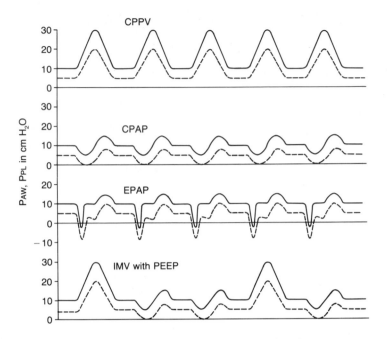

Figure 14–4. The four different forms of positive end-expiratory pressure (PEEP) therapy. Solid lines = airway pressure (PAW); dashed lines = pleural pressure (PPL). CPPV = continuous positive pressure ventilation; CPAP = continuous positive airway pressure; EPAP = expiratory positive airway pressure; IMV = intermittent mechanical or mandatory ventilation. For further explanation, see text.

considerably harder to breathe than with CPPV. This form of PEEP therapy is seldom used today.

Continuous Positive Airway Pressure. Continuous positive airway pressure (CPAP) is analogous to PEEP during spontaneous ventilation; both inspiratory and expiratory sides of the circuit are pressurized and airway pressure never falls to zero. With CPAP, each breath lowers airway pressure relative to the set level as patients inhale, but all breaths are spontaneous.

Intermittent Mandatory Ventilation. When PEEP is used during mechanical ventilation in the intermittent mandatory ventilation (IMV) mode, the patient receives CPPV during the ventilator breaths and CPAP during spontaneous breaths.

The pleural pressure tracings in Figure 14–4 illustrate important differences among CPPV, EPAP, and CPAP. As discussed in Chapter 13, mechanical ventilation can impair venous return to the thorax; this effect is accentuated during PEEP, especially with concomitant hypovolemia. Of the four PEEP modes illustrated in Figure 14–4, mean intrathoracic pressure is lowest with EPAP, somewhat higher with CPAP, progressively higher as ventilator frequency increases with IMV with PEEP, and highest with CPPV.

Importance of Circuitry and Pressurization

The foregoing definitions and descriptions of CPPV, EPAP, and CPAP are theoretical and emphasize the conceptual distinctions between these modes. In practice, the type and brand of apparatus used and the way in which the apparatus is set up determine the wave-forms and pressures to which the patient is actually exposed. Different CPAP circuits, for example, require the patient to exert more or less effort at breathing, depending upon the valves used, the physical arrangement of the tubing, and the volume of bulk gas flow through the system. A detailed description of available systems is beyond the scope of this handbook, but the clinician must become thoroughly familar with the apparatus in local use and the airway pressure actually achieved during and between breaths. As discussed in Chapter 15, circuitry and bulk flow can determine whether a given patient can be weaned from mechanical ventilation, depending upon the ventilator mode used.

Clinical Effects of Positive End-Expiratory Pressure (Table 14–2)

Effect on Lung Volume. Whether PEEP produces improvement in patient condition depends upon the physiological effect of the disease process. If lung volume is diffusely reduced, as in ARDS, increasing FRC toward normal should improve gas exchange. Further increasing FRC above normal would be expected when FRC was normal or elevated prior to adding PEEP. Barotrauma, as discussed in Chapters 10 and 13, results from overdistention of individual lung units and is likely to occur if FRC is raised above normal, particularly if large tidal volumes are used.

In the presence of localized restrictive lung disease, such as lobar pneumonia, PEEP may preferentially increase the volume of surrounding, more compliant pulmonary parenchyma. If the latter is normal to begin with, then its FRC will be increased and the chance for barotrauma will increase. As more compliant areas of lung are expanded, pulmonary vascular resistance will rise in those areas, and blood flow could be diverted to areas not affected by PEEP, e.g., the abnormal areas. With increasing PEEP, this mechanism may result in increased shunt effect through diseased areas of lung and worsening hypoxemia.

Effect on PaO_2. Increasing FRC to or toward normal would be expected to improve the matching of ventilation and perfusion and

Table 14-2. EXPECTED EFFECTS OF POSITIVE END-EXPIRATORY PRESSURE (PEEP) IN ACUTE OXYGENATION FAILURE OF DIFFERENT CAUSES

SETTING	EFFECT ON FRC	EFFECT ON COMPLIANCE	RISK OF BAROTRAUMA	EFFECT ON PULMONARY BLOOD FLOW	EFFECT ON GAS EXCHANGE	EFFECT ON PaO$_2$
Pulmonary edema (hemodynamic, increased capillary permeability)						
PEEP used appropriately	Increase toward normal	Increase toward normal	Moderate	Better matching of perfusion to ventilation	Decreased shunt	Increase
Too much PEEP	Increase above normal	Decrease	High	Increased vascular resistance	Increased dead space	None, or decrease
Localized process (lobar pneumonia or lobar atelectasis)						
Involved area	No change	None	Low	None	None	None
Surrounding normal lung	Increase above normal	Decrease	High	Increased vascular resistance	Increased shunt	Decrease
Generalized obstruction (chronic obstructive pulmonary disease; asthma)	Further increase	Decrease	High	Increased vascular resistance	Increased dead space	None, or decrease

KEY: FRC = functional residual capacity, PaO$_2$ = arterial oxygen tension.

224

to raise PaO_2. Thus, improvement in hypoxemia may be expected with judicious application of PEEP in instances of oxygenation failure associated with acute diffuse restrictive lung processes. An increase in CaO_2 with increasing PaO_2 will also occur providing SaO_2 increases as well. For example, if PEEP results in an increase in PaO_2 from 40 to 60 mmHg, as in Figure 14–1, then SaO_2 and CaO_2 will improve as shown. However, if PaO_2 is raised from 80 to 100 or even 200 mmHg, little improvement in CaO_2 will result, because at 80 to 100 mmHg hemoglobin is essentially fully saturated.

Effect on Hemodynamics. Raising lung volume substantially above normal with positive airway pressure increases pleural and intrathoracic pressure throughout both respiratory and cardiac cycles and reduces venous return to the right atrium. This largely accounts for the drop in $\dot{Q}T$ and systemic arterial pressures observed with excessive levels of PEEP. In the presence of hypovolemia or cardiac dysfunction, the degree to which lung volumes must be raised to produce this effect is reduced.

Indications for Positive End-Expiratory Pressure

There are no scientifically documented, universally agreed-upon indications for the use of PEEP. Most agree that it is a mainstay in the treatment of ARDS, although when and how it should be initiated, how much to use, what to monitor, and when to discontinue PEEP are hotly contended issues. Because the respiratory distress syndromes are characterized by widespread alveolar collapse and studies of $\dot{V}A/\dot{Q}$ indicate that many alveoli are only marginally ventilated, the expansion of overall lung volume is both theoretically and pragmatically helpful in improving gas exchange in this disorder. Whether PEEP plays any primary role in altering the natural course of these syndromes is, however, conjectural. A second and less well accepted indication for PEEP is as treatment for the patient who does not have ARDS but is at substantially increased risk for developing it. Existing data supporting this use of PEEP are flawed and much less convincing than those supporting this therapy in established ARDS.

Clinically, the main purpose of PEEP is to allow adequate oxygenation of arterial blood at a safe FiO_2. Because FiO_2 values of 0.60 and below are not proven to be harmful over periods of days to weeks, some clinicians do not initiate PEEP unless the PaO_2 is less than 60 mmHg while the patient is breathing 60 per cent O_2. Others, however, initiate PEEP in any hypoxemic patient in an attempt to reduce calculated intrapulmonary shunt to the lowest possible value. Whether the overall goal in managing hypoxemia is one of these two extremes or something in between, the following physiological criteria for the initiation of PEEP should be fulfilled:

a. Severe hypoxemia without adequate correction with supplemental O_2 (shunt effect).
b. Acute diffuse lung disease (as opposed to chronic or purely localized processes).
c. Restrictive effect (lung volumes reduced, as opposed to increased, as in obstruction).

PEEP must be applied with caution when localized or inhomogeneous disease is present and when hypovolemia, unknown volume status, or intrinsic cardiac disease exists. Although there are no absolute contraindications to PEEP in the presence of life-threatening hypoxemia, it should be used with caution in the presence of COPD, asthma, and raised intracranial pressure.

Clinical Use of Positive End-Expiratory Pressure

Effective and safe PEEP should be guided by an overall goal for its use. This goal will differ depending upon an individual's concept of "optimal PEEP." For some, optimal PEEP means that level of positive pressure at which calculated shunt is least, an approach that requires intensive fluid and often vasopressor administration to support $\dot{Q}T$. Others attempt to optimize O_2 transport, measuring both $\dot{Q}T$ and CaO_2 (rather than just PaO_2). Still others seek to keep intravascular volume low, and have as their goal adequate SaO_2 at a safe FIO_2 with no depression of $\dot{Q}T$ (an approach that permits only relatively low levels of PEEP). Obviously, the rational use of PEEP cannot begin until one of these fundamental approaches (or some other consistent approach) has been decided upon. The application of PEEP *without* such a well thought-out goal invites complications and reduces maximal effectiveness.

Rather than simply starting at an arbitrary level of PEEP, a PEEP trial, with positive pressure initiated at a low level and increased methodically until preset goals are achieved, is recommended. The PEEP trial seeks to answer two questions: (1) Is PEEP beneficial to this patient at this time? and (2) What is the best level of PEEP for this individual patient? It must be kept in mind that a given patient's PEEP requirements change as acute respiratory failure evolves and as complications or other disease processes develop. Therapeutic adjustments are necessary as dictated by respiratory and hemodynamic monitoring. It should be emphasized that, although which physiological variables to measure is controversial, careful monitoring during and after a trial of incremental PEEP is essential if the best therapeutic results are to be achieved and complications are to be avoided. Guidelines for a trial of PEEP are presented in Table 14–3.

Positive End-Expiratory Pressure Without Endotracheal Intubation

Indications and Patient Selection. Acute diffuse lung disease causing oxygenation failure which meets other criteria for use of PEEP

Table 14–3. PROTOCOL FOR THERAPEUTIC TRIAL OF POSITIVE END-EXPIRATORY PRESSURE (PEEP)

1. Change only one variable at a time; keep V_T, FIO_2, ventilator rate, and other settings the same throughout the trial.
2. Increase PEEP by increments, e.g., 3 to 5 cm H_2O, at each step, starting at zero (or starting level if already receiving PEEP).
3. Keep time intervals between changes short, e.g., 10 to 20 min at each step.
4. Make appropriate measurements after each PEEP increment:
   a. Effect on oxygenation: PaO_2 (CaO_2) ($P\bar{v}O_2$).
   b. Effect on lung/thorax compliance.
   c. Effect on cardiovascular function: MAP, $\dot{Q}_T$.
5. Monitor $\dot{Q}_T$ and pulmonary artery wedge pressure with a pulmonary artery catheter if:
   a. PEEP of greater than 10 to 15 cm H_2O is used.
   b. The patient's volume status is uncertain (e.g., unexplained tachycardia).
   c. Intrinsic cardiac disease is present.

KEY: PEEP = positive end-expiratory pressure, FIO_2 = fraction of inspired oxygen, CaO_2 = arterial oxygen content, $P\bar{v}O_2$ = mixed venous oxygen tension, V_T = tidal volume, $\dot{Q}_T$ = cardiac output, MAP = mean arterial pressure.

and which is expected to be of short duration may be treated with CPAP delivered by face mask, provided:

a. The patient is alert and cooperative.
b. The therapy is not likely to be required for more than three to four days.
c. No more than 10 to 14 cm H_2O CPAP will be required.

Mask CPAP may thus be appropriate in *Pneumocystis carinii* or viral pneumonia, smoke inhalation, and near-drowning, and in other settings in which ARDS is fairly mild and short lived. This form of therapy should not be tried in patients with altered mental status, multisystem failure, sepsis, or any other condition in which the three preceding conditions cannot be assured.

Administration. A fully cooperative patient who understands the therapy is essential. The arms must be continuously free so that the mask can be removed instantly should vomiting occur. Several soft, snugly fitting masks are now available for this application. Sedation, and any setting in which vomiting is stimulated, must be avoided. Mask CPAP should always be administered in an intensive care setting, where continuous monitoring is available. Administration of CPAP via nasal mask in the management of obstructive sleep apnea is discussed in Chapter 17.

Weaning From Positive End-Expiratory Pressure

Premature withdrawal or reduction of PEEP can worsen oxygenation and cause clinical deterioration that requires hours or days of therapy to reverse. Such reduction must therefore be undertaken carefully. Studies indicate that premature PEEP reduction can be avoided in about 80 per cent of instances if the following steps are taken prior to each withdrawal:

a. The disease process requiring PEEP should have resolved or substantially improved.
b. Condition of the patient should be clinically stable, and there should be no sepsis.
c. PaO_2 should be 80 mmHg or greater on FiO_2 of 0.40 or less.
d. These conditions should be present for 12 hours or more.

Reduction of PEEP based upon clinical judgment alone without the use of these or equivalent predictors is less likely to succeed. Once the therapeutic value of PEEP has been established in an individual patient, lowering the PEEP level more often than every 12 hours also results in more frequent failure.

Introduction of the three-minute PEEP wean has further increased the rate of success in lowering PEEP. The three-minute test is diagrammed in Figure 14–5. Once the patient meets the criteria to prevent premature PEEP withdrawal, PEEP is lowered 3 to 5 cm H_2O for three minutes. At the end of this period an arterial blood specimen is drawn for blood gas analysis and the PEEP is immediately increased to its previous level while the specimen is processed. Comparing the three-minute results to those from the specimen drawn prior to initiating PEEP reduction enables prediction of success or failure in reducing the PEEP permanently. If the PaO_2 is maintained, e.g., falls by 20 per cent of the baseline

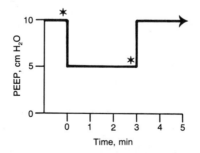

Figure 14–5. The three-minute PEEP wean test. With the patient's condition clinically stable and improving (preferably for 12 hours or more), and without changing any other aspect of management, the level of positive end-expiratory pressure (shown here initially as 10 cm H_2O) is reduced by 3 to 5 cm H_2O for three minutes. Arterial blood specimens are drawn for pH, PaO_2, and $PaCO_2$ just before each change in PEEP (see asterisks). Assuming that pH and $PaCO_2$ do not change, if the PaO_2 stays the same or drops by less than about 20 per cent after three minutes at the lower PEEP level, this lower level can be reinstituted safely. If the PaO_2 falls significantly, e.g., by 20 per cent or more, the previous PEEP level should be maintained until the next three-minute test.

value or less, there is perhaps a 90 per cent likelihood of successful PEEP reduction. If the PaO_2 falls substantially, e.g., drops by more than 20 per cent, however, the higher PEEP level should be continued and the patient's condition reassessed in another few hours.

Reducing PEEP from 5 cm H_2O to zero often causes PaO_2 to fall even if previous reductions from 10 or 15 cm H_2O were uneventful. Because of this, and also because of the belief on the part of many clinicians that low levels of PEEP are "physiological," some clinicians continue 5 cm H_2O of PEEP or CPAP until the time of extubation.

Extracorporeal Membrane Oxygenation (ECMO)

Numerous studies have shown that the membrane oxygenator can support life and oxygenate the blood of patients with profound failure of oxygenation. However, a major cooperative study (see reference 12) of ECMO in severe acute respiratory failure found no difference in eventual outcome among ECMO-supported and conventionally ventilated patients. Recent enthusiasm for partial extracorporeal gas exchange (low-frequency positive-pressure ventilation with extracorporeal CO_2 removal [$ECCO_2R$]) has been tempered by the failure of a new multicenter study to show any survival benefit from this technique, as compared with aggressive conventional management. ECMO and $ECCO_2R$ currently have no place in the routine management of patients with acute oxygenation failure. The very high mortality rate in such patients is apparently due to the disease process itself rather than to failure of any available therapy.

Hyperbaric Oxygenation

Although hyperbaric oxygenation is useful in the treatment of CO poisoning, cerebral air embolism, decompression illness, and some forms of anaerobic soft tissue infection, it is *not* useful in the management of acute respiratory failure. The main reasons for this are the logistics of its use and its toxicity in the face of disorders that usually take days to weeks to resolve.

Other Methods for Increasing O_2 Transport

Increasing Hemoglobin Concentration. At PaO_2 above about 80 mmHg the hemoglobin in blood is essentially saturated, and increasing PaO_2 further adds very little to CaO_2 unless hyperbaric conditions are used. With SaO_2 near 100 per cent, CaO_2 is mainly determined by the hemoglobin concentration in arterial blood. As shown in Figure 14–6, increasing hemoglobin from 10 to 15 gm/100 ml would increase CaO_2 by half at PaO_2 80 mmHg. On the

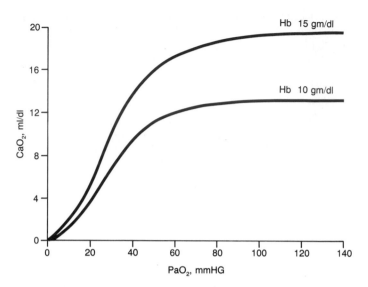

Figure 14–6. Importance of blood hemoglobin (Hb) concentration in oxygen transport. At a PaO$_2$ of 80 mmHg, arterial blood oxygen content (CaO$_2$) can be increased by 50 per cent by raising Hb from 10 to 15 gm/dl in an anemic patient.

other hand, increasing PaO$_2$ from 80 to 140 mmHg would increase CaO$_2$ by only an insignificant amount, in addition to requiring a potentially dangerous increase in FiO$_2$. Red blood cell transfusion to hematocrit values in the mid-30s or higher is often overlooked as a means of increasing CaO$_2$ in critically ill patients.

Cardiovascular Considerations. Oxygen transport depends as much on Q̇T as on CaO$_2$. Direct measurement of Q̇T often permits better adjustment of this crucial aspect of tissue oxygenation, particularly when PEEP is used or when intrinsic heart disease is present.

RECOMMENDED READING

1. Albert RK: Approach to the patient with cyanosis or hypoxemia. *In* Kelley WN (ed.): *Textbook of Internal Medicine*, 2nd ed. Philadelphia, J. B. Lippincott Co., 1992, pp. 1874–1876.
2. Glauser FL, Polatty RC, and Sessler CN: Worsening oxygenation in the mechanically ventilated patient: Causes, mechanisms, and early detection. *Am Rev Respir Dis* 138:458–465, 1988.
3. Hudson LD, et al.: Positive end-expiratory pressure: Reduction and withdrawal. *Respir Care* 33:613–619, 1988.
4. Kacmarek RM: Methods of oxygen delivery in the hospital. *Probl Respir Care* 3:563–574, 1990.

5. Kacmarek RM: Positive end-expiratory pressure. *In* Pierson DJ, and Kacmarek RM (eds.): *Foundations of Respiratory Care.* New York, Churchill Livingstone. 1992, pp. 891–920.
6. Kacmarek RM, Pierson DJ: Supplemental oxygen therapy. *In* Pierson DJ, and Kacmarek RM (eds.): *Foundations of Respiratory Care.* New York, Churchill Livingstone. 1992, pp. 859–890.
7. Maunder RJ, and Hudson LD: Management of the adult respiratory distress syndrome. *In* Kelley WN (ed.): *Textbook of Internal Medicine,* 2nd ed. Philadelphia, J. B. Lippincott Co., 1992, pp. 1861–1865.
8. Maunder RJ, et al.: Managing positive end-expiratory pressure (PEEP): The Harborview approach. *Respir Care* 31:1059–1064, 1986.
9. Pierson DJ: Indications for oxygen therapy. *Probl Respir Care* 3:549–562, 1990.
10. Positive end-expiratory pressure (PEEP). *Respir Care* 33:419–501, 539–637, 1988.
11. Rinaldo JE: Adult respiratory distress syndrome. *In* Rippe JM, et al. (eds.): *Intensive Care Medicine,* 2nd ed. Boston, Little, Brown, & Co., 1991, pp. 476–481.
12. Zapol WM, et al.: Extracorporeal membrane oxygenation in severe acute respiratory failure. *JAMA* 242:2193–2196, 1979.

15

WEANING

WEANING FROM MECHANICAL VENTILATION

DEFINITION

Ventilator weaning may be defined as the discontinuation of mechanical ventilation in patients with acute respiratory failure, based upon predetermined, objective criteria and accompanied by appropriate physiological monitoring. By analogy to the original use of the verb, to wean, ventilator weaning often implies a gradual progressive withdrawal of support. It need not have this implication, however, and many patients requiring mechanical ventilation following surgery or for other brief indications can simply have the ventilator turned off. The application of objective physiological criteria in predicting and monitoring successful ventilator discontinuation, however, is important to the best possible respiratory care of patients and central to the concept of weaning as described here.

Figure 15–1 diagrammatically shows the traditional forms of ventilator weaning. When continuous ventilation is employed in the assist/control mode (AMV), the patient receives all required minute ventilation ($\dot{V}E$) from the ventilator; when this is withdrawn (Fig. 15–1A), the patient must then supply all required $\dot{V}E$ spontaneously. This is known as traditional, or short, ventilator weaning. Using this technique, patients can also be weaned gradually through a series of brief periods of spontaneous ventilation interspersed with rest periods of AMV (Fig. 15–1B). When intermittent mandatory ventilation (IMV) is used in weaning after AMV, the proportion of machine-supplied ventilation is progressively diminished from 100 per cent to zero (Fig. 15–1C). When IMV has been the primary mode of ventilatory support, weaning is accomplished by further reducing a machine minute volume that was already only a portion of the patient's required $\dot{V}E$ (Fig. 15–1D).

Pressure support ventilation (PSV) may be added to either of the traditional weaning regimens just described and has the effect of partially supporting the patient's spontaneous breathing efforts.

232

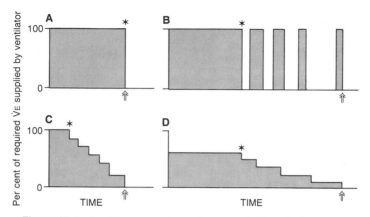

Figure 15–1. Traditional weaning techniques. *A*, Short T-piece weaning, in which full ventilatory support with assist-control (AMV) is simply stopped. *B*, Gradual weaning using the T-piece technique. Brief periods of spontaneous ventilation are gradually lengthened, with intervening rest periods with full ventilatory support (with either AMV or IMV). *C*, Weaning from full ventilatory support using the intermittent mandatory ventilation (IMV) technique. As compared with *A*, this technique starts earlier and completes weaning at about the same time. *D*, Gradual weaning from IMV (used as a primary ventilator mode) using IMV (used in weaning). Conceptually, the duration of mechanical ventilation is the same in *A* as in *C*, and the same in *B* as in *D*. Pressure support can be added to any of these scenarios and has the effect of partially supporting the patient by reducing the work of breathing. The pressure support itself must subsequently be weaned. $\dot{V}_E$ – total minute ventilation; * = weaning begun; ↑ = weaning complete.

Pressure support can also be used as a stand-alone, third basic weaning strategy: Enough PSV is added to provide a tidal volume (V_T) equivalent to that used with AMV or IMV, and then the added inspiratory pressure is progressively withdrawn as tolerated by the patient.

ASSESSMENT FOR WEANING

Oxygenation

For successful weaning from mechanical ventilation, the patient's respiratory function should be adequate to saturate arterial blood at an inspired oxygen fraction (FIO_2) of 0.50 or less. Patients with larger oxygenation defects usually require further treatment of their primary disease process before weaning can be accomplished successfully.

Ventilatory Demand

Patients requiring more than twice the normal $\dot{V}E$ in order to maintain a normal $PaCO_2$ usually have significantly elevated CO_2 production ($\dot{V}CO_2$), dead space fraction (VD/VT), or both. Therapy therefore should continue in an attempt to normalize these prior to weaning. Excessive $\dot{V}CO_2$ from sepsis, burns, or other hypermetabolic processes often prevents successful weaning despite adequate ventilatory mechanics. Similarly, a very high VD/VT, as is seen in the adult respiratory distress syndrome (ARDS), severe asthma, or massive pulmonary embolism, may prevent weaning from the ventilator despite adequate oxygenation and ventilatory mechanics.

Ventilatory Mechanics

Perhaps the best overall indicator of a patient's ability to sustain spontaneous ventilation following acute respiratory failure is the respiratory rate. Results of numerous studies show that measures of a patient's ventilatory mechanics during spontaneous breathing for a minute or two can also be used in predicting weaning success, at least following short-term ventilatory support. Although many measurements have been used, the most clinically valuable are also the easiest to do, requiring only a bedside spirometer and a manometer. These devices quantitate the strength of the respiratory muscles [maximal inspiratory force (MIF)]; the adequacy of ventilatory mechanics [vital capacity (VC)] and tidal volume (VT); the ability of the patient to match with spontaneous breathing the $\dot{V}E$ furnished by the ventilator; and the patient's capacity to increase this $\dot{V}E$ on demand. This final measurement is the maximal voluntary ventilation (MVV). To obtain the MVV, the patient is instructed to breathe as vigorously as possible for 10 or 12 seconds, and the resultant volume is multiplied to obtain a theoretical minute volume. This tests not only mechanics and muscle strength but also comprehension and cooperation, factors that also affect weaning success.

TRADITIONAL VENTILATOR WEANING

Rationale

With this weaning technique a prediction can be made that the patient no longer requires mechanical ventilatory support and the ventilator is withdrawn. If the patient is not considered able to breathe spontaneously for an unlimited period, short sojourns off the ventilator are initiated, with rest periods between, during which full ventilatory support is again provided. This technique of weaning was the first to be used and is still the standard against which newer methods are compared.

Picking the Right Time

Premature attempts at ventilator weaning and complications resulting from withdrawing support too soon can be minimized if the patient is otherwise stable and the underlying cause for acute respiratory failure has resolved or substantially improved. If significant deterioration has occurred in other organ systems—acute upper gastrointestinal bleeding or renal failure, for example—ventilator weaning may have to be delayed until these processes resolve or improve.

Technique

Prediction of Success. Table 15–1 gives a protocol for successful weaning by the traditional method. It may be used with either AMV or IMV as the baseline ventilatory support mode. Using predetermined objective measurements for judging readiness to be weaned as compared with simply deciding to proceed on clinical grounds will improve success rates. Which objective measurements and which numerical criteria are employed may be less crucial than the consistent use of the same technique with each patient.

The most helpful weaning parameters are listed under objective criteria in Table 15–1. A $\dot{V}E$ requirement during mechanical ventilation (delivered by the ventilator, or by the ventilator plus spontaneous breaths in the case of IMV) that is less than 10 or 12 L/min—or twice the patient's predicted normal resting $\dot{V}E$—indicates that the demand placed on the patient for sustained spontaneous breathing will not be too great. A VC of at least 10 ml/kg may be more useful than measurement of VT, at least following

Table 15–1. TRADITIONAL WEANING PROTOCOL

1. Satisfy some predetermined objective criteria for initiating weaning.
   a. Respiratory failure improved.
   b. FiO_2 requirement 0.50 or less.
   c. Demand for ventilation manageable ($\dot{V}E$ for normal $PaCO_2$ less than twice normal or 10–12 L/min).
   d. Spontaneous ventilatory mechanics adequate.
      i. VC at least 10 ml/kg.
      ii. MIF at least -20 cm H_2O.
      iii. MVV at least twice resting $\dot{V}E$ requirement.
2. Choose the right time of day.
3. Eliminate or minimize sedation.
4. Suction airway and position patient appropriately.
5. Switch to spontaneous ventilation (T-piece) at same FiO_2 with or without CPAP.
6. Monitor patient closely.
   a. Bedside observation/reassurance.
   b. Arterial blood gas measurement in 20–30 min.

KEY: FiO_2 = Fraction of inspired oxygen, $\dot{V}E$ = Minute ventilation, $PaCO_2$ = Arterial carbon dioxide tension, VC = Vital capacity, MIF = Maximum inspiratory force, MVV = Maximum voluntary ventilation, CPAP = Continuous positive airway pressure.

short-term ventilation (up to three to four days), and measurement of spontaneous respiratory rate (f) while the patient is momentarily off the ventilator may not be a consistently reliable predictor of weaning. An MIF of more than -20 cm H_2O indicates adequate inspiratory muscle strength. The ability to double the required resting $\dot{V}E$ during the MVV maneuver indicates sufficient ventilatory reserve to compensate for a moderate increase in demand, should this occur.

Time of Day. Several factors in addition to measurements of ventilatory function are important in successful weaning. The weaning attempt should be made at a time when staffing is maximal and other activities will not interfere. If possible, weaning attempts should be made during the day shift, and initiation of weaning at night should be avoided. The patient should not be involved in other activities, such as bathing, eating, or visiting with relatives, when the weaning attempt is made. If bronchodilator drugs are being used, the attempt should be timed so that their effects are maximal. Drugs that depress ventilation, such as narcotics and sedatives, should be withheld or cut back as much as possible. Just prior to taking the patient off the ventilator, the airway should be cleared using the techniques described in Chapter 9, and if possible the patient should be in the sitting or semiupright position, unless he or she is quadriplegic, in which case the diaphragm may function better with the patient supine.

Equipment Set-up and Personnel. Traditional weaning is accomplished by switching the patient from the ventilator circuit to a T-piece, through which humidified gas at the same FIO_2 flows at a rate sufficient to prevent rebreathing. An extension tube should be added to the expiratory side of the T-piece to prevent entrainment of room air, which can both lower the FIO_2 and dry the airway. Some clinicians add continuous positive airway pressure (CPAP) at levels of 5 cm H_2O, although the need for this approach has not been demonstrated in all patients. The transition from ventilator to spontaneous breathing should be preceded by careful explanation to the patient of what is to be done and why, along with the assurance that the person performing the weaning will remain with the patient or be immediately available. Calm reassurance by and the physical presence of physician, nurse, or respiratory therapist at the bedside during weaning prevents much patient agitation and distress that can result in abortion of the attempt.

Expected Physiological Changes. The weaning attempt should be followed by arterial blood gas measurement after 20 to 30 minutes, with success or failure determined according to the results. Mild distress and agitation can usually be managed by calmly reassuring the patient. More severe discomfort, which is more frequent the longer the patient has been ventilated prior to the weaning attempt, may necessitate temporary reinstitution of mechanical ventilation while the results of arterial blood gas analysis are awaited.

Arterial carbon dioxide tension ($PaCO_2$) often rises and arterial oxygen tension (PaO_2) falls during a trial of spontaneous ventilation; that the PaO_2 falls somewhat less in many patients receiving CPAP is a major rationale for its use. So long as arterial pH remains above 7.30 and arterial hemoglobin saturation (SaO_2) is above 90 per cent, spontaneous breathing with or without CPAP may be continued while the trend of these changes is assessed with serial measurements. The $PaCO_2$ and PaO_2 usually stabilize within a short time with continued spontaneous ventilation.

Gradual Traditional Weaning

Most patients ventilated for a few days or less can simply be disconnected from the ventilator once they meet the criteria discussed earlier, but others wean more successfully over a period of hours using alternating periods of assisted and spontaneous ventilation (see Fig. 15–1*B*). The intervals of spontaneous breathing via a T-piece are progressively lengthened until the patient is independent of the ventilator for one to several hours at a time. Clinical experience shows that, in some patients who have been ventilated for many days, gradual weaning during the day with return to full ventilatory support during the night may be more successful than abrupt weaning. Some patients receiving long-term ventilatory support are able to be independent of the ventilator throughout their waking hours, but maintain better health if they are returned to the ventilator at night.

WEANING WITH INTERMITTENT MANDATORY VENTILATION

Rationale

Intermittent mandatory ventilation was originally introduced as a weaning technique, although it is now also used as a primary mode of ventilatory support. As a weaning technique, IMV allows mechanical ventilation to be withdrawn gradually rather than abruptly. In addition, rather than relying on prediction of success prior to attempting weaning, with IMV weaning is begun empirically and allowed to proceed as far as possible using blood gas results as the major measure of success.

Picking the Right Time

Successful weaning with IMV requires adherence to the same principles discussed earlier under traditional weaning.

Technique

Weaning with IMV consists of repeating a two-step sequence until the ventilator rate is reduced to zero and the patient breathes without assistance. The machine rate is reduced, usually by one or two breaths/min, and arterial blood gas values are measured after 20 to 30 minutes. So long as the pH does not fall below a predetermined cut-off value—usually 7.30 or 7.35—these steps are repeated. Used in weaning as originally intended, IMV permits most patients to be completely off the ventilator within a few hours, as shown in Figure 15–1C. This technique is commonly misused, however, with only one or two rate reductions per day, a regimen that increases total ventilator time (and cost) in comparison with traditional weaning. Used properly, weaning with IMV after short-term ventilatory support takes about the same amount of time as traditional weaning, although it may require more ventilator adjustments and thus more blood gas measurements.

Gradual IMV Weaning

With this technique the ventilator rate is reduced more slowly and mechanical support is withdrawn over a period of days rather than hours. Although unnecessary in most patients with short-term mechanical ventilation, this regimen may be helpful in some individuals who have required prolonged ventilation prior to the weaning attempt, and perhaps in those who fail attempts at gradual traditional weaning, especially at night. Any intrinsic advantage of one weaning method over another is probably insignificant, provided the basic principles of respiratory care are followed. Whether traditional or IMV weaning is used is more a matter of individual preference than of any inherent superiority of either technique.

WEANING WITH PRESSURE SUPPORT

Rationale

With the current generation of ICU ventilators, peak inspiratory flow rates during patient-initiated breaths tend to be higher but at lower peak pressures with PSV than with AMV or IMV. The inspiratory pressure-wave form during PSV is more comfortable for many dyspneic patients than that delivered with the other modes. Use of PSV focuses on reducing the patient's overall work of breathing, and on eliminating the added (imposed) work of breathing that results from the endotracheal tube and ventilator circuit.

Picking the Right Time

This in general is the same as with T-piece and IMV weaning, as discussed above.

Technique

With PSV as a stand-alone weaning technique, the patient is switched from volume-limited ventilation (AMV or IMV) to PSV at a level sufficient to provide the same V_T (e.g., 10 to 12 ml/kg). The inspiratory pressure support level is then progressively reduced, monitoring primarily the patient's spontaneous respiratory rate as an indicator of the adequacy of support. So long as the rate remains below 30 breaths/min the pressure is sequentially lowered until it is only 5 to 10 cm H_2O, at which point the patient is extubated (assuming there is no other indication for an artificial airway—see Chapter 8). As with the other weaning techniques, arterial blood gas analysis should usually be carried out prior to extubation to confirm the success of the weaning protocol, remembering that hypoxemia and/or acute respiratory acidosis cannot reliably be detected without such analysis.

FAILURE TO WEAN

Definition

The patient who cannot be removed from mechanical ventilatory support despite application of the principles discussed in this chapter may be said to have failed a weaning attempt. The most frequent manifestation of this failure is acute respiratory acidosis, an increase in $PaCO_2$ to the degree that pH falls to 7.30 or less. Patients can also fail to be weaned because of uncontrollable agitation and respiratory distress despite correct use of equipment and technique. If gas exchange is adequate, this is usually controllable with reassurance and gentle sedation. It should be emphasized that most instances of apparent "failure" in weaning are due to neglect of one or more of the basics, either in treatment of the underlying problem or in preparation of the patient for weaning.

Weakness

Patients whose VC is less than 10 ml/kg or whose MIF is less than -20 cm H_2O on preweaning assessment are unable to keep up with ventilatory needs even if these are normal. The following causes should be sought.

Drugs. Aminoglycoside antibiotics such as polymyxin, streptomycin, or gentamycin can produce neuromuscular blockade soon after the drug is given in very large amounts, particularly if instilled in the peritoneum. Weaning should not be attempted for patients who have received neuromuscular blocking agents such as pancuronium bromide (Pavulon) or curare until all effects of the drug have disappeared.

Metabolic Abnormalities. Hypophosphatemia, hypomagnesemia, and hypokalemia can cause failure to wean because of muscular weakness. These conditions should be suspected in all patients who fail to wean because of weakness. Hypothyroidism is another potential contributor, although it is difficult to diagnose accurately in critically ill patients.

Malnutrition. Protein-calorie malnutrition in patients who have been seriously ill for weeks can produce neuromuscular weakness that interferes with weaning, although the mechanisms are unclear and this problem is difficult to document objectively. In poorly nourished patients, successful weaning sometimes becomes possible after a period of intensive nutritional repletion in conjunction with correction of metabolic and electrolyte abnormalities.

Primary Neuromuscular Disease. Conditions such as multiple sclerosis and myasthenia gravis are usually evident prior to the onset of acute respiratory failure. This cause for failure to wean is hard to document and must usually be diagnosed by exclusion of other processes. Respiratory muscle dysfunction is discussed further in Chapter 5.

Insufficient Ventilatory Drive

Respiratory Alkalosis. This is the most common cause of the failure of a patient to breathe spontaneously when disconnected from a ventilator. Especially when AMV is used, dyspneic patients may establish an acute respiratory alkalosis that effectively suppresses their drive to breathe until hypoxemia or hypercapnia intervenes. In patients with normal $\dot{V}CO_2$, $PaCO_2$ rises 8 to 10 mmHg during the first minute of apnea and about 3 mmHg per minute thereafter. With severe respiratory alkalosis, it may thus take several minutes before $PaCO_2$ rises to the usual apneic threshold—usually 36 to 38 mmHg when no metabolic component is present. When possible, respiratory alkalosis should be corrected prior to initial weaning.

Metabolic Alkalosis. As discussed in Chapter 4, metabolic alkalosis commonly results from diuretic-induced renal potassium and chloride depletion and from losses of hydrogen ion and electrolytes from the gastrointestinal tract, both of which are common in ventilated patients. The combination of metabolic and respiratory alkalosis is particularly troublesome in preventing successful weaning in many patients. These abnormalities should be corrected before another weaning attempt is made. Elimination of nasogastric suction loss and administration of potassium chloride to correct hypokalemic alkalosis are the most important measures here.

Drugs. Patients receiving narcotic analgesics and large doses of sedative drugs may fail a weaning attempt because of suppression of their ventilatory drives by these agents. Careful review of the medication sheets of patients who are difficult to wean often reveals administration of several drugs that could suppress ventilation; frequently these have been continued inadvertently even though they are no longer needed. In any case, such drugs should be discontinued or substantially cut back before another weaning attempt is made.

Other Causes. Malnutrition depresses endogenous ventilatory drives in addition to weakening the respiratory muscles. Myxedema also depresses ventilatory drives. Occasionally patients with cerebrovascular accidents or congenital abnormalities may lack hypoxic or hypercapnic sensitivity or even central respiratory drive, although such occurrences as causes of weaning failure are rare. Administration of respiratory stimulant drugs such as doxapram (Dopram) or medroxyprogesterone acetate (Provera) seldom allows an otherwise unweanable patient to become completely ventilator-independent, and weaning in cases of insufficient drive requires correction of the underlying problem, if this can be accomplished.

Excessive Work of Breathing

Small or Obstructed Endotracheal Tube. Some patients who are unable to sustain spontaneous ventilation through an endotracheal tube are capable of breathing on their own when extubated. The resistance to flow through a tube, and hence the work required to overcome it, varies with the length of the tube and also inversely with the fourth power of the tube's smallest effective radius. At a flow rate of 1 L/sec the resistance to flow through an endotracheal tube with an inside diameter of 9 mm is 0.6 cm H_2O; for an 8-mm tube, it is 1.9 cm H_2O. For a 7-mm tube the resistance increases to 4.0 cm H_2O, and it is even greater for smaller tubes. This radius effect applies to the tube's narrowest point, so that a kinked tube or one partly clogged by mucus has a smaller effective radius and much greater resistance than its caliber would suggest. Prolonged spontaneous ventilation through a 6- or 7-mm endotracheal tube may be beyond the capability of the patient, especially if the required $\dot{V}E$ is more than 10 or 12 L. For patients who are alert and who can be expected to protect their airways from aspiration, ventilator weaning and extubation can sometimes be accomplished simultaneously. If this cannot be done, the endotracheal tube should be exchanged for one at least 1 mm larger before spontaneous ventilation through a T-piece can be reattempted.

Pressure support can be added to compensate for the work of breathing imposed by the tube. For endotracheal tubes of 7.0 mm or greater inside diameter and $\dot{V}E$ requirements up to about 12 L/min, 5 cm H_2O is sufficient. If the tube is less than 7.0 mm or the

$\dot{V}E$ 12 to 16 L/min, 8 to 10 cm H_2O of pressure support should be used.

High-Resistance Pathway for Spontaneous Breathing. Because different ventilators and tubing circuits have different resistances, it is important to examine the circuit through which a patient is required to breathe spontaneously during weaning. Depending on the physical arrangement of the valves and tubing, and also on the degree of pressurization of the circuit, the effort put forth by the patient to draw spontaneous breaths may be excessive and prevent successful weaning. This consideration is technical but can be crucially important: Breathing through a ventilator circuit at a machine rate of zero may require considerably more work than breathing through a T-piece, and familiarity with the circuitry in use is essential.

Airway Obstruction. Patients with bronchospasm, thick secretions, or foreign bodies in the major airways should have these reversed or removed prior to another weaning attempt, as discussed under Traditional Ventilator Weaning.

Chest Restriction. The patient whose chest excursion is limited by bandages or restraints may be unable to be weaned until these are removed or loosened. Very obese patients or those with postoperative bowel distention may not be weaned successfully if they cannot or will not sit up.

Pain. Postoperative or postresuscitation pain can prevent weaning by causing patients to breathe rapidly and shallowly. Local or regional anesthesia may be more effective in such patients than systemic analgesia.

Anxiety. Excessively anxious or agitated patients often cannot be weaned until they can be calmed. If this cannot be accomplished without heavy sedation or paralysis, weaning will have to be deferred until the cause of the agitation can be removed.

High $\dot{V}E$ Requirement

High $\dot{V}CO_2$. Ongoing sepsis, inflammation, and occasionally excessive hyperalimentation can increase the demand for ventilation to such an extent that the patient cannot keep up without mechanical assistance. This problem can be assessed easily by collecting expired gas for three minutes in a Douglas bag and analyzing it for CO_2 on a blood gas machine, permitting calculation of $\dot{V}CO_2$ in milliliters per minute. This technique works with both AMV and IMV; with the latter the collected volume is larger, but the CO_2 produced will be the same. Carbon dioxide volume greater than the 200 to 250 ml/min expected in a normal-sized adult confirms the presence of excessive ventilatory demand due to high $\dot{V}CO_2$. When this is the case, attention should be given to correcting this excess before another weaning attempt is made.

High V_D/V_T. Patients with severe ARDS typically have high physiological dead space ventilation, and this can persist well into the phase of clinical recovery. Severe COPD, status asthmaticus, and multiple pulmonary thromboemboli are also characterized by high V_D/V_T. The V_D/V_T can be measured at the same time that $\dot{V}CO_2$ is determined if an arterial blood gas analysis is done concurrently. V_D/V_T is calculated according to the following formula:

$$V_D/V_T = \frac{PaCO_2 - P_ECO_2}{PaCO_2}$$

where P_ECO_2 is the PCO_2 in the mixed expired gas. A value for V_D/V_T exceeding 0.50 during mechanical ventilation is high, and patients usually cannot be weaned if the value exceeds 0.60.

If high V_D/V_T is documented in a patient being considered for weaning, efforts should be made to improve the condition causing the abnormality. In resolving ARDS it is often necessary to wait several days and monitor V_D/V_T and $\dot{V}CO_2$ values repeatedly before reattempting weaning.

WEANING FROM ENDOTRACHEAL INTUBATION

DEFINITION

The discontinuation of upper airway bypass by orotracheal, nasotracheal, or tracheostomy tube may be considered weaning in a sense analogous to the use of the word to describe the discontinuation of mechanical ventilation. As discussed in Chapter 8, this discontinuation can be either abrupt, as in the majority of patients when the tube is simply removed, or gradual, when transitional plugging or substitution of a button is used.

PREDICTORS OF SUCCESS

Unlike ventilator weaning, no objectively defined parameters exist to predict successful endotracheal extubation other than those assessing postextubation cough ability (see Chapter 9). No studies to date have examined the value of assessments made prior to removal in assuring that reintubation will not be required. Clinical experience shows, however, that recalling the indications for endotracheal intubation can help when assessing patients for extubation. The main reasons artificial airways are inserted are:

a. to prevent or reverse upper airway restriction.
b. to protect the lower respiratory tract from aspiration of gastric or mouth contents.
c. to facilitate the removal of secretions.
d. to provide a closed system for mechanical ventilation.

Once a patient has been weaned from mechanical ventilation, the last of these indications no longer applies, although it is occasionally useful to leave patients intubated for another day when the success of ventilator weaning of more than several hours is uncertain. The need to protect the airway against aspiration is harder to assess. The usual procedure is to stroke the posterior pharynx with a tongue depressor to see if the patient gags, although this test has neither been standardized nor studied for its protective value once the patient is extubated. Unless a discrete bulbar neurological defect is present, however, patients who are alert and mobile can usually avoid aspiration. In individuals with impaired mental status or in patients who are immobilized by disease or treatment, no firm guidelines exist. For example, whether the patient with coma after head trauma or anoxia should remain intubated to protect the airway and to prevent pneumonia has never been investigated, and the decision must rest on the experience and preference of the clinician.

When endotracheal intubation has been performed in order to facilitate the removal of secretions, extubation depends on the progress made in reversing this indication. Again, no objective measurable parameters exist other than for cough effectiveness, although it is reasonable to attempt extubation when there has been improvement in the chest roentgenogram, sputum culture, physical examination, or some other indicator of overall clinical improvement. Extubation in such instances is still an empirical trial, and the clinician must be prepared to reintubate if necessary.

TECHNIQUE

Technique and other aspects of airway care are discussed in Chapter 8.

RECOMMENDED READING

1. Boysen PG: Weaning from mechanical ventilation: Does technique make a difference? *Respir Care* 36:407–416, 1991.

2. Hall JB, and Wood LDH: Liberation of the patient from mechanical ventilation. *JAMA* 257:1621–1628, 1987.

3. Higgins TL, and Stoller JK: Discontinuing ventilatory support. *In* Pierson DJ, and Kacmarek RM (eds.): *Foundations of Respiratory Care*. New York, Churchill Livingstone, 1992, pp. 1019–1036.

4. Irwin RS: Mechanical ventilation. II: Weaning. *In* Rippe JM, et al. (eds.): Intensive Care Medicine, 2nd ed. Boston, Little, Brown Co., 1991, pp. 575–584.

5. Kacmarek RM: The role of pressure support ventilation in reducing imposed work of breathing. *Respir Care* 33:99–120, 1988.

6. Kacmarek RM, and Pierson DJ: Assessment of the adequacy of airway protection and secretion clearance. *In* Pierson DJ, and Kacmarek RM (eds.): *Foundations of Respiratory Care*. New York, Churchill Livingstone, 1992, pp. 561–570.

7. MacIntyre NR: Weaning from mechanical ventilatory support: Volume-assisting intermittent breaths versus pressure-supporting every breath. *Respir Care* 33:121–125, 1988.

8. Morganroth ML, et al.: Criteria for weaning from prolonged mechanical ventilation. *Arch Intern Med* 144:1012–1016, 1984.

9. Pierson DJ: Weaning from mechanical ventilation in acute respiratory failure: Concepts, indications, and techniques. *Respir Care* 28:646–662, 1983.

10. Pierson DJ: Overcoming nonrespiratory causes of weaning failure. *J Crit Illness* 5:267–283, 1990.

11. Wilson DO, and Rogers RM: The role of nutrition in weaning from mechanical ventilation. *J Crit Care* 4:124–133, 1989.

12. Yang KL, and Tobin MJ: A prospective study of indexes predicting the outcome of trials of weaning from mechanical ventilation. *N Engl J Med* 324:1445–1450, 1991.

16

MONITORING THE PATIENT

INTENSIVE CARE MONITORING

WHAT TO MONITOR, AND WHY

Respiratory care monitoring is performed to supply appropriate and correct physiological information about patients and to measure the effects of therapy. In order to accomplish these goals, the clinician must decide, for each patient and often on multiple occasions in the course of an illness, what variables to measure and how to measure them. General guidelines for deciding on a given monitoring procedure are outlined in Table 16–1. Implicit in the guidelines are these questions:

1. Is the procedure needed?
2. Is it safe?
3. Does it work?
4. Is it cost effective?
5. Are the data generated by the procedure accurate?
6. Will they be used?

MONITORING WITHOUT MACHINERY

No collection of numbers on a computer printout can substitute for bedside skills. In addition to such objective measures as respiratory rate, heart rate, and blood pressure, a bedside observer can assess such intangibles as patient comfort and respiratory distress. The "appropriateness" of the patient—something that encompasses mental status, communication, and cooperativeness—can be an important indicator of physiological deterioration or improvement. Observation of the patient and rapid physical examination are crucial when electronic monitoring equipment signals an abrupt change, e.g., the quick separation of physiological catastrophe from equipment malfunction or artifact. In cases of sudden patient distress during mechanical ventilation, inspection

Table 16-1. CLINICAL CONSIDERATIONS IN THE USE OF A GIVEN MONITORING PROCEDURE OR MEASUREMENT

Ease or difficulty of obtaining the measurement
Invasiveness or patient risk in obtaining the measurement
Precision and variability of the measurement technique
Baseline physiological variability of the function being measured
Relative importance of the measurement to management
    decisions in this patient
Cost of the measurement

for chest symmetry and examination for hyperresonance can be life-saving when the cause is tension pneumothorax.

Actual measurement of the work of breathing is not presently feasible for routine clinical application in seriously ill patients. However, visual estimation of minute ventilation ($\dot{V}E$) and the respiratory muscle exertion needed to maintain it can be extremely helpful, particularly if serial estimations are made. Similarly, although direct measurement of peripheral tissue perfusion is unavailable, a careful assessment of skin color, turgor, and temperature, along with mental status and urine output, may provide essential information.

Despite the value of bedside observation, this monitoring technique is limited by the clinican's skills. In addition, even the most experienced clinician may be unable to evaluate the meaning of the presence or absence of certain signs. Central cyanosis (discussed in Chapter 6) is usually suggestive of hypoxemia if present. Nevertheless, cyanosis may be evident in some patients with normal arterial oxygenation, whereas others with significant hypoxemia may not be cyanotic. Similarly, studies have demonstrated that the adequacy of alveolar ventilation cannot be reliably estimated by bedside observation, as confirmed by arterial blood gas measurements.

THE CHEST ROENTGENOGRAM AS A MONITORING TOOL

Portable chest roentgenograms are an important adjunct in noninvasive monitoring of patients in the intensive care unit (ICU). However, while this diagnostic procedure can aid management, it also has definite shortcomings. The chest roentgenogram is essential following certain invasive procedures (central venous line placement, thoracentesis, chest tube insertion) to detect complications and to confirm the results of the procedure. Pneumothorax, a common and potentially deadly complication of respiratory illness and its management, can often only be detected radiographically. In addition, the course of pneumonia or the adult respiratory distress syndrome (ARDS) can be followed by assessment of general trends over several days.

On the other hand, the bedside portable chest roentgenogram is a poor monitoring tool in numerous respects. It is expensive, and there is a tendency to read too much into it. The technical differences between portable and routine roentgenograms, discussed in Chapter 6, make interpretation of heart size difficult on a portable examination. When portable roentgenograms are taken, the patient often cannot cooperate; bandages, orthopedic devices, or other apparatus may lie in the path of the exposure; and exposure distance is hard to keep constant in serial films. Consequently, subtle abnormalities are often missed, and film-to-film variation in the appearance of pulmonary infiltrates occurs. Also, bedside roentgenograms are static, not dynamic, reflecting a patient's condition at only one moment in time. For these reasons, the portable roentgenogram should not be used to judge hour-by-hour clinical progress or to make specific diagnoses. Rather, it should be used as an adjunct to bedside examination, keeping in mind its limitations.

MONITORING VENTILATORY MECHANICS

Respiratory Rate

Spontaneous breathing frequency (f) in a patient with respiratory disease can be thought of as an index of respiratory mechanics. Counting f by visual observation is the main way this function is monitored. Respirations should be counted under comparable conditions for meaningful serial comparisons. Counting at times of external manipulation such as bathing, suctioning, and turning should be avoided. If spontaneous f is measured during a brief period off a mechanical ventilator, the interval should be the same, e.g., for 30 seconds beginning at one minute, each time.

Several methods are available for continuous mechanical monitoring of spontaneous f. These include chest impedance, utilizing two electrocardiogram leads on the chest wall; and inductance, using insulated wire coils imbedded in a mesh vest. Electromyograms and magnetometers have been tried as continuous respiratory rate monitors, but they are not accurate enough in the critically ill patient for routine use. Three techniques sometimes used to detect airflow are insertion of a thermistor or thermodilution catheter in a nasal cannula, expiratory CO_2 monitoring through such a cannula, and the use of a microphone placed over the trachea.

Lung Volumes

The lung volumes useful in management of the patient on a ventilator include expired tidal volume (V_T), vital capacity (VC), and functional residual capacity (FRC). Although some ventilators have built-in devices giving a breath-by-breath V_T readout, these must be checked for accuracy and often are only rough approximations. For V_T and VC, the time-honored Wright Respirometer, a mechanical, spinning-vane spirometer, is still the most dependable, accurate, and durable device for routine use. Hand-held electronic spirometers may also be used, although their accuracy should be checked against a known volume, and they are more easily damaged by rough use or improper cleaning. A standard water-seal or rolling-seal spirometer may be used for measuring V_T and VC, but bulk and more complicated operation make these less suitable for routine management. Lightweight pneumotachographs that have become widely available provide in-line continuous V_T measurements by integrating inspiratory or expiratory flow: These devices also register f and combine it with V_T to compute $\dot{V}_E$.

Measurements of expired V_T during mechanical ventilation must take into consideration the expansion volume of the ventilator tubing. As a rule of thumb, in standard disposable circuits this volume is approximately 3 ml/cm H_2O of static airway pressure. In patients with ARDS and other conditions producing marked lung stiffness, this compression volume can be considerable. Direct measurement rather than calculated estimation of this volume is necessary for research applications but not for day-to-day clinical management so long as the same technique is used each time V_T is measured.

Because ARDS is characterized by a reduction in FRC, and because positive end-expiratory pressure (PEEP) therapy is geared physiologically to increase FRC in order to improve arterial oxygenation, direct measurement of FRC during the course and therapy of these disorders would be a valuable monitoring tool. Unfortunately, although several devices and protocols have been published for measuring FRC in ventilated patients, none of these is simple enough for routine use. Only an indirect assessment of FRC through the chest roentgenogram is presently available outside the specialized research setting.

Auto-PEEP. During mechanical ventilation, particularly with the assisted mechanical ventilation (AMV) or controlled mechanical ventilation (CMV) modes, patients with airflow obstruction may fail to complete exhalation before the next ventilator breath begins. When this happens, progressive air trapping results, raising FRC and causing inadvertent "auto-PEEP." This auto-PEEP effect can seriously reduce cardiac filling pressures, alter vascular pressure readings, and cause cardiovascular compromise. Auto-PEEP can be measured by stopping expiratory airflow at end-expiration just prior to the next breath and allowing the pressure inside the airways and in the ventilator tubing to equilibrate; auto-PEEP is read directly from the ventilator's pressure manometer. Several currently manufactured ICU ventilators incorporate mechanisms for the semiautomated measurement of auto-PEEP.

Measures to reduce or eliminate auto-PEEP do so by increasing expiratory time and include the following:

1. Correcting respiratory alkalosis by reducing f and/or V_T.

2. Increasing inspiratory flow rate (which will increase peak inspiratory pressure as a reflection of resistance to flow in large airways, but will not increase the risk of barotrauma).

3. Replacing the standard high-compressible–volume disposable ventilator circuit with a nondisposable, low-compressible–volume circuit (which will decrease the total volume the ventilator must deliver with each breath, shortening the time required to deliver it).

Patients who are making some spontaneous breathing effort (with either AMV or IMV) in the presence of auto-PEEP must overcome the latter to initiate each breath, thus increasing breathing work. For example, if a patient has 12 cm H_2O of auto-PEEP because of incomplete lung emptying prior to the delivery of the next breath, and if it takes -3 cm H_2O to trigger that next breath, then the patient must perform sufficient ventilatory muscle work to generate $12 + 3 = 15$ cm H_2O every time a breath is taken. Adding dialed-in PEEP (external PEEP) to a level near that of the patient's own auto-PEEP may reduce this added work of breathing and relieve patient distress. However, this should not be done if it results in an increase in the total PEEP measured using the auto-PEEP maneuver.

Respiratory System Compliance

Definition. Compliance measures the change in pressure (ΔP) required to produce a certain volume (ΔV); thus, compliance $= \Delta V/\Delta P$. Respiratory system compliance (C_{RS}) is the pressure required to inflate the lungs and move the chest wall with a given volume of gas. Its two components, lung compliance and chest wall compliance, are altered by many disease processes but are difficult to measure separately, especially in sick, mechanically ventilated patients. For this reason, approximations of C_{RS} under dynamic and static conditions are used.

Dynamic Compliance. Dynamic respiratory system compliance (C_{DYN}) is a measure of the maximum airway pressure (P_{MAX}) required to deliver a given V_T to a ventilated patient, minus the amount of PEEP also used to expand the lungs. Thus, $C_{DYN} = V_T/(P_{MAX} - PEEP)$. As dynamic measurements, C_{DYN} and P_{MAX} reflect the resistance to gas flow in the airways and ventilator tubing as well as the compliance characteristics of the lungs and chest wall. Peak airway pressure will rise and C_{DYN} will fall in the presence of bronchospasm, airway secretions, a small endotracheal tube, an agitated patient, or any combination of these.

Static Compliance. Static respiratory system compliance (CSTAT) is a measure of the airway pressure (PSTAT) required to hold the lungs and chest wall at end-inspiration after a VT has been delivered and gas flow is not present. The amount of PEEP being used should be subtracted; thus, $C_{STAT} = V_T/(P_{STAT} - PEEP)$. A normal value is 60 to 90 ml/cm H_2O. As static measurements, CSTAT and PSTAT reflect only the compliance of the lungs and chest wall and are not affected by resistance to gas flow. Static airway pressure will rise, and CSTAT will fall, in the presence of lung stiffness, which is most pronounced in ARDS, and also with abnormalities of the chest wall, such as obesity, vigorous respiratory muscle contraction, and casts and bandages that limit movement. Tension pneumothorax and large pleural effusions also make CSTAT fall.

Serial Compliance Measurements. Although single determinations of CDYN and CSTAT provide some information, serial measurements are more helpful. Abrupt increases in CDYN but not CSTAT may provide important clues as to the presence of airflow obstruction; on the other hand, decreases in CSTAT but not CDYN may reflect increased lung stiffness as found in pulmonary edema. Multiple-breath volume-pressure curves may also be generated at the bedside using serial measurements of dynamic airway pressure (PDYN) and PSTAT at different VTs. Plotting VTs against PDYNs produces a dynamic compliance curve; plotting VTs against PSTATs produces a static compliance curve. In the presence of increased airways resistance, the dynamic curve is shifted to the right and flattened, indicating a much higher PMAX with increasing VT, but the static curve is unchanged. The static wave is shifted to the right when pneumothorax occurs.

Flow Rates

Measurements of expiratory volume in the first second of a forced vital capacity maneuver (FEV$_1$) are possible in intubated patients but are rarely made. Spontaneously breathing, nonintubated patients with severe airflow obstruction, such as individuals with status asthmaticus, may be able to perform this maneuver, and serial FEV$_1$ determinations are sometimes used in following these patients acutely. More commonly employed in this setting is the measurement of peak flow, which is often better tolerated and can be done with convenient portable devices such as the Mini-Wright Peak Flow Meter.

Respiratory Muscle Function

Although diaphragmatic and intercostal electromyc
used in research, clinical respiratory functic
assessed by bedside observation and measurement

inspiratory force (MIF), as discussed in Chapter 6. Discoordination of chest and abdominal muscles during spontaneous breathing or patient-initiated breathing during mechanical ventilation produces a pattern similar to that seen with bilateral diaphragmatic paralysis, as described in Chapter 5. This finding is predictive of risk for acute ventilatory failure and of difficulty in weaning from the ventilator.

MONITORING GAS EXCHANGE

Oxygenation of the Arterial Blood

General Considerations. The maintenance of adequate arterial oxygenation, as reflected in the arterial oxygen tension (PaO_2), is one of the fundamental goals of respiratory intensive care. Arterial oxygenation can be monitored either intermittently or continuously, and several different techniques are available.

Inspired Oxygen Fraction. Measurement or approximation of the PaO_2 is most useful when compared with the concurrent fraction of inspired O_2 (FIO_2). Some ventilators have built-in sensors to measure FIO_2, although the accuracy of these devices varies and must be checked against a more reliable O_2 analyzer. Various analyzers are available; some have rapid response time, although this is not necessary for routine clinical measurement. The introduction of mass spectrometry into some intensive care units has made rapid, continuous, accurate FIO_2 monitoring possible in routine patient care, although the overall need for this outside the research setting remains to be seen.

Arterial Oxygen Tension. The PaO_2 may be measured in a 2- to 3-ml sample obtained from either percutaneous arterial puncture or indwelling arterial catheter. Repeated percutaneous sticks, if done with skill using a small-bore (25-gauge) needle, are safe even when repeated dozens of times over the course of a week. Their disadvantages are inconvenience, the risk of bleeding if the site is not held under pressure or if the patient is anticoagulated, and the pain they cause. Arterial catheters are convenient once in place and allow rapid, reliable arterial access for multiple specimens. They carry a higher risk for complications such as ischemia and embolization than do percutaneous sticks, however, and may be overused. Arterial lines are necessary when hemodynamic instability demands continuous arterial pressure monitoring, and are justified when multiple blood samples must be obtained in critically ill patients, for example, during PEEP trials. Although indwelling continuous arterial blood gas samplers with either fine catheters or intra-arterial electrodes are available, they are not yet sufficiently accurate or reliable for routine use.

Capillary and Venous Oxygen Tension. Systemic capillary or arterialized peripheral venous blood can be used in certain settings to reflect arterial pH and carbon dioxide tension (PCO_2). However, the oxygen tension (PO_2) of these sources is lower than that of arterial blood, especially if local blood flow is impaired. These measurements do not have a significant role in the management of adult patients in the ICU.

Transcutaneous Oxygen Tensions. Transcutaneous PO_2 ($PtcO_2$) monitors accurately reflect PaO_2 in neonates and small children, but not in adults because of their thicker dermis; they also are inaccurate in the presence of varying peripheral perfusion. Thus, $PtcO_2$ monitoring is not acceptable as a sole index of oxygenation in adult patients whose condition is unstable.

Pulse Oximetry. The availability of accurate, reliable pulse oximeters has made continuous monitoring of arterial O_2 saturation (SaO_2) practical in several clinical settings. These devices are important in the evaluation of sleep disorders, in regulating low-flow O_2 therapy in some patients with severe chronic obstructive pulmonary disease (COPD), and in clinical exercise testing. They may also be helpful in the continuous assessment of patients whose PaO_2 values are below about 65 mmHg. Above this PaO_2, because of the flat shape of the O_2-hemoglobin dissociation curve, the pulse oximeter is less useful as a monitoring tool. Its accuracy is about $\pm$ 3 per cent, and hemoglobin is effectively completely saturated at PaO_2 values in excess of about 80 mmHg, so that its value in continuous monitoring is mainly in the detection of falls in PaO_2 below this level. The pulse oximeter cannot distinguish between PaO_2 values of 100 and 300 mmHg. It may also be inaccurate in the presence of high serum bilirubin concentrations, green dye (used in some determinations of cardiac output by indicator dilution), and poor ear perfusion.

Alveolar-Arterial Oxygen Differences. The adequacy of oxygen transfer from alveolus to arterial blood can be assessed precisely only when both alveolar and arterial PO_2 are known. Alveolar PO_2 can be estimated using the measured FiO_2 and the alveolar air equation (see Chapter 2) and from this an alveolar-arterial O_2 difference or gradient $[P(A-a)O_2]$ can be calculated.

A rough approximation of the $P(A-a)O_2$ can be derived from the ratio of PaO_2 to FiO_2 (P/F ratio). This easy calculation allows comparison of serial PO_2 determinations even when FiO_2 varies, and is acceptably accurate over the range of FiO_2 of 0.40 to 0.70. Thus, if a patient has a PaO_2 of 80 mmHg on an FiO_2 of 0.40, *t* P/F ratio is 200, which would be the same if this patient *k*

PaO_2 of 120 mmHg on an FIO_2 of 0.60. A worsening of arterial blood oxygenation may be detected using P/F ratios even when FIO_2 has been changed since the previous specimen was obtained.

Alveolar Ventilation

General Considerations. As discussed in Chapter 2, the body normally maintains an alveolar and arterial PCO_2 of approximately 40 mmHg by adjusting alveolar ventilation ($\dot{V}A$) to meet its CO_2 production ($\dot{V}CO_2$). This process is symbolized in the alveolar ventilation equation: $PACO_2 = PaCO_2 = \dot{V}CO_2/\dot{V}A$. Assuming a near-constant $\dot{V}CO_2$, the $PaCO_2$ is an accurate reflection of $\dot{V}A$, and hyperventilation and hypoventilation are defined by this measurement.

Arterial Carbon Dioxide Tension. Monitoring $PaCO_2$ is subject to the same constraints as with PaO_2: An arterial sample is required, and with present technology this means intermittent rather than continuous assessment.

Transcutaneous Carbon Dioxide Tension. Transcutaneous PCO_2 ($PtcCO_2$), although slightly higher than $PaCO_2$, is a reflection of the latter in hemodynamically stable patients. Although subject to limitations similar to those for $PtcO_2$, the cutaneous monitoring of PCO_2 may become more useful in detecting acute changes and trends in $\dot{V}A$ while allowing fewer arterial blood specimens to be drawn. At present, however, the $PtcCO_2$ should be thought of as a supplement to, but not a replacement for, the $PaCO_2$.

Expired Gas Tension. Measuring PCO_2 in expired gas rather than in blood (capnography) currently is an adjunct to other monitoring techniques and in certain circumstances can replace repeated arterial sampling. In normal individuals, end-tidal expired PCO_2 ($PETCO_2$) is approximately the same as $PACO_2$ and $PaCO_2$. However, in patients with a large physiological dead space ($\dot{V}D$), with extensive ventilation and perfusion ($\dot{V}A/\dot{Q}$) mismatching, or with prolonged expiration due to severe COPD or asthma, $PETCO_2$ is not an accurate measure of $\dot{V}A$. Because changes in either $PaCO_2$ or $\dot{V}A/\dot{Q}$ distribution can change $PETCO_2$, this measure can also be misleading if used to follow trends between arterial samplings. Thus, patients with severe respiratory insufficiency of any cause and patients whose condition is acutely unstable from either a cardiovascular or a respiratory standpoint are not candidates for continuous end-tidal CO_2 monitoring as a primary surveillance technique.

Mixed expired CO_2 tension ($PECO_2$) is also a useful measurement in respiratory care. It reflects overall ventilatory efficiency in that the lower the $PECO_2$ in relation to $PaCO_2$, the higher the patient's

V_D. The $P_{E}CO_2$ in pooled expiratory gas samples is necessary for measuring $\dot{V}CO_2$ and the dead space to tidal volume ratio (V_D/V_T) in assessment for ventilator weaning.

pH

Arterial pH is an index of the body's acid-base status as affected by respiratory and metabolic processes. The pH is necessary in judging whether abnormal $PaCO_2$ values are acute or chronic and whether they threaten life, as described in Chapter 7. At present, arterial pH can be monitored only by repeated arterial blood gas sampling.

MONITORING OXYGEN TRANSPORT

General Considerations

Systemic O_2 transport, as discussed in Chapters 2 and 7, is equal to the product of the amount of O_2 carried in arterial blood, the arterial O_2 content (CaO_2), and the total blood flow to the tissues, the cardiac (left ventricular) output ($\dot{Q}_T$). Thus, systemic O_2 transport $= CaO_2 \times \dot{Q}_T$.

Arterial Oxygen Content

The CaO_2 is equal to the hemoglobin concentration in grams per 100 ml of blood times the O_2 carrying capacity of the hemoglobin (normally 1.34 ml O_2/gm) times the SaO_2, plus the small amount of O_2 normally dissolved in blood (0.003 ml/100 ml) times the PaO_2. All these variables can be measured; the most important are the hemoglobin concentration and the SaO_2.

Cardiac Output

Calculated Values. The $\dot{Q}_T$ is the product of heart rate (HR) and stroke volume (SV); it also may be calculated by dividing the systemic perfusion pressure [mean arterial pressure (MAP) minus right atrial pressure] by the systemic vascular resistance (SVR). Although HR is easily counted and SV can be measured by echocardiographic techniques, determinations of the latter variables are relatively crude so far. The SVR cannot be measured directly, although MAP and right atrial pressure can be, so other methods are used to measure $\dot{Q}_T$.

Indicator Dilution. The most commonly used clinical method for measuring $\dot{Q}_T$ is the indicator dilution technique. Although dyes may be used for this purpose, thermodilution is usually employed.

Thermodilution requires a catheter with openings in the right atrium and in the pulmonary artery. A bolus of cold liquid is injected rapidly into the right atrium, causing its negative heat to be diluted by mixing with blood as it passes from the right atrium, through the right ventricle, and into the pulmonary artery. A thermistor senses the temperature of the blood passing the distal catheter opening, and with the aid of a computer, the area under the cooling curve caused by the injected bolus can be calculated and expressed as $\dot{Q}T$ in liters per second. Five per cent glucose in water, 10 ml at $0°$ C, is used for the cold injection in adult patients. Care is taken to inject the bolus at a constant, reproducible rate, and the average of three measurements is used as the $\dot{Q}T$.

The thermodilution technique has several potential limitations, the most important of which is that it measures right ventricular output, which may differ from that of the left ventricle from beat to beat. Thermodilution also has several possible sources of error, on the part of the person performing the measurements and the instruments used. (The references listed at the end of this chapter provide further information.)

The Fick Method. The Fick equation holds that $\dot{Q}T$ is equal to the body's O_2 consumption $(\dot{V}O_2)$ divided by the amount of O_2 extracted by the peripheral tissues, which is the difference between the arterial and mixed venous O_2 contents $[CaO_2 - C\bar{v}O_2$ or $C(a-\bar{v})O_2]$. The CaO_2 and $C\bar{v}O_2$ can be calculated from simultaneously obtained samples of arterial and mixed venous blood; a pulmonary artery catheter is required for the latter. The $\dot{V}O_2$ may be calculated from the differences between the inspired and expired fractions of O_2 (FIO_2, FEO_2) in a sampling of expired gas. However, gas samples are technically difficult to collect in mechanically ventilated patients, and the difference between FIO_2 and FEO_2 approaches the measurement error for most O_2 analyzers when $\dot{V}E$ exceeds 10 L/min, as it often does in patients. One way around these logistical difficulties is to assume that $\dot{V}O_2$ is constant and equal to the normal value of 250 ml/min. Unfortunately, however, these assumptions rarely apply to sick patients. Thus, although the Fick principle provides conceptual insights (as discussed later in this chapter), it is difficult to use in intensive care monitoring.

INVASIVE HEMODYNAMIC MONITORING TECHNIQUES

Arterial Catheters

As noted previously, the need for continuous pressure monitoring and for repeated sampling of arterial blood often mandates that indwelling arterial catheters be used in critically ill patients. The main complications of arterial catheters—thrombosis and infection—can be minimized if care is taken in insertion and maintenance and if the catheter is removed promptly when no longer essential.

Central Venous Catheters

Passage of a catheter into the right atrium via the superior or inferior vena cava permits measurement of right ventricular end-diastolic pressure (preload) and hence systemic return to the heart. However, in acute respiratory failure of any etiology, or in the presence of intrinsic cardiac disease, right atrial pressure cannot be assumed to reflect left atrial end-diastolic pressure, that is, left-sided filling pressure and left-ventricular preload. Elevated left atrial pressure can coexist with normal or even low right atrial pressures and vice versa because of differences in the compliance characteristic of the two ventricles. In addition, vena caval or right atrial blood cannot be used to represent mixed venous blood; the latter must be sampled from the pulmonary artery to avoid error from inadequate mixing. Thus, central venous catheters cannot provide adequate pressure monitoring or blood sampling for critically ill patients, and their use has diminished significantly.

Balloon-Tipped Pulmonary Artery (Swan-Ganz) Catheters

General Considerations. Although direct measurement of left atrial pressures would permit monitoring of left ventricular preload, this is not done because of the difficulty and danger of the direct left-sided approach. However, if a catheter with an inflated balloon just proximal to the distal tip is carried by the flow of blood into a branch of a pulmonary artery as far as it will go until it "wedges" there, so that the branch is momentarily occluded and blood flow in it and its downstream pulmonary vein ceases, then the pressure sensed by the catheter tip will be that transmitted back through the pulmonary veins from the left atrium. In other words, during peripheral pulmonary artery occlusion, the pulmonary artery wedge pressure (PPAW) reflects left atrial pressure, which is the same as left ventricular pressure at end-diastole, when the mitral valve is open. Left-sided filling pressures can thus be monitored by a series of brief pulmonary artery occlusions, achieving access to left ventricular preload measurements without actually entering the left side of the heart.

In addition to supplying information about PPAW, the pulmonary artery catheter also can be used to determine pressures in the central veins, the right atrium and ventricle, and the pulmonary artery as it is being inserted. When the balloon is deflated and flow is present through the pulmonary artery, samples of mixed venous blood may be obtained through the tip. A hole at the right atrial level provides a site for the cold injection used for the thermodilution measurement of $\dot{Q}T$. Pulmonary artery catheters are also available with additional ports for assessing right ventricular function, and with fiberoptic bundles for continuous monitoring of mixed venous oxygen saturation.

Indications. The major indications for passage of a pulmonary artery catheter are:

1. To guide fluid management in critically ill patients, especially those with shock, ARDS, severe cardiac disease, and acute renal failure.

2. To optimize O_2 transport and prevent cardiovascular compromise in PEEP therapy (especially important when levels above 10 to 15 cm H_2O are used).

3. To separate cor pulmonale from left ventricular failure when this cannot be done with certainty using conventional clinical signs.

4. To assess the response to O_2 therapy and exercise in patients with severe pulmonary hypertension.

5. To determine a patient's ability to withstand pulmonary resection when other evaluation gives inconclusive results.

Insertion. Pulmonary artery catheters can be inserted through the internal jugular, subclavian, antecubital, and femoral approaches. Internal jugular and subclavian approaches offer large vessels, ease in maintaining sterility of the skin site, and a short path. The internal jugular route is less likely to cause pneumothorax; the subclavian approach has the advantage of stability in avoiding inadvertent catheter movement. Left brachial and left subclavian approaches offer the easiest route because of their unidirectional bend, whereas the femoral route can be more difficult, especially if the right ventricle is enlarged. Catheter placement is easy in the femoral vein; this location also can be useful in patients with low $\dot{Q}T$, although it is the hardest site to keep clean. The antecubital fossa gives easy access but usually requires a cutdown and thus damages the vein. It is often more difficult to thread the catheter from this insertion site, and arm movement can change the position of the catheter tip.

Figure 16–1 shows how a catheter is passed into the pulmonary artery and illustrates the characteristic pressure tracings obtained at each site. The catheter is inserted through the skin and advanced until its tip enters the thorax, as indicated by the appearance of pressure swings with respiration. The balloon is then filled with air to the volume prescribed by the manufacturer. The catheter is advanced via the superior or inferior vena cava into and through the right atrium (Fig. 16–1A), past the tricuspid valve, and into the right ventricle. Arrival in the ventricle is signaled by an increase in the systolic and pulse pressures on the tracing, with the normal 20 to 35 mmHg over zero (Fig. 16–1B). The catheter is advanced further, through the pulmonic valve and into the pulmonary artery, at which point the diastolic component of the pressure tracing rises as compared with that of the right ventricle (normal = 20/5 mmHg,

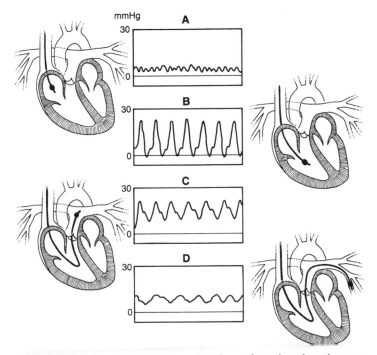

Figure 16–1. Insertion of a balloon flotation catheter into the pulmonary artery, with accompanying pressure tracings at each step. *A*, Right atrium. *B*, Right ventricle. *C*, Pulmonary artery. *D*, Pulmonary artery "wedge" position.

mean 15 mmHg) (Fig. 16–1*C*). Finally, the catheter is passed further into the pulmonary artery until its tip, surrounded by the balloon, impacts a smaller branch and a typical "wedged" tracing appears (Fig. 16–1*D*).

Several tips may facilitate passage of a pulmonary artery catheter. A number 7 French catheter is easier to pass than are smaller sizes, its greater stiffness preventing kinking and its larger lumen providing better quality tracings. The right lateral position may facilitate entry into the pulmonary outflow tract. Because catheter material can soften at body temperature, squirting a small quantity of iced saline through the lumen may restore enough stiffness to complete passage if this has taken longer than about 10 minutes. If a digital readout is used in guiding insertion, the "systole" reading should be used when passing from right atrium to right ventricle, the "diastole" reading when in the right ventricle, and "systole" again when attempting to wedge the catheter tip. The distance from ventricle to pulmonary artery outflow tract is not more than 15 cm, so the catheter should be withdrawn and another pass made if more than this has been advanced in the attempt. When the catheter is in the pulmonary artery, a wedge position should be achieved within 8 to 10 cm. The insertion of approximately 0.8 ml of air into the balloon should be all that is required to wedge the catheter.

Fluoroscopy can be of considerable help during catheter passage but is usually not necessary. When the procedure is complete and the catheter tip has been withdrawn from the wedge position to prevent ischemia and thrombosis in the distal vessel, a portable chest roentgenogram should be obtained promptly to confirm appropriate placement and to assure that no pneumothorax has occurred. If the catheter tip is more than about 3 cm beyond the hilum, an increased chance of pulmonary infarction develops, and the tip should be pulled back. This may not be required if the catheter continues to wedge with a 0.8-ml volume.

Catheters usually go to areas with the greatest flow, which in a supine patient means into a pulmonary artery directed posteriorly. They are thus usually placed in a lung region in which vascular pressures are always greater than airway pressures and the catheter "sees" pulmonary arterial or Ppaw pressure as intended. Sometimes, however, the catheter may rest in a pulmonary artery whose flow is interrupted by the surrounding airway (alveolar) pressure during all or part of the respiratory cycle. This is more likely to occur during PEEP therapy or in the presence of severe obstructive lung disease or hypovolemia. In such circumstances the pressures registered from the catheter reflect alveolar pressure and may be erroneously high. This can usually be detected by examining the pressure tracing (rather than just a digital readout) for the characteristic vascular patterns (see Fig. 16–1). A significant respiratory variation should be present if the catheter is measuring alveolar pressure. If there is a suspicion of malpositioning of the catheter as described here, a cross-bed lateral roentgenogram, taken with the patient in the same position in which pressure readings were obtained, will clarify the catheter's location in the chest's anterior-posterior dimension. It is more likely to give artifactual readings if it lies above the level of the left atrium.

These factors can help to confirm that a pulmonary artery catheter is "wedged." In this position, the phasic pulmonary artery tracing flattens into a characteristic left atrial pattern. The mean Ppaw is lower than mean pulmonary artery pressure. Also, blood aspirated very slowly from the catheter in the "wedge" position should be fully saturated pulmonary venous blood. This last rule, however, may not hold in the presence of ARDS.

Interpretation. Several practical factors are crucial to obtaining meaningful information from a pulmonary artery catheter. The pressures measured are dynamic, not static, and the values used should be the average of at least two separate readings. Wedge pressures should not be recorded until distal venous runoff ceases, which may take 5 to 10 seconds in some patients. The PPAW should be measured at the same point in the respiratory cycle each time (end-expiration is best, as there are no superimposed pressures and it is easily identified). Also, the patient should always be in the same position, although elevation of the backrest to 20 degrees does not affect the measurement. Uncontrollable agitation renders all pressure readings erroneous, and in such situations a valid PPAW reading may simply not be possible. Fundamental to clinically useful data collection are careful zeroing of the pressure transducer to the same (left atrial) level on the patient's chest every time, and reading of the PPAW from a calibrated tracing, rather than a digital readout, in order to be sure the numbers are not artifactual.

Measurements of vascular pressures, and especially PPAW during therapy with PEEP, are an area of confusion and controversy. A common question is whether a PPAW value obtained during PEEP accurately reflects true intracavitary left atrial pressure. The answer is that it does, so long as the pressure tracing shows the characteristic "wedge" pattern. But does it correspond to what the PPAW would be without the PEEP? Probably not, because PEEP physiologically alters intrathoracic hemodynamics. If taken off PEEP the patient would quickly manifest a different set of cardiovascular and airway pressures reflecting increased venous return to the thorax and other changes; these too would be accurate if correctly measured, but they would not necessarily reflect the situation present during PEEP. It seems most reasonable to measure the pressures that apply to the patient during therapy rather than during a brief interval without it, and for this reason mechanical ventilation or PEEP is not discontinued when making measurements.

The amount of PEEP should not be subtracted from the PPAW reading. Instead, a valid rule of thumb for estimating the effect of PEEP is to assume that approximately one-half the PEEP is transmitted to the left atrium, or about 1.5 mmHg for every 5 cm H_2O of PEEP. Because PPAW is usually measured in millimeters of mercury and PEEP in centimeters of water, both must be seen in the same units. Thus, about half of the converted PEEP magnitude is then subtracted from the PPAW reading to give an approximation of true intracavitary left atrial distending pressure. As an example, if in a given patient on 20 cm H_2O PEEP, a PPAW reading of 26 mmHg is obtained, subtracting 6 mmHg (1.5 mmHg/5 cm H_2O PEEP) yields an intracavitary true left atrial pressure of 19 mmHg. When PEEP is increased, the measured PPAW should never increase by more than half the amount; if this happens, airway pressure is probably being detected rather than left atrial pressure.

Measurement of PPAW in patients with severe airflow obstruction is technically difficult to perform with accuracy because of coexistent wide intrathoracic pressure swings when these patients breathe spontaneously. Readings should be made at end-expiration, and the mean of several separate measurements should be used. In addition, "auto PEEP" should be looked for and the wedge pressure corrected in the same manner used for PEEP. In some patients with agitation or severe distress, valid PPAW measurements simply cannot be made until these resolve or improve.

Fluid Challenge. The pulmonary artery catheter makes possible the direct assessment of circulatory dynamics in patients whose volume status is unclear. However, a single measurement may not completely clarify the issue. In such instances a fluid challenge can be employed as a monitoring tool. Having assessed the patient's cardiovascular function as extensively as the clinical situation dictates—by using MAP, urine output, PPAW, and thermodilution $\dot{Q}T$—the clinician rapidly infuses a bolus of fluid, usually 50 to 200 ml over 15 to 20 minutes, and repeats the assessment after 5 to 10 minutes. Using this procedure the appropriate fluid therapy for the individual patient can be judged according to the response elicited. An abrupt rise in PPAW of 5 to 7 mmHg or more, or the onset of dyspnea, signals excessive fluid administration, whereas an improvement in the parameters measured, along with a lesser increment in PPAW, suggests that the infusion of more fluid will further improve circulatory dynamics.

Complications. Numerous complications can result from the insertion, maintenance, and use of a pulmonary artery catheter. Perhaps the most frequent of these are the generation of erroneous, artifactual, or improperly collected data and the misuse of good data by staff who do not fully understand the measurements. These detriments to good patient care can be eliminated by scrupulous attention to technique and thorough familiarity with the physiology underlying the use of the catheter. Several other complications occur, including bleeding, infection, pneumothorax, and local trauma to nerves and other tissues at the insertion site. Once inside the thorax, a catheter can produce serious dysrhythmias, air embolism, direct valve damage, laceration or rupture of a pulmonary artery, and pulmonary infarction distal to a catheter left too long in the wedged position. Familiarity with these and other potential complications will help decrease the likelihood of their occurrence.

Infection at the catheter insertion site can be minimized if special effort is made to keep the area sterile. Dressings should be changed daily. As a general principle, a pulmonary artery catheter should be removed or changed in 72 hours; lack of other access sites may occasionally demand extension of this period, although this may increase the risk of infection.

MONITORING TISSUE OXYGENATION

Therapy to improve tissue oxygenation (see Chapter 14) is aimed at providing a steady supply of O_2 to the tissues that is adequate for their metabolic needs. According to the Fick equation, these needs—the $\dot{V}O_2$—are the product of $\dot{Q}T$ and the peripheral O_2 extraction, $CaO_2 - C\bar{v}O_2$ or $C(a-\bar{v})O_2$. Oxygen supply—O_2 transport—is identified by the terms $\dot{Q}T$ and CaO_2 in this equation. The Fick equation predicts that $\dot{Q}T$, $C(a-\bar{v})O_2$, or both must increase to maintain an increasing $\dot{V}O_2$. It has been assumed, therefore, that O_2 supply is set by O_2 demand.

In keeping with this assumption, the $C(a-\bar{v})O_2$ or the $C\bar{v}O_2$ has been used as an indicator of the adequacy of tissue oxygenation. Even more popular indicators are the PO_2 of mixed venous blood ($P\bar{v}O_2$) and the mixed venous O_2 saturation ($S\bar{v}O_2$) obtained by pulmonary artery catheterizations. It generally is accepted that a marked decline in the $P\bar{v}O_2$ from the normal level of 40 mmHg or an SaO_2 below 75 per cent indicates inadequate tissue oxygenation. This inadequacy is attributed to the CaO_2 and especially the $\dot{Q}T$, because it is believed that the peripheral tissues are extracting more O_2 from their diminished supply of oxygenated blood. In fact, the $P\bar{v}O_2$ and $S\bar{v}O_2$ frequently are used to estimate $\dot{Q}T$, especially when thermodilution techniques are not available.

Although this is appropriate in many patients, it may not apply to those with severe ARDS. Recent studies have shown that $\dot{V}O_2$ varies directly with $\dot{Q}T$ and CaO_2 in certain patients with ARDS; in other words, $\dot{V}O_2$ may be set by O_2 supply rather than vice versa. As a result, in these individuals, $C(a-\bar{v})O_2$ may not vary with changes in $\dot{Q}T$ to the degree expected if $\dot{V}O_2$ remains constant, especially in the setting of a very low $\dot{Q}T$. The mechanisms accounting for these findings are not clear, although alterations in regional blood flow or O_2 extraction or both may be responsible. It also is not clear whether the findings are due to ARDS, to PEEP, or to both. Nevertheless, the link between O_2 supply and demand implies that the $C\bar{v}O_2$, $P\bar{v}O_2$, and $S\bar{v}O_2$ may not accurately reflect the adequacy of tissue oxygenation in patients with severe ARDS. Of course, the same is true in cyanide poisoning, in which severe tissue hypoxia exists in the presence of an elevated $P\bar{v}O_2$, owing to a paralysis of intracellular respiration.

Given the limitations of the $P\bar{v}O_2$, what is the optimal indicator of tissue oxygenation? Ideally, the clinician requires some measurement of tissue activity or performance: lactate to pyruvate ratios from key tissue beds as reflections of alveolar metabolism, for example, or sophisticated tests of brain function. Yet these are not generally available. Until they are, the clinician must assess all hemodynamic and clinical data in concert with simple bedside observation, including a careful mental status exam.

RECOMMENDED READING

1. Balk RA, and Bone RC: Patient monitoring in the intensive care unit. *In* Burton GG, et al. (eds.): *Respiratory Care: A Guide to Clinical Practice.* 3rd ed. Philadelphia, J. B. Lippincott Co., 1991, pp. 705–717.

2. Benson MS, and Pierson DJ: Auto-PEEP during mechanical ventilation of adults. *Respir Care* 33:557–565, 1988.

3. Conference on Monitoring Critically Ill Patients. *Respir Care* 30:406–499, 549–636, 1985.

4. Glauser FL, et al.: Worsening oxygenation in the mechanically ventilated patient: Causes, mechanisms, and early detection. *Am Rev Respir Dis* 138:458–465, 1988.

5. Kacmarek RM: Assessment and monitoring of ventilatory muscle function. *In* Pierson DJ, and Kacmarek RM (eds.): *Foundations of Respiratory Care.* New York, Churchill Livingstone, 1992, pp. 555–560.

6. Kacmarek RM: Assessment of gas exchange and acid-base status. *In* Pierson DJ, and Kacmarek RM (eds.): *Foundations of Respiratory Care.* New York, Churchill Livingstone, 1992, pp. 477–504.

7. Luce JM: Hemodynamic and respiratory monitoring in critical care medicine. *In* Kelley WN (ed.): *Textbook of Internal Medicine.* 2nd ed. Philadelphia, J. B. Lippincott Co., 1992, pp. 1845–1849.

8. Noninvasive monitoring. *Respir Care* 35:482–601, 640–746, 1990.

9. Pierson DJ: Alveolar rupture during mechanical ventilation: Role of PEEP, peak airway pressure, and distending volume. *Respir Care* 33:472–484, 1988.

10. Tobin MJ: Respiratory monitoring in the intensive care unit. *Am Rev Respir Dis* 138:1625–1642, 1988.

11. Voyce SJ, et al.: Pulmonary artery catheters. *In* Rippe JM, et al. (eds.): *Intensive Care Medicine.* 2nd ed. Boston, Little, Brown and Co., 1991, pp. 48–72.

12. Wiedemann HP: Assessment and monitoring of cardiovascular function. *In* Pierson DJ, and Kacmarek RM (eds.): *Foundations of Respiratory Care.* New York, Churchill Livingstone, 1992, pp. 525–540.

17

HOME RESPIRATORY CARE

Home care is the provision of health care services in a patient's home rather than in the hospital or a physician's office. Respiratory home care has assumed an increasingly important role as stricter reimbursement policies have shortened hospital stays and the cost-effectiveness of managing patients in their own homes has been documented. In-home management of sicker, often technology-dependent patients has led to development of sophisticated home care delivery systems and the emergence of the respiratory home care specialist—usually a respiratory care practitioner (respiratory therapist)—as a key liaison between physicians and patients. Unfortunately, to date the training of physicians in current respiratory home care practice has lagged behind that offered to nurses and respiratory care practitioners.

Although the field includes an expanding array of treatments and home care services, this chapter focuses on four: long-term oxygen therapy (for treatment of chronic hypoxemia and cor pulmonale), long-term ventilatory assistance (for individuals unable to breathe spontaneously or to rest the ventilatory muscles in patients with chronic respiratory insufficiency), nocturnal continuous positive airway pressure (for management of obstructive sleep apnea), and pulmonary rehabilitation (to increase functional capability in patients with a variety of chronic respiratory disorders). Information on other aspects of respiratory home care, as well as more comprehensive coverage of the modalities discussed here, can be found in the recommended reading listed at the end of this chapter.

LONG-TERM OXYGEN THERAPY

THERAPEUTIC RATIONALE

Supplemental oxygen therapy is administered to hospitalized, acutely ill, hypoxemic patients to restore adequate tissue oxygenation and to prevent cardiac dysrhythmias and other potentially serious complications of tissue hypoxia. At the time of discharge from the hospital following an infection or other acute illness, some patients may still be hypoxemic and may be prescribed supplemental oxygen therapy for use in the home for a few days or weeks during convalescence. Such short-term oxygen therapy should not be confused with long-term oxygen therapy (LTOT), which is an elective treatment prescribed for the purpose of improving hemodynamics, increasing long-term survival, and enhancing functional capabilities in patients with chronic hypoxemia whose condition is clinically stable.

Figure 17–1 shows the pathophysiologic sequence through which sustained alveolar hypoxia (along with other factors) increases pulmonary vascular resistance and leads to right ventricular hypertrophy and eventual frank cardiac failure. Although it does not normalize pulmonary arterial pressures in patients with chronic obstructive pulmonary disease (COPD), LTOT does improve hemodynamics in such individuals. If used correctly, LTOT alleviates excess mortality due to chronic hypoxemia in COPD, so that survival for any given severity of airflow obstruction (as measured by forced expiratory volume in 1 second—FEV_1) is roughly the same as in individuals without hypoxemia. In addition, LTOT can reduce the need for hospitalization, improve sleep and neuropsychological function, increase exercise capabilities, and enhance overall well-being in appropriately selected patients.

There is little evidence that breathing supplemental oxygen for less than 12 hours a day improves survival or affords other health benefits. Multicenter studies have shown that such benefits increase with the number of hours per day the oxygen is used beyond the minimum 12 to 15 hours. Accordingly, except for patients who develop hypoxemia only during sleep or exercise, the goal of therapy is continuous (24 hours/day) use, with sufficient oxygen flow to raise arterial PO_2 above 60 mmHg or arterial oxyhemoglobin saturation (SaO_2) above 90 per cent. Oxygen therapy offers merely a placebo effect for individuals without hypoxemia or when used only for short periods during dyspnea.

INDICATIONS AND PATIENT SELECTION

Improvements in survival and other benefits from LTOT have been shown only in specific clinical settings, and it is important that this expensive therapy (typically $200 to $400 a month) be prescribed only for documented indications. These indications are summarized in Table 17–1. For LTOT to be justifiable, patients should meet all the criteria listed in the table, not just some of them.

Data on the benefits of LTOT have come almost exclusively from patients with COPD; its use in cystic fibrosis, interstitial pulmonary fibrosis, kyphoscoliosis, and chronic neuromuscular

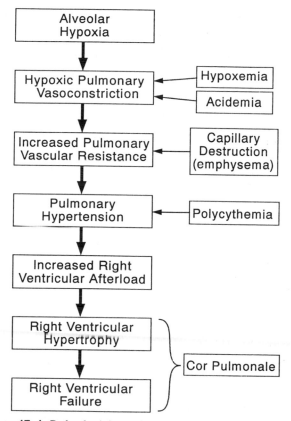

Figure 17-1. Pathophysiology of pulmonary hypertension and cor pulmonale in chronic obstructive pulmonary disease. Therapy directed at end manifestations (e.g., inotropic agents, diuretics) is only partly effective at best, and the primary focus of management is to alleviate the alveolar hypoxia through long-term oxygen therapy. (Weiss SM, and Pierson DJ. Disorders of the pulmonary circulation. *In* Pierson DJ, and Kacmarek RM (eds.): *Foundations of Respiratory Care.* New York, Churchill Livingstone, 1992, pp. 233–248. With permission.)

diseases is based on inference rather than on actual studies. The diagnosis of COPD requires a history of longstanding exertional dyspnea and/or productive cough *plus* demonstration of airflow obstruction by spirometry, typically with FEV_1 less than 60 per cent of the predicted value and FEV_1/forced vital capacity less than 0.60.

Assessment of arterial hypoxemia should be by arterial blood gas analysis. The use of pulse oximetry to determine SaO_2 is acceptable under current Medicare reimbursement guidelines in

Table 17–1. INDICATIONS FOR LONG-TERM OXYGEN THERAPY IN CHRONIC OBSTRUCTIVE PULMONARY DISEASE*

Clinical stability

Other aspects of medical management optimized (e.g., bronchodilator therapy, diuretics, chest physiotherapy, reconditioning exercise, etc.) according to individual needs of patient

Documentation of hypoxemia, while awake, at rest†

PaO_2 < 55 mmHg,‡ *or*

PaO_2 55–59 mmHg,‡ *plus* evidence of significant end-organ dysfunction due to chronic hypoxia, as shown by one or more of the following:

    a. Clinical right-sided heart failure (pedal edema)

    b. P-pulmonale (P waves 3 mm or more in leads II, III, or aVF of ECG)

    c. Erythrocytosis (hematocrit over 55%)

Demonstration that hypoxemia is chronic, by follow-up assessment, breathing room air, at least 3–4 weeks after above criteria are met, by:

    Persistence of above PaO_2 findings, *or*

    SaO_2 < 89% to correspond to PaO_2 < 55 mmHg as above§

    SaO_2 89% to correspond to PaO_2 55–59 mmHg as above§

Availability of appropriate social and economic resources

Physical and psychological capability of patient to use apparatus appropriately and safely

Willingness of patient to comply with prescribed regimen

---

*These may also apply to patients with other chronic pulmonary conditions (e.g., cystic fibrosis, interstitial pulmonary fibrosis, kyphoscoliosis), although this has not been proven by controlled clinical studies.

†If the patient does not meet these arterial oxygenation criteria at rest, while awake, but does so during exercise or while asleep, LTOT is indicated during those circumstances but not continuously.

‡Although arterial oxyhemoglobin saturation measurements using pulse or ear oximetry are currently acceptable for reimbursement purposes in the U.S., these do not provide sufficient physiological assessment for *initiation* of therapy. They may be used in follow-up, as shown later in table.

§If criteria are not met according to results of oximetry at follow-up, arterial blood gas measurements should be obtained.

the United States but does not provide sufficient physiological information for initiation of therapy (as opposed to dose titration and follow-up) and may exclude some patients who otherwise qualify for LTOT. If patients do not meet the oxygenation criteria shown in Table 17–1 while awake and at rest, but do so during sleep and/or exercise, LTOT is probably indicated. However, whether such patients benefit from oxygen use while awake and at rest is unproven, and third-party payers in the United States will generally not reimburse them for this.

Follow-up assessment of arterial oxygenation after approximately one month is crucial, since as many as half of all patients assessed for LTOT following an acute exacerbation will continue to improve and no longer be hypoxemic enough to qualify after three or four weeks. If pulse oximetry is used for this follow-up evaluation and the SaO_2 is 90 per cent or greater, an arterial blood specimen should be drawn. If the arterial PO_2 is 60 mmHg or greater, there is no evidence that LTOT will benefit the patient and it should not be prescribed.

Patients who continue to smoke are denied LTOT by some physicians. However, because of the addictive aspects of smoking, some individuals may not be capable of stopping despite earnest efforts, and this life-extending therapy should not be withheld so long as it can be used properly and never while the patient smokes.

CONTRAINDICATIONS AND ADVERSE EFFECTS

LTOT is contraindicated in any patient who is not hypoxemic. This intrusive, expensive therapy should also not be prescribed for patients who do not want it, will not use it, have altered mental status, or who cannot comprehend the instructions for its safe use.

Clinically significant pulmonary oxygen toxicity from the low flows used for LTOT has not been documented. CO_2 retention and acidemia from depression of hypoxic ventilatory drive are potential problems with administration of oxygen during acute respiratory insufficiency, but seldom occur to a clinically important degree in patients whose condition is stable. Hypercapnia can occur if excessive flows are used (e.g., producing PaO_2 values > 80 to 90 mmHg) but should not be a problem if a therapeutic goal of 60 to 70 mmHg (SaO_2 90 to 94 per cent) is employed. The great majority of patients (95 per cent in one large study) require 3 L/min or less to achieve this level of oxygenation.

Oxygen does not burn, but will enhance combustion and increase the rate and vigor with which combustible materials burn. Facial burns (corresponding to the path of the plastic cannula from nose across cheeks to ears) are uncommon and occur almost exclusively in patients who smoke while wearing their oxygen apparatus. Patients should, however, avoid open flames (stove tops and the like) when breathing oxygen.

AVAILABLE SYSTEMS FOR OXYGEN ADMINISTRATION IN THE HOME

Oxygen may be administered in the home by three types of systems: compressed gas cylinders, liquid oxygen reservoirs, and oxygen concentrators. Although "oxygen is oxygen" in the sense that there are no physical or physiologic differences among the three systems once the patient breathes the oxygen, there are substantial differences in terms of portability, convenience, and costs (Table 17–2).

Compressed Gas Cylinders. The standard delivery system utilizes 130-pound H tanks, which hold 6600 L of gaseous oxygen (55 hours at 2 L/min). Smaller E cylinders, commonly supplied as back-up supplies or for ambulation, weigh 12 pounds, hold 622 L, and last 5.5 hours at 2 L/min. They can be moved from place to place by the patient, but when combined with the necessary sturdy, wheeled cart they are too heavy to be truly portable. Still smaller cylinders weigh 5.25 to 9.0 pounds and can provide 1.5 to 3.0

Table 17–2. COMPARISON OF AVAILABLE HOME OXYGEN SOURCES

SOURCE/SYSTEM	ADVANTAGES	DISADVANTAGES
Compressed gas cylinder	No O_2 loss on storage Best source for emergency back-up O_2 supply Widely available	Heavy; cumbersome Must be taken out of home to refill Requires frequent replacement with continuous use Least visually appealing source
Liquid O_2 system	Most convenient portable units for ambulatory use (refilled in home by patient) Requires less frequent filling than cylinders Can be refilled in home	Most expensive system Continuous O_2 loss from system through evaporation when not in use Not available in all areas
Concentrator	No periodic refilling* Least expensive source for continuous use, especially with flows >2–3 L/min Most visually appealing source	Not portable Noise; heat production Expense to patient for electricity May malfunction (↓ FiO_2) without patient's knowledge

*Requires regular maintenance, however.

hours of oxygen at 2 L/min; in addition to this limited duration, these units have the disadvantage of having to be taken away to be refilled.

Liquid Oxygen Systems. These consist of a stationary reservoir (essentially a large Thermos bottle) containing liquid oxygen at −297.3°F and weighing 70 to 160 pounds when full. Each pound of liquid oxygen evaporates to produce 342 L of gaseous oxygen. The reservoir is filled directly at appropriate intervals by the durable medical equipment provider from a larger reservoir housed in a delivery truck. When not in use, these systems lose oxygen continuously through evaporation; thus, when patients are hospitalized for more than a few days, a fresh delivery should be arranged on their return home. Portable units weighing 5.0 to 13.5 pounds can be filled by the patient in the home from the stationary reservoir and provide 2.75 to 13.0 hours of oxygen flow at 2 L/min. With pulsed oxygen delivery (see below) equivalent to 2 L/min continuous flow, these portable units can provide up to 25 hours' supply. Liquid oxygen is the most expensive system, but provides the most practical system for ambulatory oxygen therapy.

Oxygen Concentrators. These are electrically powered devices that filter nitrogen out of room air by means of molecular-sieve technology, concentrating the oxygen from 21 per cent to 90 to 95 per cent at flows of up to about 5 L/min. Concentrators provide the least expensive oxygen source, particularly for patients using higher flows, since cost is unrelated to oxygen flow. Although the rental of these devices is usually reimbursed, in the United States the cost of electricity (up to $50 a month) must be borne by the patient. Current concentrator and battery technology does not permit the manufacture of units small enough for portable use, although concentrators weighing about 30 pounds that can run on an automobile cigarette lighter are commercially available.

Oxygen for LTOT is administered by nasal cannulas (prongs), or in some instances via an oxygen-conserving device (see below), rather than by mask. Many clinicians (and patients) believe that humidifying the oxygen decreases discomfort from nasal drying, nosebleeds, and skin irritation, but this is probably a placebo effect, since controlled studies have been unable to demonstrate either objective or subjective benefit from such humidification. In fact, passing the oxygen through a bubble humidifier at room temperature adds very little moisture, and patients must generally bear the added cost of the apparatus required.

OXYGEN-CONSERVING TECHNIQUES AND DEVICES

Three methods are available for achieving arterial oxygenation comparable to that from continuous oxygen flow but using less oxygen. All three approaches work, in that they reduce the number of liters required per minute. They do not necessarily reduce the overall cost of LTOT; instead, their potential usefulness is primarily from lighter portable units and increased ambulation time. In addition, transtracheal oxygen may improve patient compliance and enable severely hypoxemic patients to be more effectively and consistently oxygenated than with nasal prongs.

Reservoir devices (e.g., Oxymizer pendant and mustache cannula) utilize a low continuous oxygen flow that fills a reservoir during exhalation and then provides a bolus of oxygen during inhalation. They are larger devices than the standard cannulas, and their cumbersomeness affects patient acceptance. The cost for regular replacement must generally be borne by the patient.

Intermittent flow devices (e.g., Pulsair, Oxymatic) utilize a thermistor or pressure transducer to sense inspiration, and provide pulses of oxygen only during the inhalation phase of the respiratory cycle. They may be used with any oxygen source, and when attached to a portable oxygen unit they can markedly increase the patient's time away from home. Coverage for the costs of these electronic and/or mechanical devices is variable.

Transtracheal oxygen delivery is accomplished by means of a flexible cathether inserted percutaneously into the patient's trachea (Fig. 17–2). Dead space and wastage of oxygen during exhalation are eliminated, and the oxygen flow for the same blood oxygenation at rest is generally about half that required with nasal prongs. The cosmetic advantages of less conspicuous oxygen use in public (the catheter can be concealed under a sweater or cravat and the source

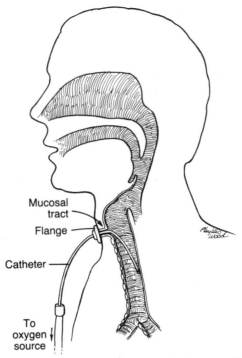

Figure 17–2. Catheter placement for transtracheal oxygen therapy. After establishment of "minitracheostomy" tract and appropriate patient education, the catheter can be irrigated and changed at home as needed.

in a handbag or satchel) are of considerable psychological benefit to some patients, and true 24-hour-a-day oxygen use becomes easier to achieve. However, transtracheal oxygen administration requires a surgical procedure, lengthy training, compliance with an ongoing maintenance regimen, and considerable expense, so that this delivery technique is appropriate for only highly motivated patients with adequate psychosocial and financial resources.

OXYGEN PRESCRIPTION

In the United States, any licensed physician can prescribe home oxygen therapy. In the past, home oxygen therapy was often prescribed for reasons that would not be accepted as indications today, and many patients were given this therapy without appropriate documentation of hypoxemia. Partly as a result of these factors, and because reimbursement for oxygen therapy and equipment is the largest single component of the annual federal Medicare expenditure for home care, specific, detailed documentation of the need for and administration of oxygen in the home is now required. Table 17–3 outlines the information required by Medicare and other third-party payers in the United States for reimbursement for home oxygen therapy; because few patients can afford to pay for LTOT out of their own pockets, these requirements essentially define the use of this therapy in this country.

LONG-TERM MECHANICAL VENTILATION

Although far fewer patients receive ventilatory assistance in the home as compared with LTOT (perhaps 5000 vs. 500,000 in the United States), this labor- and technology-intensive form of therapy occupies a position of disproportionate importance in home respiratory care. Long-term mechanical ventilation (LTMV) refers to mechanical ventilatory assistance administered to individuals who are not in acute respiratory failure. It is done in two distinct clinical settings: (1) LTMV as life support. This is the traditional setting

Table 17–3. COMPONENTS OF A PRESCRIPTION FOR HOME OXYGEN THERAPY

Documentation of need
  Diagnosis (e.g., COPD)
  Estimated length of need
    Short-term oxygen therapy following acute illness (> 3 months)
    Long-term oxygen therapy (presumably lifelong)*
  Arterial PO_2 (SaO_2 also acceptable for Medicare certification, but see Table 17–1)
    Conditions under which obtained (at rest; walking; exercising; sleeping)
    Oxygen supplementation if not obtained breathing air
    Date of measurement
Quantity of oxygen prescribed
  Oxygen flow rate (L/min)
  Hours per day of intended use†
Oxygen equipment prescribed
  Supply system
    Stationary source (compressed gas cylinder; liquid oxygen; concentrator)
    Portable or ambulatory source (liquid oxygen; compressed gas cylinder)
  Delivery system (nasal cannula; transtracheal catheter; reservoir oxygen-
    conserving device; intermittent flow oxygen-conserving device)
Justification for portable or ambulatory system
  Description of activities requiring portable or ambulatory oxygen
  Frequency of activities (e.g., number of trips per day or per week)

Based on U.S. Medicare form HCFA–484 (5–90)
*Should not be ordered after acute illness without reassessment after one month (see Table 17–1).
†If less than 24 hours a day, specify number of hours and conditions (e.g., sleeping, walking, exercising).

for home ventilation, in which a patient is unable to be weaned from the ventilator after a bout of acute respiratory failure and would presumably die if this support were withdrawn. (2) LTMV as elective therapy. Both more recent and more controversial, this is part-time ventilatory assistance initiated in a patient whose chronic respiratory insufficiency is progressively but not acutely worsening, for the purpose of preserving function and forestalling the development of frank respiratory failure. The following discussion of LTMV in these two settings refers to the care of adult patients rather than of infants with bronchopulmonary dysplasia following the infantile respiratory distress syndrome.

LONG-TERM MECHANICAL VENTILATION AS LIFE SUPPORT

Diagnosis and Patient Selection. Extensive experience in North America and Europe has shown that LTMV is much more successful in terms of both survival and functional status in some conditions than in others. It is most successful in neuromuscular disorders such as quadriplegia secondary to high cervical spinal cord injury, central hypoventilation syndromes, poliomyelitis, muscular dystrophy and other myopathies, and peripheral nerve disorders such as bilateral diaphragmatic paralysis and the Guillian-Barré syndrome. Patients with these diagnoses receiving LTMV typically become more independent, leave the home more often, and are more likely to return to work or school than those with other conditions. A few patients with kyphoscoliosis and post-thoracoplasty respiratory insufficiency have also done well, but experience in other diseases has generally been disappointing. In the latter category are COPD, interstitial lung disease, bronchiectasis, and amyotrophic lateral sclerosis. Patients with these conditions, who tend to be older with progressive pulmonary disease and complicating medical illnesses, generally do not achieve prolonged survival or an improved quality of life with LTMV.

Numerous factors in addition to the primary diagnosis must be considered in patient selection (Table 17–4).

Preparation for Discharge. The patient must be medically ready for discharge from the hospital, and the need for readmission should not be anticipated for at least a month. Ventilator settings (on full, not partial, ventilatory support) should be stable without need for adjustment. Gas exchange, metabolic and acid-base status, and nutritional status should be adequate and stable. Infections, dysrhythmias and other cardiovascular instability, and any other active medical problems need to be corrected or controlled prior to discharge to the home setting. The patient should have a tracheostomy, not an endotracheal tube. Adequate management of the airway and of respiratory tract secretions should be estab-

Table 17–4. PATIENT CHARACTERISTICS THAT MAY DETERMINE SUCCESS IN HOME VENTILATOR CARE

	IDEAL	ACCEPTABLE	UNACCEPTABLE
Individual coping styles	Optimistic Motivated Resourceful Flexible Adaptable Sense of humor Directive	Optimistic Motivated Sense of humor	None
Support systems	Close family and social supports	Social supports	Lack of family and social supports
Education	College degree Ability to learn	Ability to learn Mechanically astute	Altered mental status Inability to learn
Financial resources	Adequate personal assets Optimal health insurance coverage	Adequate health insurance coverage	Lack of personal assets Lack of health insurance
Medical condition	Stable neuromuscular disease Significant "free time" off ventilator No other medical illnesses	Stable neuromuscular or obstructive airway disease Limited or no "free time" off ventilator	Medically unstable
Self-Care ability	Ability to provide self-care and/or direct others	Able to provide self-care	Unable to care for self or direct others

From Gilmartin ME: Long-term mechanical ventilation: Patient selection and discharge planning. Resp Care 36:205–216, 1991.

lished, with the patient and/or home caregiver able to clear and maintain the airway.

LTMV for the ventilator-dependent patient requires a team effort. The discharge planning coordinator, who may be a respiratory care practitioner, a nurse, or some other member of the team, is the key individual, who must serve as liaison among four categories of participants in the patient's management: the patient and his or her family; the patient's physician; the hospital team (respiratory care, nursing, rehabilitation services, speech therapy, social services, psychiatry/psychology, and nutritional services); and the home care team (durable medical equipment company, community nursing agencies, community services, schools, and the like).

One thing that must be established before the patient can go home is who will be carrying out the actual care of the patient, and this will vary according to the patient's medical condition, age, socioeconomic status, and numerous other factors. Some patients can perform most of their own care, while others require a dedicated caregiver, who may or may not be a family member. This individual must acquire a set of specific skills prior to the patient's arrival in the home (Table 17–5).

Ventilators and Equipment. The needs of patients receiving LTMV differ markedly from those encountered in the intensive care unit (ICU), and a special home care ventilator should be used. Although all home care ventilators manufactured in the United States have several modes, controlled mechanical ventilation (CMV) or assist-control (A/C or AMV) are preferable to intermittent mandatory ventilation (IMV) or pressure-limited ventilation for home use. Unlike most modern ICU ventilators, home ventilators are unable to compensate for the markedly increased work the patient must do to breathe spontaneously through the system, and humidification may also be inadequate during the spontaneous component of ventilation with IMV. Some patients require supplemental oxygen, but this can generally be bled into the system at 1 to 3 L/min without the necessity of a high-pressure, ICU-type blender system. Patients receiving LTMV as life support will almost always have been endotracheally intubated initially, followed by tracheostomy, and this route of ventilation should generally be continued in the home setting.

Table 17–5. LONG-TERM VENTILATION: SKILLS NEEDED BY PATIENT AND/OR CAREGIVERS BEFORE DISCHARGE

A. Self-Care Techniques
   Airway management:
     Tracheostomy and stoma care
     Cuff care
     Tracheal suctioning
     Changing tracheostomy tube
     Changing tracheostomy ties
   Chest physical therapy techniques:
     Percussion
     Vibration
     Coughing
   Medication administration:
     Oral
     Inhaled
   Bed-to-chair transfers
   Feeding tube care
   Indwelling catheter care
   Implantable IV line care
   Bowel care
   Switching from ventilator to weaning
       device

B. Equipment Maintenance
   Ventilator care
   Humidifier
   Suction machines
   Battery and charger
   Oxygen administration
   Manual resuscitator
   Troubleshooting for problems
   Cleaning and disinfection

C. Emergency Measures
   Ventilator failure
   Power failure
   Dislodged tracheostomy tube
   Obstructed airway
   Cuff leaks
   Shortness of breath
   Ventilator circuitry problems
   Infection
   Falls
   Bleeding
   Cardiac arrest

From Gilmartin ME: Long-term mechanical ventilation: Patient selection and discharge planning. Resp Care 36:205–216, 1991.

LONG-TERM MECHANICAL VENTILATION AS ELECTIVE THERAPY

Rationale. Muscle fatigue is a condition in which there is a loss in the capacity for developing force and/or velocity of muscle contraction, resulting from muscle activity under load, that is reversible by rest. Much attention has focused on the ventilatory muscles during the last decade, and it is currently believed that progressive muscle fatigue is an important contributor to the development of acute ventilatory failure in patients with chronic respiratory insufficiency. It is further believed, although not proven, that unloading (resting) the ventilatory muscles will enable them to recover from the fatigued state, thereby improving their contractility and endurance. In addition, it is known that ventilatory drives and other aspects of respiratory function change during sleep and that chronic ventilatory insufficiency may be exacerbated during sleep.

Studies have shown that signs of ventilatory muscle fatigue can be reduced or eliminated following a period of controlled ventilation. In view of this, there is considerable current interest in electively resting the ventilatory muscles, for a few hours on a daily basis, with the hope that this could improve ventilatory function between these periods of rest. If such were the case, and if ventilatory muscle fatigue were important in the genesis of progressive deterioration in patients with chronic ventilatory insufficiency, then LTMV as elective therapy might improve function, reduce the need for hospitalization, forestall the development of acute ventilatory failure, and even increase survival. While convincing proof of these beneficial effects is not yet at hand, a number of investigators have obtained encouraging results in certain patient groups, and recommendations can be made about which patients would be expected to benefit most from this therapy.

Diagnosis and Patient Selection. With the exception of acute cervical spinal cord transection and other paralytic states, the diagnostic groups best suited to LTMV as elective therapy are the same ones listed above for LTMV as life support: muscular dystrophy, post-polio chronic respiratory insufficiency, kyphoscoliosis, and the late sequelae of thoracoplasty. Patients with these problems have respiratory insufficiency in the setting of restrictive disease that does not primarily affect the lung parenchyma. Individuals with obstructive lung disease (e.g., COPD) or with primary restrictive pulmonary disease are not good candidates, and clinical experience with this therapy in such settings has been disappointing.

Because it is an elective treatment applied to patients who are less seriously ill than those discussed in the preceding section, part-time ventilatory assistance does not require such extensive resources and training. Patients can usually initiate and terminate the session of mechanically assisted breathing by themselves, it is unnecessary to have a caregiver in attendance, and no back-up ventilator is required. In most instances the period of ventilatory assistance is timed to coincide with or include the patient's hours of sleep.

Ventilators and Equipment. A wider array of apparatus can potentially be used for part-time ventilatory support than when such support is required 24 hours a day. Most patients who receive LTMV as elective therapy do not have a tracheostomy, and direct airway access can be avoided in most instances. Positive pressure ventilation, using a standard home care ventilator, can be delivered via mouthpiece or full-face mask, but is most commonly done today with a nasal mask. Air leaks around the mask are usual, and a period of close observation and adjustment in the clinic or hospital may be required to obtain an acceptable, consistent tidal volume. Bi-PAP, a new system that alternates high and low levels of continuous positive airway pressure (CPAP), may also prove effective for part-time ventilatory assistance, although its efficacy and patient preferability in comparison with standard intermittent positive-pressure ventilation have not been established.

Negative-pressure ventilation can be used successfully in some patients, either by cuirass or poncho-type wrap ventilator; tank ventilators (iron lungs) are also effective but are poorly suited to elective therapy because an assistant/observer is required. As with positive-pressure ventilators, careful, sometimes lengthy individual adjustment is required to achieve successful ventilation with settings acceptable to the patient. Another type of device that can be employed successfully in this situation is the rocking bed, a mechanized bed that is pivoted in the middle to rock back and forth up to about 30 times a minute, through an arc of up to 60 degrees. This device relies on shifting of the abdominal contents to inflate and deflate the lungs; it works best in slightly overweight patients whose lung compliance is normal.

NASAL CONTINUOUS POSITIVE AIRWAY PRESSURE

Therapeutic Rationale. Obstructive sleep apnea (OSA) is primarily a disorder of men with a long history of loud snoring, and affects 1 to 4 per cent of the adult male population. Patients with OSA periodically stop breathing during sleep, primarily because an abnormally lax upper airway is sucked closed by the negative pressure of inspiration; although inspiratory efforts continue, there is no air movement, and progressive hypoxemia and respiratory acidosis develop. After a period of apnea that can vary from 10 to 60 seconds or more, the patient overcomes the obstruction with an intense inspiratory effort accompanied by arousal and loud snoring. This sequence may be repeated 30 to 60 times per hour or more throughout the night. OSA produces sleep deprivation and daytime hypersomnolence, can lead to cor pulmonale and right-sided cardiac failure, and is often accompanied by systemic arterial hypertension, behavioral disturbances, and other disabling clinical manifestations.

Although there are other types of sleep apnea that may respond to respiratory stimulant drugs, these are generally ineffective in OSA. Therapy for OSA is primarily directed at relieving the physical obstruction to airflow during sleep. Tracheostomy and weight loss are the "gold standards" of therapy, although the intrusiveness and complications of the former and typical lack of success of the latter make them far from ideal. Surgical procedures aimed at enlarging the upper airway to prevent obstruction, which are successful in a variable number of patients, include uveopalatopharyngoplasty (debulking of the hypopharynx) and mandibular advancement (pulling the tongue forward). Nasal CPAP is a much less invasive approach to therapy that attempts to maintain upper airway patency by preventing intraluminal pressure from dropping low enough for closure to occur.

Patient Selection. Although snoring occurs in as many as one fourth of all men and a lesser number of women, OSA is much less common. Accurate diagnosis of clinically significant OSA requires a formal sleep study (polysomnography). In most sleep laboratories, once OSA is detected, the effects of different levels of nasal CPAP will automatically be assessed, so that both diagnosis and determination of the appropriate therapy can be accomplished at the same time. However, even among patients with polysomnographically documented OSA and individualized prescriptions for nasal CPAP, successful use of this therapy requires motivation and consistent compliance with the regimen as prescribed.

Equipment and Practical Considerations. Several commercial CPAP systems are available for home use. Most are small, portable, and reasonably straightforward to use. The nasal mask must fit the patient's face and be held in place by straps or a harness (Fig. 17–3). Most patients require 7.5 to 15.0 cm H_2O of CPAP for elimination of apneas. For some patients the improvement in symptoms is so dramatic that regular use of the device is no problem; for others it becomes unacceptably intrusive, and long-term compliance cannot be obtained. Patient selection is obviously an important determinant of success, but in one large series, more than two thirds of patients adhered to the therapy for up to 25 months. Minor side effects such as dryness of nose and throat and soreness of eyes were common, but more serious adverse effects (e.g., pneumothorax) did not occur.

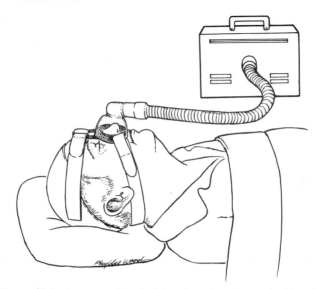

Figure 17–3. Apparatus for administration of continuous positive airway pressure via nasal mask. Several commercial versions of this basic design are available.

PULMONARY REHABILITATION

Definition and Goals. The American College of Chest Physicians defines pulmonary rehabilitation as "an art of medical practice wherein an individually tailored, multidisciplinary program is formulated which, through accurate diagnosis, therapy, emotional support, and education stabilizes or reverses both the physio- and the psychopathology of pulmonary diseases and attempts to return the patient to the highest possible functional capacity allowed by his or her pulmonary handicap and overall life situation." Pulmonary rehabilitation is based on the assumption that patient disability and physical impairment need not be synonymous and that ability to function may be increased even though pulmonary handicap remains.

Pulmonary rehabilitation generally is administered to patients with chronic respiratory insufficiency, the overwhelming majority of whom have COPD. Most of these patients suffer from severe dyspnea, and prevention, control, and tolerance of this dyspnea is a primary goal for the program. Rehabilitation is most likely to succeed in patients whose airflow obstruction is at least partially reversible. The absence of other serious medical conditions is also a favorable prognostic factor. Most important are such personality factors as optimism and an ability to participate in organized programs. Rehabilitation is unlikely to be of benefit in patients whose status is medically unstable or in those who are not motivated to participate.

Components of a Successful Program. Table 17–6 summarizes the main components of a comprehensive pulmonary rehabilitation program. Such a program does not require particular categories of participants so much as access to the array of services and capabilities shown in the table—it may involve as many as 10 or 15 health professionals or as few as 3 or 4. The "main movers" of a rehabilitation program are usually a physician, a respiratory care practitioner, and/or a respiratory nurse specialist, with access to the skills of dietitians, physical therapists, occupational therapists, social workers, psychologists, and psychiatrists.

Exercise Reconditioning. Pulmonary rehabilitation patients often have coexistent cardiac disease and other medical conditions and are in poor general physical condition. Their avoidance of exercise often reflects an ever-worsening progression from dyspnea to decreased activity, increasing debility, social withdrawal, and feelings of fear and hopelessness. Reconditioning exercises are aimed at slowing or stopping this progression on a psychological and physiological basis. From a psychological position, regular exercise can enhance one's ability to perform the activities of daily living more efficiently and can engender a sense of optimism and a greater enjoyment of life. From a physiological standpoint, reconditioning can result in decreased heart rate, blood pressure, and serum lactate concentration and increased blood flow to and oxygen extraction from working muscles at a given level of work. Although rehabilitation patients may not be able to achieve the same degree of physiological improvement as healthy individuals (e.g., increases in maximum oxygen consumption of 10 to 20 per cent), objective improvement can be anticipated in some, and subjective benefit in most, of the patients who participate.

Reconditioning programs for pulmonary patients are modeled after those created for persons with heart disease and need to be individualized for a given patient's degree of impairment. They should also be based on an accurate assessment of pulmonary function and cardiac reserve as part of a progressive exercise testing protocol. Arterial oxygenation should be assessed at rest and during exercise, and supplemental oxygen administered if necessary to keep arterial PO_2 greater than 55 to 60 mmHg (SaO_2 more than 85 to 90 per cent) under these conditions. From this and other information, an exercise prescription should be derived. This prescription should focus not on activities requiring short bursts of energy, but rather on gradually progressive exercises involving warm-up, work, and cool-down periods.

Table 17–6. COMPONENTS OF A PULMONARY REHABILITATION PROGRAM

COMPONENT	DESCRIPTION	PURPOSE/RATIONALE	COMMENTS
Patient and family education	Individual and/or group instruction; printed materials; videotapes	Increase understanding and adaptation to illness; improve compliance with management regimen	Often neglected; other aspects of program may be ineffective as a result of failure here; need not involve formalized program
Smoking cessation	Counseling; various structured and individualized programs; supplementation with nicotine gum as necessary	Decrease rate of loss of pulmonary function; extend survival; decrease sputum production	Requires active involvement of physician as well as others in program; should be part of management for all smoking patients
Avoidance of inhaled irritants	Avoidance of smoke, fumes, dusts, and other exposures that increase patient's symptoms	Prevention of acute exacerbations; improvement in functional status; decrease medication use	Often requires assistance from spouse, employer, etc.
Prevention of infection	Influenza vaccine; pneumococcal vaccine; avoidance of persons with respiratory infections	Avoidance of complicating infections, especially in winter months; prevention of acute exacerbations; reduce morbidity and mortality	Yearly influenza vaccination required, usually in fall; patients with severe disease should avoid crowds and persons with respiratory infections, especially during influenza season
Medications	Bronchodilators; corticosteroids; antibiotics; diuretics; antidepressants, etc.	Maximize pulmonary function; improve functional status	Improvement in airflow limited in most patients, but empirical trials warranted; role of antibiotics controversial; inhaled steroids probably ineffective in COPD; depression common and often unrecognized
Long-term O_2 therapy	Continuous administration of O_2 via nasal cannulas or transtracheal catheter to keep PaO_2 >60 mmHg (SaO_2 >90%)	Reduce excess mortality due to chronic hypoxemia and cor pulmonale; decrease need for hospitalization; improve neuropsychiatric function; improve quality of life	For selected patients only (see text and Table 17–1)

Secretion clearance therapy	Therapeutic coughing; systemic hydration; postural drainage; chest percussion	Improve airway function; facilitate expectoration; reduce symptoms	Regimen must be individualized; not necessary for all patients
Breathing exercises; breathing retraining	Instruction and assistance with slow, deep breathing; pursed-lip breathing; focus on abdominal/diaphragmatic breathing	Reduce dyspnea during exercise and other activities of daily living; control and prevent panic attacks; decrease work of breathing	Can improve gas exchange ($\uparrow PaO_2$, $\downarrow PcCO_2$), but only while being performed; especially helpful in patients with episodes of acute severe dyspnea and anxiety
Ventilatory muscle endurance training	Training regimen involving frequent sessions of inspiration against resistance	Increase ventilatory muscle strength and resistance to fatigue; improve exercise capacity; improve activities of daily living	Whether and how this works are uncertain; any lasting benefit requires continuation of training regimen
Exercise reconditioning	Training regimen focused on somatic muscle exercise, e.g., walking, stationary bicycle, shoulder-girdle/upper extremity exercises	Improve exercise capacity; increase functional status and activities of daily living	May also benefit socialization; effective in reducing morbidity for many patients, but regimen must be ongoing
Diet modification	Counseling on size, contents, and scheduling of meals; provision of adequate caloric intake and appropriate nutritional composition	Reverse or prevent protein-calorie malnutrition; correct nutritional deficiencies	Special (expensive) pulmonary dietary products and regimens of unproven value; weight gain often difficult to achieve
Psychosocial management	Assessment and management of interpersonal, social, and economic aspects of chronic pulmonary impairment; requires access to social worker, clinical psychologist, psychiatrist, etc.	Address nonphysiological aspects of patient's disability; improve functional status and compliance with regimen; improve quality of life	Main obstacles to function and compliance with regimen often financial, family related, or emotional; failure to address these may render other components of program ineffective
Vocational rehabilitation	Assessment and modification of work environment in accordance with disease limitation; vocational counseling and job placement for employable patients who are not working	Keep patient as functional in society as possible; lessen economic burden of illness	Even patients too impaired to work can be helped at home or in special centers through assistance of occupational therapist.

Table 17–7. PHYSIOLOGICAL PARAMETERS IN VARIOUS DEGREES OF PHYSICAL EXERCISE*

CLASSIFICATION OF EXERCISE	EXAMPLES OF EXERCISE	PULSE RATE/MIN	METABOLIC RATE $\dot{V}O_2$ L/min	METABOLIC RATE Cal/min	VENTILATION Volume $\dot{V}E$	VENTILATION Rate f	VENTILATION RQ	LACTIC ACID IN MULTIPLES OF RESTING VALUE	METABOLIC EQUIVALENTS (mets)	TIME OF DURATION EXERCISE CAN BE SUSTAINED
Light Very light	Eating, washing hands and face	80	0.5		10			Normal	2.5	
Mild	Walking downstairs, propelling wheelchair	<100	0.5–1.0	<4	10–20	<14	0.85	Normal	2.5–5.0	Indefinite
Moderate	Walking 4 mph, golfing	<120	1.0–1.5	<7.5	20–35	<15	0.85	Normal	5.0–7.5	8 hours daily on the job
Optimal	Ambulating with crutches, downhill skiing	<140	1.5–2.0	<10	35–50	<16	0.90	1.5×	7.5–10.0	8 hours daily for a few weeks (seasonal work, military maneuvers)
Heavy Strenuous	Cycling 13 mph, tending furnace	<160	2.0–2.5	<12.5	50–65	<20	0.95	2×	10.0–12.5	4 hours, 2 or 3 times a week for a few weeks (special physical training)
Maximal	Ascending stairs, cross-country skiing	<180	2.5–3.0	<15	60–86	<25	1.00	5–6×	12.5–15.0	1 to 2 hours, occasionally (usually in competitive sports)
Severe Exhausting	Running upstairs	180+	3.0	15+	85	30+	2.00+	6× or more	15.0	A few minutes, rarely

*Adapted from Parmley, LF Jr. (ed.): Proceedings of the National Workshop on Exercise in the Prevention, Evaluation, and Treatment of Heart Disease. S Car Med Assoc J, 65:5, 1969. KEY: $\dot{V}O_2$ = oxygen consumption, $\dot{V}E$ = minute ventilation, f = respiratory rate, RQ = respiratory quotient, Metabolic Equivalents = multiples of resting $\dot{V}O_2$, assuming 3.5–4.0 ml/O_2/kg/min.

Stationary bicycles and treadmills are useful in assessing exercise potential and providing prolonged workouts, particularly under medical supervision, but whenever possible conditioning should involve walking and other activities that can be performed in the context of the patient's lifestyle. Exercises should be designed to stress large-muscle groups such as those of the trunk, legs, and upper extremities. Patients should be taught to analyze activities and specific exercises in terms of the expected energy expenditure so that they can modify their expectations. A brief summary of the physiological parameters associated with such activities is outlined in Table 17–7.

RECOMMENDED READING

1. Casaburi R, and Petty TL (eds.): *Principles and Practice of Pulmonary Rehabilitation.* Philadelphia, W. B. Saunders Co., 1992.
2. Christopher KL (ed.): The current status of oxygen therapy. *Probl Respir Care,* 3:549, 1990.
3. Christopher KL: Long-term oxygen therapy. *In* Pierson DJ, and Kacmarek RM (eds.): *Foundations of Respiratory Care.* New York, Churchill Livingstone, 1992, pp. 1155–1174.
4. Christopher KL, et al.: A program for transtracheal oxygen delivery. *Ann Intern Med,* 107:802–808, 1987.
5. Gilmartin ME: Long-term mechanical ventilation outside the hospital. *In* Pierson DJ, and Kacmarek RM (eds.): *Foundations of Respiratory Care.* New York, Churchill Livingstone, 1992, pp. 1185–1204.
6. Goldstein RS, and Avendano MA: Long-term mechanical ventilation as elective therapy: Clinical status and future prospects. *Respir Care,* 36:297–304, 1991.
7. Lucas J, et al.: *Home Respiratory Care.* Norwalk, Conn., Appleton & Lange, 1988.
8. Make BJ, and Gilmartin ME (eds.): Mechanical ventilation in the home. *Probl Respir Care,* 1:1988.
9. Nino-Murcia G, et al.: Compliance and side effects in sleep apnea patients treated with nasal continuous positive airway pressure. *West J Med,* 150:165–169, 1989.
10. Sullivan CE, et al.: Reversal of obstructive sleep apnea by continuous positive airway pressure applied through the nares. *Lancet,* 1:862–865, 1981.

18

CHEST TRAUMA AND SURGERY

CHEST TRAUMA

In the United States, chest injuries cause one out of every four deaths due to trauma. Two thirds of these deaths occur after patients reach the hospital and can be prevented by prompt diagnosis and correct management. Guided by a high index of suspicion for specific injuries, emergency care personnel should perform a primary survey and resuscitation of trauma patients. Only after immediately life-threatening injuries have been treated should a secondary survey and definitive care be performed.

INJURIES OF THE THORACIC CAGE

Rib Fractures

Rib fractures usually follow blunt chest trauma but also may result from forceful coughing. The fractures generally involve the third through tenth ribs and occur laterally where the ribs are not protected by chest muscles (see Fig. 1–2). Fractures of the first and second ribs require great force to the chest and are often associated with other intrathoracic damage. Fractures of the lower ribs often are associated with damage to intra-abdominal organs, especially the liver and spleen. Patients with rib fractures may manifest crepitation, swelling, and tenderness at the site of injury. Definitive diagnosis is made by physical examination aided by chest roentgenograms that may be taken from an oblique angle to highlight the ribs. Even with this roentgenographic technique, anterior fractures may be hard to see.

The most common complications of fractures are pain and limited diaphragmatic and chest wall motion, or splinting, that result in atelectasis of the underlying lung and hypoxemia through ventilation-perfusion ($\dot{V}A/\dot{Q}$) mismatching. The pain may be relieved by systemic analgesics, at the risk of ventilatory depression; by the instillation of narcotic analgesics in the epidural space of the spinal cord; or by intercostal nerve blocks in which local anesthetics are infiltrated into the intercostal nerve roots. Taping the chest to limit its movement compounds the physiological problem, worsens atelectasis, and should be avoided. The most serious initial complications of rib fracture are pneumothorax and hemothorax resulting from penetration of the pleura by the jagged ends of broken ribs. In the hours to days following rib fracture, atelectasis and pneumonia are the main complications.

Flail Chest

Flail chest occurs when three or more ribs, or the junction of ribs and the sternum, are each fractured at two points. This injury is suggested by paradoxical inward movement of the flail segment during inspiration, when the rest of the thoracic cage expands but the flail segment is pulled in. The flail fracture sites may be confirmed by routine posterior-anterior chest roentgenograms, although the sternum itself is best viewed obliquely or with tomography.

At one time, the paradoxical motion of flail segments was thought to cause a condition called pendelluft, in which inhaled gases were shifted from one lung to the other, resulting in hypoxemia through hypoventilation. In accord with this erroneous physiological model, flails were stabilized either externally, with taping or rods, or internally, with mechanical ventilation and positive end-expiration pressure (PEEP) delivered to intubated patients who were sedated, paralyzed, or hyperventilated to restrict spontaneous ventilation.

In recent years, however, clinicians have realized that the hypoxemia associated with flail chest results not from pendelluft but from a combination of many conditions, including atelectasis due to pain and splinting and contusion of the lung underlying the flail segment. These conditions may be more severe if the flail is large, but they do not necessarily require stabilization of the segment. Thus, therapy is aimed at relieving pain through the measures suggested above, correcting hypoxemia, and supporting patients while waiting for the contused lung to heal. Mechanical ventilation and PEEP are reserved for patients with acute respiratory failure, which is called post-traumatic respiratory failure in this setting and is discussed at length below.

ABERRANT AIR AND OTHER PLEURAL INJURIES

Aberrant Air

The terms *aberrant* and *extrarespiratory* are used to describe air (or some other gas) that appears where it is not normally seen following a variety of disease processes, including chest trauma. If the air is found under the skin, commonly in areas such as the thorax, head, and neck, it is called subcutaneous emphysema.

Mediastinal emphysema or pneumomediastinum refers to air in the mediastinum, which envelops the upper trachea and includes the pericardium. Pneumothorax describes air in the pleural space; pneumoperitoneum is air in the peritoneum; pneumatocele is air in the lung parenchyma.

Although air may reach these locations from an external source, as might occur when the lung is lacerated by a jagged rib end or a foreign object, it usually results from internal rupture of a bronchus or the alveoli. Such rupture may result either from trauma or from overdistention related to position pressure ventilation. When alveolar rupture occurs, the air may remain localized in the form of pneumatocele. More commonly, it may enter the distal bronchovascular space and track to the mediastinum, where it may cause pneumomediastinum or decompress into the subcutaneous tissue, the retroperitoneal space and from there into the peritoneum, or into the pleural space via the mediastinal pleura.

Although subcutaneous emphysema usually does no more than alter patient appearance, it also may prevent eye-opening and interfere with respiration. Similarly, pneumomediastinum may rarely compress the trachea, great vessels, and heart. Impaired cardiac output secondary to pneumopericardium has been reported, as has intracranial hypertension due to impaired central venous return in a patient with pneumomediastinum. Pneumoperitoneum, on the other hand, may prompt unnecessary surgical exploration of the abdomen. And pneumothorax, especially if large amounts of air enter but cannot leave the pleural space and thus are under tension, may cause respiratory failure and cardiovascular collapse.

Subcutaneous emphysema is easily diagnosed by the disfigurement it causes and by skin crepitation. Pneumomediastinum also may be reflected as a sound during the cardiac cycle that is called mediastinal crunch. The physical signs of pneumothorax are ipsilateral hyper-resonance with diminution of breath sounds and fremitus and contralateral tracheal deviation. Aberrant air also may be visualized by a variety of radiographic procedures, including the routine chest radiograph.

Pneumothorax may resolve spontaneously as the air is dissipated and the ruptured alveoli or airways heal themselves. The resolution will be accelerated if patients breath 100 per cent oxygen, which lowers the partial presence of nitrogen in circulating blood, facilitating reabsorption of aberrant air. However, because the air leak may continue and because it may be associated with severe underlying conditions, tube thoracostomy drainage frequently is required. Indeed, bilateral chest tubes often are placed empirically in trauma patients who have subcutaneous emphysema and are suspected of having tracheobronchial rupture or tension pneumothorax and who are likely to receive positive pressure ventilation. The treatment of pneumothorax is discussed more fully in Chapter 19.

Systemic Air Embolism. Another form of aberrant air is systemic air embolism, which has been reported after both penetrating and blunt chest injury. Air embolism results when a traumatic fistula is created between a bronchus and a pulmonary vein. Air enters the vein during either spontaneous or, more likely, mechanical ventilation and then may pass through the left ventricle into the cardiac or cerebral arteries or further into the systemic circulation. Air embolism should be suspected after chest trauma in patients who develop focal neurological findings in the absence of obvious head injury, patients who manifest cardiovascular collapse after the initiation of intermittent positive pressure ventilation, and patients in whom air is recovered from the left ventricle or is visualized in the coronary arteries. Therapy includes the administration of 100 per cent oxygen, insertion of intravascular catheters to remove air, and surgery to isolate the injured lung and repair fistulas. Obtaining frothy blood from systemic arterial catheters associated with air embolism is an ominous prognostic sign.

OTHER PLEURAL INJURIES

Hemothorax

Hemothorax frequently accompanies pneumothorax in patients with chest trauma. Pleural blood accumulation generally is limited when it results from lung lacerations or capillary rupture because the pulmonary circulation is a low pressure system. However, massive hemothorax may occur if intercostal or internal mammary vessels or the great vessels of the chest are torn. Therefore, before or after hemothorax has been confirmed on chest radiography, early placement of chest tubes is indicated in patients who have experienced intrathoracic blood loss on the order of 500 to 1000 ml/hour. Autotransfusion should be considered in such circumstances, and the rate of continued blood loss should be monitored closely. Thoracotomy usually is recommended if the rate of bleeding exceeds 500 ml over the subsequent six to eight hours. Whether or not surgery is performed, the chest tubes should remain in place until the bleeding falls below approximately 100 ml in 24 hours, or until a concurrent air leak is resolved.

Early thoracotomy once was recommended to evacuate clotted blood and prevent sequelae in patients with traumatic hemothorax who either did not require immediate exploration or whose pleural spaces were not drained completely with chest tubes. Subsequent studies have shown that residual hemothoraces usually are reabsorbed on their own and rarely cause persistent lung restriction. Similarly, pleural empyema is not a common consequence of residual hemothorax. It is therefore accepted today that chest tube drainage is sufficient to drain most hemothoraces and that their early decortication is not generally required.

Chylothorax

Chylothorax may not be obvious immediately following chest trauma because the flow of chyle through the thoracic duct is depressed when activity and diet are restricted. When they do occur, chylous pleural effusion may be diagnosed by the presence of milky fluid rich in lymphocytes and refractile fat droplets under the microscope. Such effusions usually resolve spontaneously or in response to chest tube drainage and a low fat diet. Surgical ligation of the thoracic duct is indicated if the effusions do not clear, if they interfere with lung function, or if they are associated with extreme nutritional loss.

INJURY TO THE AIRWAYS AND LUNGS

Laryngeal Fracture

Fracture of the larynx may occur during severe trauma to the neck or upper chest. It leads to an alteration in voice, upper airway obstruction, or subcutaneous emphysema. Diagnosis is confirmed by laryngoscopy or bronchoscopy. Airway patency must be assessed, followed by surgical repair. Since manipulation and attempts at intubation may cause sudden airway compromise, such procedures are best carried out in the operating room.

Tracheobronchial Rupture

Although the cervical trachea may rupture, the commonest site of injury is the main bronchus (right more often than left) within three centimeters of the tracheal bifurcation at the carina. The pathophysiology of tracheobronchial rupture is uncertain. One theory holds that the lungs expand laterally as the chest is crushed and distort the airways. Rupture occurs below the carina because the trachea is relatively fixed at this site but is free to swing below. Alternatively, it is thought that intraluminal airway pressure may increase significantly during trauma because patients exhale against a closed glottis (Valsalva maneuver) in anticipation of being struck.

Whatever its exact mechanism(s), tracheobronchial rupture presents in one of two ways depending on whether or not the involved airway communicates with the pleural space. Patients presenting acutely may have cough, hemoptysis, and subcutaneous emphysema followed by pneumothorax as gas escapes from the ruptured airway into the pleural cavity. When the gas leak is treated with a chest tube, the ipsilateral lung fails to re-expand and even may collapse downward owing to traction on the severed bronchus on chest roentgenogram when the patient is upright; this condition ed the *falling lung sign*. In chronic bronchial rupture, on the nd, the escape of gas from the lacerated airway is impeded by peribronchial tissue. A small pneumothorax may be present, but most of the gas is reabsorbed, leaving only residual atelectasis. Granulation tissue growing over the injury site may lead to airway stenosis and further atelectasis without pneumothorax on the chest roentgenogram. Bronchoscopy should be performed to establish the diagnosis of both types of tracheobronchial rupture before surgical repair. Tears of the tracheobronchial tree should be suspected if the first or second ribs are broken during severe chest trauma.

Lung Contusion

The most common initial pulmonary complication of blunt chest trauma is lung contusion. Such contusion may occur under the site of a flail chest or independently of obvious external injury. Alveoli in the contused area fill with fluid and blood, and severe hypoxemia may result from subsequent shunt and $\dot{V}A/\dot{Q}$ mismatching. A localized infiltrate is usually present on admission or at least becomes evident within a few hours. Contused lung may heal in an irregular pattern and look like a cavitating lung abscess on chest roentgenogram. It may be confused with hematoma, which is a more circumscribed area of parenchymal bleeding that also clears several days to weeks after trauma, and traumatic lung cyst, which is a collection of air following laceration of lung tissue.

CARDIOVASCULAR INJURIES

MYOCARDIAL CONTUSION

Myocardial contusion results from sudden deceleration or the application of great pressure to the chest and is commonly seen in patients with steering wheel injuries, including sternal fracture. Although coronary artery lacerations and thrombosis may occur in this situation, contusion usually represents an intramural hematoma in the myocardial wall. This may either cause no complication or may lead to supraventricular or ventricular dysrhythmias or to congestive failure related to decreased compliance and dyskinesia of the ventricular wall.

The true incidence of myocardial contusion is unknown because diagnostic criteria are both insensitive and nonspecific. Patients in whom the diagnosis is most likely to be made have anterior chest pain and electrocardiographic abnormalities such as ST-T wave changes. The MB fraction of creatine phosphokinase (CPK) will be increased, although the amount of myocardial damage does not correlate with CPK MB levels. Abnormal wall motion or a decreased ejection fraction may be demonstrated on two-dimensional (2-D) echocardiographic or radionuclide cineangiographic examination of the heart. Patients with known contusion who manifest potentially lethal dysrhythmias should be treated with lidocaine, procainamide hydrochloride (Pronestyl), or other agents. Inotropic agents and intra-aortic balloon counterpulsation have been used for severe congestive heart failure. The long-term care of patients who survive these problems is uncertain because myocardial contusion is not an ischemic injury related to coronary artery disease. Similarly, the optional management of patients with anterior chest pain but no other symptom is unclear. Although intensive care unit (ICU) admission has been recommended for all patients with suspected contusion, those who have no electrocardiographic changes or evidence of impaired cardiac function probably can be monitored outside the ICU.

CARDIAC RUPTURE AND PENETRATION

Cardiac rupture and penetration are seen infrequently in the ICU because patients with these problems usually die outside the hospital. However, patients may survive both conditions, especially if the right ventricle is less than fully injured or the atrium leaks blood slowly. Patients with cardiac rupture or penetration have either shock or signs of pericardial tamponade. Evidence of valvular disruption or an intraventricular septal defect also may be present. The treatment is surgical, although temporary measures such as pericardiocentesis may be used.

CARDIAC TAMPONADE

Cardiac tamponade in trauma patients usually results from rupture, penetrating wounds in the heart, or retrograde aortic rupture. These conditions allow a collection of blood in the pericardium sufficient to interfere with diastolic filling of the ventricles and, as blood pressure falls, so does perfusion of the coronary circulation. The rate of formation of hemopericardium varies among patients; many patients with tamponade secondary to cardiac rupture or penetration die immediately, whereas in a few with slow bleeding diagnosis may not be made until surgery for other problems has been completed and they are in the ICU.

Depending on the rate of bleeding and other factors, the well-known Beck's triad of arterial hypotension, central venous hypertension, and distant heart sounds may or may not be present in patients with cardiac tamponade. Nevertheless, the significance of elevated central venous pressure (CVP) after chest trauma is such that a CVP line probably should be placed in most patients who sustain major thoracic injury. Exaggerated pulsus paradoxus, the fall in systolic blood pressure that normally occurs as cardiac output declines in inspiration, also is an inconsistent finding. A widened cardiac silhouette rarely is present on the chest radiograph because the pericardium has not been stretched sufficiently to accommodate large volumes of blood in acute tamponade. Because of these factors, tamponade often must be diagnosed by 2-D echocardiography or empirical pericardiocentesis. When tamponade is known to exist, pericardiocentesis should be performed or a subxiphoid pericardial window created to stabilize the patient's condition before definitive surgery.

AORTIC RUPTURE

Aortic rupture is the most common cause of immediate death among accident victims who do not survive long enough to reach the hospital. In those patients who are alive on arrival, intrathoracic bleeding is prevented by either the aortic adventitia or the pleura creating a false aneurysm that usually leaks gradually or massively within the next few days. In survivors and nonsurvivors of motor vehicle accidents, the aorta usually ruptures at its isthmus just distal to the descending aortic origin of the subclavian artery, although the ascending aortic root also may rupture during falls. It is thought that during deceleration, the heart and proximal aorta move forward and twist while the descending aorta is held in place, at a time when intraluminal pressure is greatly elevated.

Patients with aortic rupture classically have shock or signs of cardiac tamponade. If conscious, they may complain of intense interscapular pain. Hoarseness from recurrent laryngeal nerve compression may occur, as may hypertension in the upper extremities and hypotension below, a sign of acute coarctation. The chest radiograph may reveal fractures of the upper three ribs, apical capping due to subpleural blood, and especially a widened mediastinum. Computed tomography may identify aortic rupture, but aortography usually is required to confirm the diagnosis and guide surgical repair.

INJURY OF OTHER STRUCTURES

Esophageal Rupture

Rupture of the esophagus is usually manifested by mediastinal widening and pleural effusion on chest roentgenograms and may be indistinguishable from aortic laceration. However, whereas the pleural fluid should be grossly bloody in the latter circumstance, it is more likely to be serosanguineous and to contain a low pH and a high amylase level when the esophagus is involved. Concurrent pneumothorax may be due to air entering the pleural space from the esophagus. The origin of the gas leak can usually be determined by esophagography. Esophageal rupture will progress to massive mediastinal infection and death if not treated with systemic antibiotics and, usually, open drainage and surgical repair.

Diaphragmatic Injury

Unilateral or bilateral diaphragmatic paralysis may result from disruption of the phrenic nerve(s) by chest trauma. Another possible complication is hemidiaphragmatic rupture related to the high intra-abdominal pressure generated during crush injuries. The liver prevents transmission of this pressure to the right hemidiaphragm, so the left hemidiaphragm ruptures in the majority of cases. The affected hemidiaphragm may appear elevated on chest roentgenogram, or herniated loops of bowel may be visible above it. Passage of a nasogastric tube into the stomach may help determine the stomach's presence in the chest, especially if radiopaque contrast material is injected into the tube. If the herniation is not diagnosed or surgically treated, bowel strangulation may occur. Furthermore, as many as two thirds of patients with diaphragmatic rupture following trauma have an associated intra-abdominal injury requiring repair.

Abdominal Visceral Injury

Traumatic damage to the liver, spleen, and other abdominal organs should be suspected after chest trauma, particularly in hypotensive patients and in patients with abdominal swelling or pain, and patients with lower rib injuries.

Skeletal Injuries

Neutral fat composed of triglycerides is released from many skeletal sites during trauma, including those not directly injured. Such release is uncommon after intramedullary reaming or nailing of fractured bones but is seen during total hip replacement and reaming of intact bones. Although neutral fat can be seen in the blood and urine of many trauma patients, only a small number go on to develop the *fat embolism syndrome*. The fat embolism syndrome is usually heralded within one to two days after injury by restlessness, confusion, and other central nervous system abnormalities. Petechiae appear on the upper thorax, axillae, and palate; tachypnea develops; diffuse infiltrates are found on the chest roentgenogram; and inadequate oxygenation may ensue.

Although investigators once believed that neutral fat blocking the cerebral and pulmonary circulations was responsible for these findings, it now is believed that the fat embolism syndrome results from the breakdown of the neutral fat to free fatty acids that cause an intense inflammatory reaction in the lungs and elsewhere.

Heparin, which activates lipase and may enhance the breakdown of neutral fat, is contraindicated in this disorder. Corticosteroids appear to benefit certain patients as well as experimental animals given intravenous oleic acid, the major free fatty acid implicated in the fat embolism syndrome in humans.

Central Nervous System Injury

Spinal Cord Injury. Cord injury sustained during chest trauma may result in paraplegia or quadriplegia; the effects of quadriplegia on respiratory muscle function are discussed in Chapter 5. The neck and thorax should be immobilized in all patients until nervous system injury can be evaluated. Related laryngeal, tracheal, or esophageal injury should be looked for as indicated.

Head Trauma. Central nervous system injury frequently accompanies injury of the chest and may complicate its management. Cerebral perfusion pressure, the pressure providing blood flow to the brain, especially where cerebral autoregulation is impaired, represents the difference between mean arterial pressure (MAP) and intracranial pressure (ICP). Cerebral resuscitation therefore is aimed at maintaining MAP and ICP within their normal ranges. Intracranial pressure can be lowered by hyperventilation, which causes cerebral vasoconstriction and decreased cerebral blood flow. Most patients with head injury who also have post-traumatic respiratory failure require mechanical ventilation with PEEP. This increases pleural pressure, which may increase right atrial pressure, impede cerebral venous drainage, and increase ICP.

Fortunately, although significant increases in ICP have been observed in some patients on PEEP, this response is not universal. Furthermore, patients with concurrent head injury and post-traumatic respiratory failure usually have noncompliant lungs that prevent the full transmission of airway pressure to the pleural space and right atrium, so ICP rise on PEEP is limited. Finally, even if ICP does increase with PEEP, cerebral perfusion pressure can usually be maintained by volume infusion to raise MAP and by sitting patients at a 30-degree angle to reduce cerebral venous pressure and lower ICP. Intracranial pressure also may be decreased by intravenous mannitol and by corticosteroids.

POST-TRAUMATIC RESPIRATORY FAILURE

The hypoxemic respiratory failure that follows trauma has been called by a variety of names, including shock lung, Da Nang lung, the adult respiratory distress syndrome, and post-traumatic respiratory failure. These terms are necessarily vague because the respiratory failure may have many causes and because its exact mechanism is unknown. Trauma patients may experience pulmonary contusion, aspiration pneumonia, hypotension, bacterial sepsis, air embolism, fat embolism syndrome, neurogenic pulmonary edema, and many other conditions that individually or in concert result in respiratory failure. Patients should receive the general measures for failure of arterial oxygenation outlined in Chapter 7 until a more specific diagnosis and therapeutic regimen can be achieved.

CHEST SURGERY

RESPIRATORY EFFECTS OF GENERAL ANESTHESIA AND SURGERY

The respiratory system is altered by every form of general anesthesia and surgery. For example, analgesics and drying agents administered during the preoperative period may depress ventilation and impair the clearance of secretions. Intubation bypasses normal upper airway defense mechanisms and may trigger bronchospasm. General anesthesia affects diaphragmatic position and predisposes the patient to the aspiration of gastric contents. Surgery on the upper abdomen and thorax produces pain and splinting. These in turn impair cough, reduce the functional residual capacity (FRC), and cause atelectasis and hypoxemia. In addition, pneumonia and deep venous thrombosis with pulmonary embolism may complicate the postoperative period.

GENERAL AND PULMONARY RISK FACTORS

Although respiratory complications may occur in all patients undergoing general anesthesia and surgery, they are more common in individuals with the following conditions and disorders: advancing age, obesity, general debility, alcohol or drug abuse, bleeding or clotting disorders, cardiac disease, and metabolic derangements (Table 18–1). Specific pulmonary risk factors include acute respiratory infection, a history of heavy cigarette smoking, pulmonary hypertension, forced expiratory volume in one second (FEV_1) of less than 2 liters or approximately 50 per cent of the predicted volume, maximal voluntary ventilation (MVV) of less than 50 liters or less than 50 per cent of that predicted, and arterial carbon dioxide tension ($PaCO_2$) of 45 mmHg or more (Table 18–2). Hypoxemia has not been identified as an independent risk factor, presumably because of its potential reversibility and its many causes.

Table 18–1. GENERAL RISK FACTORS FOR ANESTHESIA AND SURGERY

Age > 70 years
Obesity
General debility
Alcohol or drug abuse
Hematological abnormalities
Cardiac disease
    Congestive heart failure
    Myocardial infarction within preceding 6 months
Metabolic disorders

PREOPERATIVE EVALUATION AND PERIOPERATIVE MANAGEMENT TO PREVENT RESPIRATORY COMPLICATIONS

A thorough medical history must be taken and a physical examination performed on all patients before general anesthesia and surgery. From a general standpoint, questions regarding previous illnesses and surgical procedures and their outcome must be asked. A detailed respiratory history with reference to cigarette smoking, respiratory infections, and diseases such as asthma is indicated. Physical examination of the respiratory system should focus on lung sounds, cyanosis, digital clubbing, and the other findings discussed in Chapter 6. Full pulmonary function testing is desirable in certain patients. All patients with pulmonary risk factors should have arterial blood gas determination and spirometry (with an MVV maneuver) before general anesthesia and surgery. These tests can be performed at the bedside.

Patients found to have significant pulmonary disease should receive bronchodilators, corticosteroids, antibiotics, and other medications as indicated during the perioperative period. Cigarette smoking must be discontinued. Patients should be instructed preoperatively in the use of incentive spirometers and other devices to aid lung inflation, and those with mucus hypersecretion should be shown how to cough effectively despite upper abdominal or chest pain. Pain relief should be afforded postoperatively unless it compromises ventilation. This may be achieved by intercostal or epidural blocks in place of or in addition to systemic analgesia.

Table 18–2. PULMONARY RISK FACTORS FOR ANESTHESIA AND SURGERY

Forced expiratory volume in 1 second (FEV_1) <2 liters or 50 per cent of predicted volume
Maximum voluntary ventilation (MVV) 50 liters or <50% of that predicted or <50 liters/minute
Arterial carbon dioxide tension ($PaCO_2$) 45 mmHg or greater
Pulmonary hypertension
Heavy cigarette smoking
Acute respiratory infection

Chest percussion and postural drainage may help mobilize secretions in some individuals. Supplemental oxygen, adequate fluids and electrolytes, and nutrition should be provided. Deep venous thrombosis and pulmonary embolism can be prevented by heparin administered subcutaneously in 5000-unit doses two or three times daily. High-risk patients should be monitored in an ICU whenever possible. Early ambulation should be strived for. Several aspects of this approach that are useful in patients with pulmonary diseases are outlined in Table 18–3.

SPECIAL EVALUATION OF PATIENTS UNDERGOING LUNG RESECTION

The respiratory consequences and potential risk of general anesthesia and surgery are increased in patients who will lose

Table 18–3. PREOPERATIVE PREPARATION AND PERIOPERATIVE MANAGEMENT IN PATIENTS WITH PULMONARY DISEASE

A. Month before operation:
  1. Identify the high-risk patient.
  2. Assess pulmonary function.
  3. Control weight if necessary.
  4. Stop smoking.
B. Week before operation:
  1. Select appropriate measures for increasing lung volumes in perioperative period:
    a. Exercises.
    b. Incentive spirometry.
    c. Intermittent positive pressure breathing.
  2. Control bronchial infection if present.
  3. Optimize bronchodilator regimen.
  4. Select appropriate measures for secretion clearance.
  5. Alert anesthesiologist to high-risk patient.
  6. (Stop smoking.)
C. Day of operation:
  1. Schedule procedure for late in day, not as first case.
  2. Mobilize patient several hours before operation.
  3. Perform complete bronchial hygiene treatment prior to preoperative medication:
    a. Bronchodilator inhalation.
    b. Cough and deep breathe.
    c. Chest physiotherapy if necessary.
D. During operation:
  1. Minimize anesthesia time.
  2. Avoid hyperventilation.
  3. Maintain airway humidification.
  4. Continue bronchodilator therapy.
E. After operation:
  1. Continue all aspects of regimen tailored preoperatively to patient's needs.
  2. Mobilize as soon as possible:
    a. In bed.
    b. Out of bed.
  3. Provide adequate analgesia while avoiding respiratory depression:
    a. Local anesthesia.
    b. Epidural/peridural anesthesia.
    c. Lowest possible doses of narcotics, sedatives, and hypnotics.

functioning lung tissue. Although insignificant amounts of tissue are removed during open lung biopsy, entire segments, lobes, or lungs may be resected for the treatment of arteriovenous malformations, bullae, or, more commonly, lung cancer. Normal persons can tolerate the removal of one lung, assuming that the blood vessels of the remaining lung can accommodate the entire right ventricular output after pneumonectomy. The diffusing capacity decreases by less than 50 per cent in such individuals, reflecting the recruitment of previously unused vessels in the remaining lung for gas exchange.

However, the pulmonary vascular bed may be so limited in patients with emphysema and other diseases that pulmonary hypertension and cor pulmonale may develop at rest or during moderate exercise after lung resection. Emphysema is common in cigarette smokers, the individuals who are most likely to be surgical candidates for lung cancer. Therefore, the function of the lung tissue that will remain after surgery should be known before any lung tissue is resected in such individuals. Although a partial resection may be possible, the patients usually should be evaluated as if they will undergo pneumonectomy, because this affords the surgeon the greatest operative latitude.

The technique most commonly used to determine separate lung function before surgery is perfusion lung scanning. An FEV_1 in the lung expected to remain after surgery is calculated by multiplying the preoperative FEV_1 for both lungs by the fraction of perfusion distributed on lung scan to the lung to be removed. If the predicted postsurgical FEV_1 is 800 ml or greater, the patient is considered appropriate for pneumonectomy; the same criterion applies to bronchospirometry. In addition to determining whether patients can tolerate the loss of a lung, perfusion lung scanning is useful in estimating the consequences of losing smaller amounts of tissue.

THE CHEST AFTER PNEUMONECTOMY

Total lung capacity does not decrease by 50 per cent after lung removal because the remaining lung expands somewhat. Pleural pressures are considerably more negative, however, because a smaller amount of lung tissue recoils within a chest cavity that has changed little in volume. The negative pleural pressure helps draw fluid from vessels of the chest wall and mediastinum into the pleural space, and the space usually fills with fluid and fibrin. Because of this, chest tubes are not used after pneumonectomy (they are used after lobectomy, however, owing to air leaks from lung fissures). The trachea remains in the midline position or shifts towards the resected pleural space as a result of contralateral lung expansion after pneumonectomy. If the space does not fill, it remains a potential site of infection by organisms entering the space from the blood or, more commonly, via a persistent bronchopleural gas leak at the stump of the removed lung.

Bronchopleural gas leaks announce their presence by an air-fluid level on chest roentgenogram. The pleural fluid is assumed to be infected if a fistula is present. Systemic antibiotics must be given; the stump is usually repaired unless the bronchopleural fistula heals spontaneously; and the pleural space may be obliterated by removing several ribs and collapsing the thoracic cage around it, a procedure called a thoracoplasty. In contrast to this situation, if the pleural space fills initially and the trachea is shifted to the contralateral side, bleeding into the space should be suspected. A tracheal shift occurring months to years after pneumonectomy may herald the return of cancer for which surgery was initially performed.

SURGERY ON THE UPPER ABDOMEN

A REMINDER

Although a full discussion of abdominal surgery is beyond the scope of this chapter, it is worth noting that respiratory complications are even more common after upper abdominal operations than those involving the chest. This occurs in part because upper abdominal incisions cause pain and splinting, reduce functional residual capacity, and interfere with defense mechanisms, especially coughing. Awareness of those changes is essential in keeping complications to a minimum.

RECOMMENDED READING

1. Ali J, et al.: Consequences of postoperative alterations in respiratory mechanics. Am J Surg, 128:376–382, 1974.
2. Burchiel KJ, et al.: Intracranial pressure changes in brain-injured patients requiring positive end-expiratory pressure ventilation. Neurosurgery, 8:443–449, 1981.
3. Burrows B, et al.: The postpneumonectomy state: clinical and physiologic observations in thirty-six cases. Am J Med, 28:281–297, 1960.
4. Chayen MS, et al.: Pain control with epidural injection of morphine. Anesthesiology, 53:338–339, 1980.
5. Cullen P, et al.: Treatment of flail chest. Use of intermittent mandatory ventilation and positive end-expiratory pressure. Arch Surg, 11:1099–1103, 1975.
6. Hara KS, Prakash UB: Fiberoptic bronchoscopy in the evaluation of acute chest and upper airway trauma. Chest, 96:627–630, 1989.
7. Kakkar VV, et al.: Prevention of fatal postoperative pulmonary embolism by low doses of heparin. An international multicentre trial. Lancet 2:45–51, 1975.
8. Lewis FR Jr, et al.: Incidence and outcome of posttraumatic respiratory failure. Arch Surg, 113:436–443, 1977.
9. Martin TD, et al.: Blunt cardiac rupture. J Trauma, 24:287–290, 1984.

10. Maunder RJ, et al.: Subcutaneous and mediastinal emphysema. *Arch Intern Med*, 144:1447–1453, 1984.
11. Olsen GN, et al.: Pulmonary function evaluation of the lung resection candidate: a prospective study. *Am Rev Respir Dis*, 111:379–388, 1975.
12. Pierson DJ: Pneumomediastinum. *In* Murray JF, and Nadel JA (eds.): *Textbook of Respiratory Medicine*. Philadelphia, W. B. Saunders Co., 1988, pp. 1795–1809.
13. Potkin RT, et al.: Evaluation of noninvasive tests of cardiac damage in suspected cardiac contusion. *Circulation*, 66:627–637, 1982.
14. Shackford SR: Blunt chest trauma: The intensivist's perspective. *J Intern Care Med*, 1:125–130, 1986.
15. Thomas AN, and Stephens BG: Air embolism: A cause of morbidity and death after penetrating chest trauma. *J Trauma*, 14:633–638, 1974.
16. Tisi GM: Preoperative evaluation of pulmonary function. Validity, indications, and benefits. *Am Rev Respir Dis*, 119:293–310, 1979.
17. Waldschmidt ML, and Laws HL: Injuries of the diaphragm. *J Trauma*, 20:587–592, 1980.

19

DRAINAGE, OBLITERATION, AND DECORTICATION OF THE PLEURAL SPACE

THE PLEURAL SPACE

NORMAL FUNCTION

The pleura is a membrane that separates the lung from the chest wall, diaphragm, and mediastinum (see Chapter 1, Fig. 1–2). The parietal pleura adheres to the inside of the chest wall; the visceral pleura surrounds the lungs except at the hili, where the bronchi and major blood vessels enter the lungs. The pleural membranes are lined with mesothelial cells. Normally the space between the pleurae contains approximately 5 ml of lubricating fluid and is free of air. The pleural membranes are functionally adherent owing to the negative pressure in the pleural space.

At functional residual capacity (FRC), the natural tendency of the chest wall to recoil outward and that of the lungs to recoil inward are balanced. Pressure in the pleural space at FRC is 755 mmHg compared with an atmospheric pressure of 760 mmHg, so the pleural pressure is said to be negative (-5 mmHg) relative to that at the mouth. During inspiration from FRC, as the diaphragm and the other respiratory muscles contract, the chest wall moves outward. Pleural pressure becomes more negative (approximately -20 mmHg at total lung capacity) because of the seal created between the pleural surfaces by the presence of water that is both incompressible and inexpandable. The inward recoil of the lungs is overcome, and they expand. Alveolar pressure becomes negative relative to atmospheric pressure during inspiration because gas molecules in the alveoli move further apart. Gas then flows into the alveoli from the atmosphere until a pressure gradient between the alveoli and the mouth no longer exists.

Expiration normally is a passive process during which pleural pressure remains negative relative to atmospheric pressure because the chest wall is below the resting position it would take if it were not joined with the lungs and because it still has a small outward recoil force. Alveolar pressure becomes positive owing to gas compression, however, so gas flows from the alveoli to the mouth until the pressure gradient between them no longer exists. During forced expiration, as the abdominal muscles contract, pleural pressure becomes slightly positive relative to the atmosphere, although it always is less than alveolar pressure. Nevertheless, the pleural surfaces remain apposed, and gas does not accumulate in the pleural space during the ventilatory cycle. This also is true if the surfaces are permanently applied to one another by the procedures discussed later.

ABNORMAL FUNCTION

In contrast to the normal situation, entry of gas (pneumothorax) or fluid (pleural effusion) allows the pleural membranes to separate. The tendency of the chest wall to recoil outward and that of the lungs to recoil inward now are less opposed because pleural pressure is less negative, so the thoracic cage expands and the lungs collapse. Because of this collapse, the lung can no longer maintain efficient gas exchange, and hypoxemia due to ventilation-perfusion ($\dot{V}A/\dot{Q}$) mismatching ensues.

DISEASES OF THE PLEURAL SPACE

PNEUMOTHORAX

Simple Pneumothorax

Simple pneumothorax occurs when gas accumulates in the pleural space but pleural pressure does not significantly exceed atmospheric pressure. Gas can enter the space from outside the chest wall, as occurs with wounds or therapeutic procedures that penetrate the parietal pleura, via the lung through a breach in the visceral pleura, or through the mediastinal pleura.

Spontaneous pneumothoraces are thought to begin with the rupture of distended alveolar walls. When this occurs, alveolar gas takes the path of least resistance and usually tracks along the peribronchial interstitial tissues towards the hilum, where it enters the pleura surrounding the mediastinum and causes a pneumomediastinum. Since the mediastinal pleura is continuous with fascial planes in the neck, the gas may accumulate under the skin and create subcutaneous emphysema. The mediastinal pleura is also continuous with the pericardium, so a pneumopericardium may result. In some cases mediastinal, subcutaneous, or pericardial air accumulates in the absence of pneumothorax. Nevertheless, the alveolar gas most often ruptures through the mediastinal pleura to cause a pneumothorax. Pneumothorax also may occur if alveolar gas travels towards the periphery of the lung and collects in subpleural blebs that become distended and rupture directly into the pleural space.

Pain generally is felt as the gas irritates the parietal pleura, and dyspnea is common because of the activation of pulmonary stretch receptors. Small amounts of gas cause pleural pressure to increase slightly, but it remains subatmospheric during inspiration because it is in equilibrium with alveolar pressure, which is negative. Although pleural and alveolar pressures become positive during forced expiration, slight separation of the pleural surfaces does not compromise ventilation. If the pneumothorax is small and the pleural leak seals itself, the gas will be absorbed at a rate dependent on the partial pressure differences between the gas in the pleural space and in the blood. If the gas is air, approximately 10 per cent of it will be absorbed each day. Absorption will increase if the patient breathes 100 per cent O_2 because nitrogen will be washed out of inhaled air and circulating blood, so the partial pressure of nitrogen will be higher in the pleural space than in blood, favoring its uptake. Larger pneumothoraces that compromise ventilation can be evacuated by closed pleural drainage, as discussed later.

Spontaneous pneumothoraces occur in healthy individuals, most commonly in slender young men, and occasionally in patients with emphysema or in patients whose alveolar walls are altered by interstitial fluid or fibrosis. Because of their abnormal ventilatory mechanics, such patients often must generate more negative pleural pressures to inspire than do people with normal lungs. They cannot do this if their pleural seal is broken, so their ventilation may be severely compromised by even a small pneumothorax. Spontaneous pneumothorax occurs in 5 per cent of persons receiving intermittent positive pressure ventilation, especially if high tidal volumes are used. Continuous positive pressure ventilation carries an even greater risk of pneumothorax because of its greater risk of alveolar overdistention.

Tension Pneumothorax

In contrast to simple pneumothorax, tension pneumothorax is characterized not only by abnormal gas exchange but also by a progressive increase in pleural pressure sufficient to impair circulation. This occurs as gas enters the pleural space during spontaneous negative pressure inspiration (or a positive pressure machine breath) and remains there during expiration because tissue occludes the rent in whichever pleural surface is torn; this is called a ball-valve effect. The accumulating gas not only collapses the ipsilateral lung but also shifts the mediastinum and its contents into the opposite chest. This mechanical distortion may interfere with venous return to the right ventricle and compromise contralateral lung functions; at the same time the continuous positive pleural pressure will decrease the pressure gradient necessary for venous flow into the thorax. Tension pneumothorax usually causes intense dyspnea followed by cardiopulmonary arrest. The condition may be fatal, especially if it occurs during mechanical ventilation, unless the gas is immediately evacuated by means of a large-bore needle or a thoracostomy tube.

PLEURAL EFFUSION

Transudates and Exudates

Pleural effusion is the accumulation of fluid in the pleural space. The fluid continually seeps from capillaries lining the parietal and visceral pleurae and is reabsorbed by lymphatics. Secretion and reabsorption of pleural fluid are affected by capillary hydrostatic and oncotic pressure, capillary permeability, and the availability of lymphatics for drainage.

Pleural fluid tends to accumulate in four basic circumstances: (1) when the normal hydrostatic gradient is altered by an increase in pulmonary capillary pressure, as occurs in left heart failure; (2) when capillary oncotic pressure is severely reduced, as in cirrhosis or nephrosis; (3) when the pleural surfaces and their underlying vessels are inflamed by infection or tumor; and (4) when lymphatic drainage is impaired by local or generalized obstruction. In the first two circumstances the pleural effusion is largely water and its protein concentration is less than half that of serum; this fluid is called a transudate. In the latter two circumstances the pleural fluid to serum protein ratio is greater than 0.5, indicating that the fluid is an exudate. An elevation of pleural fluid lactic dehydrogenase (LDH) to 200 units or greater than two thirds of the upper limit of normal values or a fluid to serum LDH ratio of 0.6 also signifies the presence of exudative fluid.

Diagnosis of Pleural Effusions

Pleural fluid may be sampled by inserting a thin needle through the chest wall. This procedure, called thoracentesis, is described in Chapter 6. Analysis of the fluid for protein and LDH concentration allows determination of whether a transudate or exudate is present. This information can then be used to establish a differential diagnosis of the effusion's etiology, as outlined in Table 19–1. A low glucose level in the fluid, compared with the serum glucose, suggests utilization by metabolizing cells and indicates that infection or another cause of severe inflammation is responsible for the fluid accumulation. A high amylase level is found in effusions that originate in the esophagus or result from pancreatitis. Esophageal

Table 19–1. TYPES AND CAUSES OF PLEURAL EFFUSIONS

TYPE	CAUSES
Transudative (pleural fluid protein:serum protein < 0.5, LDH < 200 IU or greater than 2/3 upper limits of normal, pleural fluid LDH:serum LDH < 0.6)	Pulmonary capillary hypertension in left ventricular failure, hypoalbuminemia due to cirrhosis or nephrosis, passage of subdiaphragmatic transudative effusions related to Meigs' syndrome or peritoneal dialysis
Exudative (pleural fluid protein:serum protein > 0.5, LDH > 200 IU or greater than 2/3 upper limits of normal, pleural fluid LDH:serum LDH > 0.6)	Pleural inflammation caused by tumor, infection (bacterial, tuberculous, mycoplasmal, viral), pulmonary embolism with infarction, connective tissue diseases, subdiaphragmatic inflammatory conditions such as pancreatitis, general or localized lymphatic obstruction
Hemorrhagic	Tumor, trauma, pulmonary embolism with infarction
Chylous	Lymphatic obstruction, trauma to thoracic duct
Cholesterol-rich	Chronic exudative effusion from tuberculous rheumatoid arthritis

LDH = lactic dehydrogenase.

rupture is also suggested by a low fluid pH, by the presence of food particles, or by both. Blood in the pleural space is indicated by a red blood cell count greater than 100,000 cells per cubic millimeter (mm^3). Empyema, or pus accumulation, is suggested by a low glucose concentration and white blood cell count of 15,000 cells/mm^3 or higher, in addition to infectious organisms.

A high white blood cell count or a pleural fluid pH of 7.0 or lower suggests the presence of severe inflammation that will cause the fluid to congeal in certain places and form adhesions between the pleural surfaces. Separate pockets of fluid then form, a process called loculation. Loculated effusions are difficult, if not impossible, to drain with a single chest tube. A diagnostic thoracentesis should be performed promptly on any unexplained collection of pleural fluid, especially if empyema is suspected and loculation might occur.

Common Causes of Pleural Effusion

Pneumothorax. This abnormality is associated with a small pleural effusion in approximately 25 per cent of cases. The fluid usually is an exudate caused by irritation of the pleura by air. Large amounts of fluid suggest another source, such as a bleeding vessel or ruptured esophagus.

Parapneumonic Effusions. Pleural effusions accompany up to one half of all cases of pneumonia. They usually are exudative, reflecting pleural inflammation, and they clear as the pneumonia resolves. If they do not, the fluid may have become infected.

Empyema. Empyema is present if the pleural fluid is grossly purulent or if its white blood cell count is high, as noted above. Some authors also require that infectious organisms be seen on Gram stain or grown on culture, although strictly speaking pus can be present in the absence of organisms. A large collection of pus in the pleural space is called pyothorax. Empyema of any size generally requires prompt drainage in addition to systemic antibiotic therapy if infection is documented or suspected. Undrained fluid becomes loculated and may congeal into a semisolid mass, called fibrothorax, that limits lung expansion and may require decortication, which is discussed below.

Exudative Tuberculous Effusions. These fluid collections represent hypersensitivity reactions in the pleural space and usually are seen in patients with positive tuberculin skin tests. Presumptive diagnosis of tuberculous effusions can be made by seeing noncaseating granulomas on pleural biopsy, a procedure discussed in Chapter 6, whereas definitive diagnosis is made by observing acid-fast bacilli on stains or culture of the pleural fluid. Unlike tuberculous empyemas, which usually are teeming with mycobacteria and white blood cells, tuberculous effusions have few microorganisms. They generally respond to systemic antituberculous agents and do not require drainage.

Malignant Effusions. These effusions usually are due to primary or metastatic pleural tumor implants, although lymphoma characteristically causes pleural fluid to accumulate through lymphatic obstruction. The major primary pleural malignancy, mesothelioma, is discussed below. Pleural metastases most often originate from tumors of the lung, breast, ovary, and stomach. These tumors usually are adenocarcinomas and may be difficult to distinguish histologically from mesothelioma. The prognosis is poor for patients with malignant effusions; such persons have a mean survival of only three months, and 50 per cent die within a year. The effusions also tend to be large and to reaccumulate after initial drainage, even if the primary tumor is treated. A low pleural fluid pH is a poor prognostic sign.

Bloody Effusions. Blood in the pleural space suggests trauma, tumor, or pulmonary embolism with infarction. The blood causes an exudation from the pleural surfaces that dilutes the blood and lowers its hematocrit. The inflammatory reaction also consumes clotting factors, so blood remaining in the pleural space for longer than a few minutes will not coagulate. This means that clotted blood encountered during a thoracentesis performed for the diagnosis of pleural effusion usually stems not from the effusion but from a traumatic tap. A small amount of pleural blood will be reabsorbed in time, but a larger amount (hemothorax) usually must be removed to avoid the formation of a fibrothorax. A thoracostomy tube usually is adequate.

Chylothorax. A collection of lymph within a pleural space is called a chylothorax. This may be caused by diffuse lymphatic obstruction in a rare condition called pulmonary lymphangiomyomatosis, by localized obstruction due to lymphoma, or by traumatic disruption of the thoracic duct. The duct, a major lymphatic vessel, originates in the cisterna chyli beneath the right hemidiaphragm and ascends adjacent to the right vertebral column until the fifth or sixth thoracic vertebra, where it courses to the left side of the chest to join the azygos vein. Disruption along its course causes a chylous effusion on the ipsilateral side. Chylous fluid is milky white in color and contains large amounts of fat but no cholesterol. Chylothorax usually can be controlled with closed drainage and reduction of the formation of fluid.

Cholesterol-Rich Effusions. These effusions, which are also called pseudochylous effusions, also are white in color but contain cholesterol rather than fat. They are seen in chronic inflammatory conditions, including tuberculosis and rheumatoid arthritis.

PLEURAL MALIGNANCIES

Malignant mesothelioma is the most common primary tumor arising from the pleural surfaces. It is seen for the most part in patients with a history of asbestos exposure who present with pleural effusion and pain. Diagnosis can be made only rarely by thoracentesis and in perhaps 20 per cent of patients by closed pleural biopsy; open biopsy is usually necessary for a larger sample size. Effective therapy for malignant mesothelioma is not available.

CLOSED PLEURAL DRAINAGE

GENERAL CONSIDERATIONS

Correction of a pneumothorax or pleural effusion must be accomplished swiftly if life is threatened. However, chronic collections of air or fluid need not be removed at once, and the rapid evacuation of large collections should generally be avoided lest reexpansion pulmonary edema occur. This condition causes edema and massive fluid loss in the ipsilateral and, occasionally, the contralateral lung. Although its etiology is unclear, re-expansion edema can generally be prevented if no more than 1000 ml of air or fluid are withdrawn at one time. When greater drainage is necessary, patients should be followed closely.

THORACENTESIS

Although thoracentesis is most often performed for diagnostic purposes, it may be done therapeutically to remove large amounts of air or fluid. If air or fluid is accumulating rapidly or if repeated procedures cause the patient undue discomfort, thoracostomy tube drainage is preferred.

THORACOSTOMY

General Principles

A thoracostomy tube, or chest tube, allows rapid, continuous evacuation of air or fluid from the pleural space. Chest tubes often cause pain at the time of insertion and may be poorly tolerated. They also are a potential source of infection and other complications unless they are used properly.

Insertion

Before thoracostomy tube insertion the skin is cleansed and locally anesthetized. For gas drainage, a small incision for insertion of a tube is made in the second or third intercostal space along the anterior midclavicular line or in the fourth to fifth intercostal space along the midaxillary line. A lower intercostal space along the midaxillary line is usually preferred for evacuation of fluid. Blunt dissection of the chest wall soft tissue and the parietal pleura is then performed with a hemostat, and the tube is inserted through this channel so that its most proximal holes are well inside the chest. The blunt method may lead to chest wall infections in patients with empyema and should be avoided in this disorder. The tube usually remains clamped when introduced to prevent passage of air from the atmosphere into the pleural space. The tube is sutured in place and secured with tape. A gauze dressing is applied to the entry site. When the tube is connected to a drainage system, the clamp is removed.

Connection

Thoracostomy tubes are connected with the drainage systems described below through several feet of flexible tubing. This prevents kinking of the chest tube and traction on patients as they roll from side to side or sit upright in bed. All connection sites should be secured with tape. The drainage tube is generally coiled and secured to the bottom bed sheet to prevent formation of a loop below the level of the mattress, lest fluid in the dependent loop impede flow into the drainage system.

Drainage System

One-Bottle System. The one-bottle system, or underwater seal, is the simplest kind of drainage device (Fig. 19–1). It is created by placing the distal end of the rubber connecting tube 2 cm beneath the surface of a solution of normal saline in a bottle that is open to the atmosphere. The tube then functions like a straw placed under water. As gas pressure builds in the pleural space, gas is forced out the end of the tubing when its pressure exceeds that of the column of water above the distal end of the tube. However, if pleural pressure becomes negative, gas cannot enter the tubing because the water creates a seal. Transmission of pleural pressure forces the water level to rise and fall like a manometer, allowing the pressure to be measured, and confirms that the tube is functioning properly. Venting the drainage bottle to air is required to prevent pressure from mounting in the bottle as gas or drainage accumulates. *The major disadvantage with this system is that drainage collecting in the bottle increases the length of the submerged tubing and hence the pressure that must be overcome to evacuate the pleural space.* Thus, the one-bottle system can be used only when the pleural space contains primarily air.

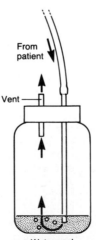

Figure 19–1. One-bottle pleural drainage system.

Two-Bottle System. In the two-bottle system, the underwater seal is separated from the patient by a collection bottle that traps fluid, allowing the fluid level in the underwater-seal bottle to remain constant (Fig. 19–2). Although this set-up is adequate for draining small amounts of air and fluid, large leaks require that a system with suction be used.

Three-Bottle System. The three-bottle system with suction enhances the pressure differences between the pleural space and the collection bottle. Only small amounts of negative pressure, such as -20 cm H_2O in adults, are applied to the pleural space. This is because larger amounts are generally unnecessary and may perpetuate a bronchopleural gas leak or cause lung tissue to be sucked into the "eyes" of the thoracostomy tube. However, most hospital wall vacuum outlets and portable suction pumps are capable of generating very great amounts of negative pressure. To regulate this pressure, a suction-control bottle is interposed between the suction device and the underwater seal in the three-bottle system (Fig. 19–3).

The suction-control bottle contains a long tube, one end of which is open to air; the other end is under a column of water 10 to 25 cm high. When negative pressure is applied to the suction-control bottle, it will be applied to the pleural space only in an amount slightly less than the column of water because greater amounts of negative pressure will draw atmospheric air into the tube, creating bubbles in the bottle. Thus, the height of the water column in the suction-control bottle determines the maximum suction in the

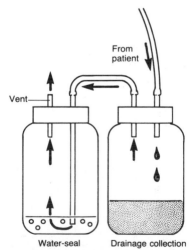

Figure 19–2. Two-bottle pleural drainage system.

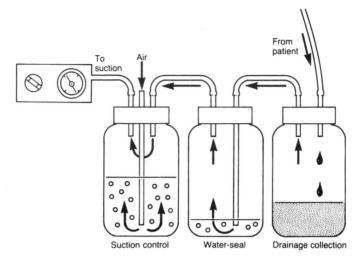

Figure 19–3. Three-bottle pleural drainage system.

system. Bubbling in the control bottle indicates that the suction is on but not necessarily that gas is being drained from the pleural space; if drainage is occurring, bubbles will be seen in the underwater-seal bottle as well. The underwater-seal bottle functions as a manometer of pleural pressure only if the suction is turned off. When this is done, the suction-control bottle must be vented to air to prevent pressure from building up in the system.

Commercial Systems. Several commercial systems are based on the preceding models. The Pleur-evac is a three-bottle system with a self-contained air vent that prevents a back-up of pressure (Fig. 19–4). The Argyle Double-Seal, which provides a similar function, adds another underwater-seal bottle open to air (Fig. 19–5). Both systems are portable and can be used with or without suction.

Monitoring

A chest roentgenogram should be taken after the patient and drainage system are connected to see if the lung has re-expanded and to confirm the thoracostomy tube's location. Confirmation of placement cannot always be achieved with a posterior-anterior film alone, inasmuch as the tube may lie in a fissure or protrude through lung and still appear normal. Therefore, a lateral view should be routinely obtained. Chest tubes, drainage tubing, and drainage bottles should be checked regularly—perhaps every hour—for patency. Bottles should be kept below the level of the chest to prevent fluid reflux. Pleural fluid drainage should be recorded on

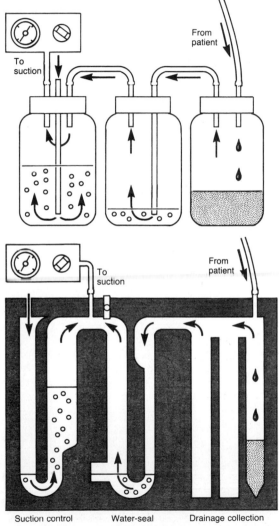

Figure 19–4. Pleur-evac pleural drainage system. Air vent is shown.

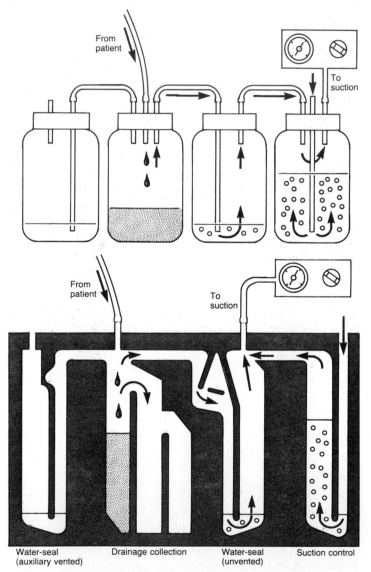

Figure 19–5. Argyle Double-Seal pleural drainage system. Second water-seal bottle is pictured at left.

the collection bottle and in the chart. Lack of fluctuation in the underwater-seal bottle with the suction off and open to air suggests a lack of communication with the pleural space. Patency can be demonstrated by asking the patient to take a deep breath. A chest tube whose patency has been lost should be replaced or removed, since it no longer prevents pneumothorax.

Stripping

If fresh bleeding occurs, clots of blood and fibrin may form in the drainage tubing and obstruct its lumen. To clear clots, the proximal end of the tubing may be temporarily clamped and the clots pushed distally either with the thumb and forefinger or with special stripping devices. However, this can generate high negative pressures, up to -400 mmHg, and injure the lung when the clamp is removed. Stripping should therefore be done with caution and only when fresh bleeding occurs. It should not be done if there is a bronchopleural gas leak.

Clamping

Clamping a chest tube will lead to tension pneumothorax if air continues to leak through either the parietal or the visceral pleura into the pleural space. Because of this, if an air leak is present, tubes should be clamped only when looking for its source. Stripping should not be done in this situation. Bubbling in the underwater-seal bottle when the patient is on suction indicates a source of gas somewhere between the seal and the pleural space. Assuming that the air does not come from the alveoli, the next most likely place is around the insertion site of the thoracostomy tube. This can be confirmed if the bubbling stops once the tube is clamped just distal to its exit from the chest. If the bubbling does not stop after this maneuver, the tubing and drainage system should be clamped in a stepwise fashion moving toward the underwater-seal bottle. If the leak is found to arise from the drainage system, the system should be replaced.

Removal

Chest tubes generally are removed when the pleural leak has sealed and the lung has re-expanded, when fluid drainage has ceased or is less than approximately 75 ml/day in an adult, or when the first and either of the second conditions occur. This usually occurs three to four days after lung resection but may take up to several weeks in patients with spontaneous pneumothorax, especially in those who require continuous mechanical ventilation. Physical examination and chest roentgenograms are used to determine the suitability of chest tube removal. Dressings around the tube insertion site are then removed, and the anchoring sutures are cut. The patient then is instructed to take a deep breath and exhale against a closed glottis (Valsalva maneuver), which provides positive pleural pressure and prevents air from entering the pleural space. The tube is quickly withdrawn and sterile Vaseline-impregnated gauze is held over the site, or a pursestring suture already in place is pulled on as the tube is removed to close the hole. The wound is dressed to absorb fluid that may seep from the insertion site over the next several days.

FLAP VALVE

Drainage from a chronic pneumothorax or effusion may be provided with a flap valve that allows gas and fluid to escape but prevents air from entering the pleural space. The valve is generally mounted on the stump of a chest tube cut off near the chest wall. Chronic infection in the tube track is inevitable if the apparatus is left in place for prolonged periods, but the infection generally remains localized.

OPEN CHEST DRAINAGE

Pleural drainage is occasionaly accomplished by removing a portion of a thoracic rib, tacking the parietal pleura to the skin (a process called marsupialization), and leaving the pleural space open to air. This procedure impairs lung function and is performed only if the lung is extensively diseased, if the pleural space cannot be adequately treated by chest tubes alone because of a persistent space, or if pleural infection persists after pneumonectomy.

PERSISTENT BRONCHOPLEURAL GAS LEAK DURING MECHANICAL VENTILATION

A persistent bronchopleural gas leak (PBL) or bronchopleural fistula results when communication between the airways and the pleural space does not heal spontaneously or in response to therapy. This condition occurs most commonly in patients receiving mechanical ventilation and may cause several adverse effects (Table 19–2). If the leak is large, the involved lung may not be ade-

Table 19–2. ADVERSE EFFECTS OF PERSISTENT BRONCHOPLEURAL AIR LEAK DURING
MECHANICAL VENTILATION

1. Incomplete lung expansion
2. Loss of tidal volume
3. Loss of PEEP
4. Infection of pleural space
5. Factitious ventilator cycling
6. Inability to remove CO_2 in some cases

PEEP = positive end-expiratory pressure.

quately ventilated, resulting in gas exchange abnormalities due to $\dot{V}A/\dot{Q}$ mismatching and shunt; however, a recent study has shown that carbon dioxide may be removed in large quantities through a PBL. Positive end-expiratory pressure (PEEP) also may be difficult to maintain, and removal of pleural gas by suction may trigger the ventilator by transmitting the negative pressure through the proximal airways to the machine. A final problem is infection of the pleural space.

As outlined in Table 19–2, the general goals of PBL management are to minimize the pressure gradient among the airways, the alveoli, and the pleural space while maintaining lung inflation and gas exchange, if possible, and correcting the underlying cause or causes of the leak. This can usually be accomplished by using the pleural drainage systems described previously while following the conservative techniques listed in Table 19–3. The pressure gradient from the airways and the alveoli to the pleural space is much less during spontaneous breathing than during mechanical ventilation, as described in Chapter 13. The ventilator should be adjusted to minimize the time spent in inspiration by keeping the inspiration

Table 19–3. PERSISTENT BRONCHOPLEURAL AIR LEAK DURING MECHANICAL VENTILATION:
CONSERVATIVE MANAGEMENT

1. Use lowest number of mechanical breaths compatible with adequate ventilation (spontaneous ventilation if possible; IMV at a low rate is preferable to continuous ventilation).
2. Reduce effective (returned) tidal volume to 10 ml/kg or less.
3. Minimize inspiratory time (keep I:E low) (high inspiratory flow; no inflation hold).
4. Avoid expiratory retard.
5. Avoid or minimize PEEP.
6. Use lowest effective chest tube suction.
7. Explore positional differences.
8. Sedate patient, with or without paralysis, if spontaneous movements accentuate leak.
9. Treat underlying cause of respiratory failure while maintaining nutritional and respiratory care support.

IMV = intermittent mechanical ventilation, I:E = ratio of inspiration to expiration, PEEP = positive end-expiratory pressure.

Table 19–4. PERSISTENT BRONCHOPLEURAL AIR LEAK DURING MECHANICAL VENTILATION:
AGGRESSIVE MANAGEMENT

1. Apply PEEP to chest tube.
2. Occlude chest tube during inspiration.
3. Ventilate lungs independently.
4. Use high-frequency jet ventilation.
5. Repair leak site directly.

PEEP = positive end-expiratory pressure.

to expiration ratio as low as possible, and expiratory retard should not be used. Positive end-expiratory pressure should be administered at the lowest possible levels. Chest tube suction also should be maintained at the lowest level that will guarantee lung expansion. Sedation, paralysis, and control of fever may lower CO_2 production in some patients while allowing time for the pleural leak to seal.

If these measures prove unsuccessful, more aggressive approaches, outlined in Table 19–4, should be considered. One such approach is the application of PEEP to the chest tube in patients with PBL who require PEEP for oxygenation. This reduces the bronchopleural pressure gradient by equalizing pleural and end-expiratory pressures via a PEEP device inserted between the ventilator circuit and the chest tube. It should be noted that the chest tube pressure is thus increased with the PEEP, increasing the intrapleural pressure necessary for escape of air and in turn increasing the risk of tension pneumothorax. In addition, because the effective chest tube suction is reduced, complete re-expansion of the affected lung may not be possible when the leak is large.

Pressurization of the chest tube during inspiration by placement of an exhalation valve in line with the chest tube reduces escape of air through the tube during part, but not all, of the ventilatory cycle. However, this is technically difficult. Alternatively, the two lungs can be ventilated separately using double-lumen endotracheal tubes and separate ventilators. This approach may help patients in acute distress but is not applicable to many patients with chronic PBL because both lungs are diseased. High-frequency ventilation reduces the bronchopleural gradient by reducing mean airway pressure. This technique allows for adequate ventilation but may not be suitable in hypoxemic patients.

Direct surgical repair would appear to be the definitive therapy for PBL, but this approach is usually not feasible because the pleura leaks from multiple sites or the underlying process precludes satisfactory closure. A related technique is obliteration of the pleural space, as described below, which frequently is not successful. Indeed, all the aggressive approaches have major limitations, and their usefulness is supported only by anecdotal experience. Conservative management suffices in most patients with PBL who

Table 19–5. PREVENTION OF BRONCHOPLEURAL AIR LEAK DURING MECHANICAL VENTILATION

1. Scrupulous medical, nursing, and respiratory care:
   a. Careful central line placement, thoracentesis, and other invasive intervention
   b. Sterile technique in chest tube care and procedures to avoid pleural space infection
   c. Avoidance of airway contamination and other sources of nosocomial infection
   d. Avoidance of chest tube stripping
2. Early vigorous management of acute respiratory failure and conditions predisposing to it
3. Low tidal volumes (10 ml/kg or less)
4. Avoidance of high airway pressures during inspiration and coughing
5. Delivery of lowest number of mechanical breaths compatible with adequate alveolar ventilation and lung expansion
6. Use of lowest effective PEEP

PEEP = positive end-expiratory pressure.

are likely to benefit from any form of treatment. Ideally, PBL should be prevented in the first place by the measures outlined in Table 19–5.

OBLITERATION OF THE PLEURAL SPACE

GENERAL CONSIDERATIONS

Recurrent accumulations of pleural air or fluid that cause discomfort or compromise lung function may require obliteration of the pleural space. As discussed above, such obliteration should not interfere with ventilatory mechanics. It is usually painful, however, and anticipated physiologic benefits must be weighed against the morbidity of the procedure. Furthermore, some restrictive defect generally follows obliterative procedures.

SPECIFIC APPROACHES

Obliteration of the pleural space is achieved by fusion of the pleural surfaces. Such fusion may be partial if only adhesions are created, or may be complete, in which case a pleurodesis is formed. Pleurodesis can be accomplished surgically by abrading the pleural surfaces through a thoracotomy site. It may also result from pleurectomy, in which the parietal pleura is stripped away to create an intense inflammatory reaction that seals the visceral pleura to the chest wall. Pleurodesis may be achieved in a less traumatic fashion by instilling agents that elicit an inflammatory response. These are injected between the pleural surfaces via a thoracentesis needle or, more commonly, a thoracostomy tube. This approach is not likely to succeed if effusions are loculated and prevent free passage of the agents across the pleurae or if persistent pneumothorax prevents a close approximation of the pleural surfaces.

Among the agents used for pleural symphysis are antineoplastic drugs (nitrogen mustard, 0.4 mg/kg), antibiotics (quinacrine, 800 mg), and radioisotopes (^{198}Ac/75 mCi). Although these agents produce symphysis in 75 per cent of patients, they cause significant side effects. The most widely used agent at present is unbuffered tetracycline, which is thought to incite inflammation because of its low pH. One protocol calls for administering 500 to 1000 mg of tetracycline mixed with 50 to 100 ml normal saline and 50 ml of 1 per cent lidocaine through a chest tube after the ipsilateral lung has been all but completely re-expanded. Better anesthesia often may be obtained by injecting the lidocaine before the tetracycline, and systemic analgesic with drugs such as morphine may be desirable. The patient is put in various positions over a 1- to 3-hour period to ensure complete distribution of the agent, and the tube is then pulled. This protocol is associated with a high success rate and minimal discomfort in most individuals.

At the time of this writing, unbuffered tetracycline had become unavailable in the United States. Many clinicians were reporting good results from doxycycline.

DECORTICATION OF THE PLEURA

Fibrothoraces that cause significant restriction may be treated by decortication, in which the mass of fibrin and inflammatory cells encasing the lung is removed surgically. Decortication is a difficult process that should be attempted only when the fibrothorax has matured into a solid and well-demarcated structure, which usually takes several months. Care is taken to avoid traumatizing the visceral pleura and compromising lung function. Early drainage of empyema or hemothorax should obviate the need for this approach.

RECOMMENDED READING

1. Bishop MG, et al.: Carbon dioxide excretion via bronchopleural fistulas in adult respiratory distress syndrome. *Chest*, 91:400–402, 1987.
2. Broaddus C, and Staub NC: Pleural liquid and protein turnover in health and disease. *Semin Respir Med*, 9:7–12, 1987.
3. Chernow B, and Sahn SA: Carcinomatous involvement of the pleura. An analysis of 96 patients. *Am J Med*, 63:695–702, 1977.
4. Erickson R: Chest tubes: They're really not that complicated. *Nursing*, 11:34–43 (May), 11:62–68 (June), 1981.

5. Leff A, et al.: Pleural effusion from malignancy. *Ann Intern Med*, 88:532–537, 1978.
6. Light RW: Pleural effusions. *Med Clin N Am*, 61:1339–1352, 1977.
7. Light RW, et al.: Pleural effusions: the diagnostic separation of transudates and exudates. *Ann Intern Med*, 77:507–513, 1972.
8. Pierson DJ: Persistent bronchopleural air leak during mechanical ventilation: a review. *Respir Care*, 27:408–416, 1982.
9. Sabiston D, and Spencer F: *Gibbon's Surgery of the Chest*, 4th ed. Philadelphia, W. B. Saunders Co., 1983.
10. Sahn SA, and Good JT: Pleural fluid pH in malignant effusions: Diagnostic, prognostic, and therapeutic implication. *Ann Intern Med*, 108:345–349, 1988.
11. Sherman S, et al.: Optimum anesthesia with intrapleural lidocaine during chemical pleurodesis with tetracycline. *Chest*, 93:533–536, 1988.
12. Weiner-Kromish JP, et al.: Lack of association of pleural effusion with chronic pulmonary arterial and right atrial hypertension. *Chest*, 92:967–970, 1987.

20

PREVENTING RESPIRATORY INFECTIONS IN HOSPITALIZED PATIENTS

NOSOCOMIAL PNEUMONIA

OVERVIEW

Incidence

Nosocomial or hospital-acquired infections occur in five to ten per cent of hospitalized patients and are a major source of morbidity and mortality in the intensive care unit (ICU). Urinary tract infections and infections associated with intravascular catheters occur with increased frequency in this patient population, but the most common and potentially fatal nosocomial infections are those of the respiratory system. Hospital-acquired pneumonia was reported in 22 per cent of all ICU patients from one center, one quarter of whom died from their infections.

Colonization Versus Infection

The nasopharynx and oropharynx are normally populated by a varied yet relatively constant population of aerobic and anaerobic bacteria. Gram-negative rods and other potential pathogens are absent or are present only in small amounts in the oral secretions of normal individuals, and healthy subjects will clear larger amounts of these bacteria if they are deposited in the mouth under experimental conditions. In contrast, shortly after admission to the hospital and especially to the ICU, seriously ill patients readily develop pharyngeal colonization, in which the normally absent bacteria increase in number until they suppress the growth of other organisms.

Although colonization is the rule in ICU patients, only one fourth of them go on to develop clinically apparent infection in which bacteria invade body tissues and provoke an inflammatory response. Such infection includes tracheobronchitis, in which the epithelial cells lining the airways are invaded, and pneumonia, in which lung parenchyma is involved. The progression of colonization to nosocomial infection relates to the pathogenicity of the responsible organisms, the ability of human hosts to withstand infection, and the role of the hospital in thwarting host defense mechanisms.

Responsible Organisms

Respiratory system colonization and infection are most often caused by gram-negative rod-shaped aerobic bacilli such as *Escherichia coli, Klebsiella, Pseudomonas, Proteus, Enterobacter, Serratia,* and the relatively recently identified *Legionella* species. *Staphylococcus aureus,* a pathogenic gram-positive coccus, also may be responsible. Certain viruses, especially the respiratory syncytial virus, fungi, and parasites may infect severely immuno-compromised patients as well as the elderly and the very young. These organisms rarely cause community-acquired infections because they do not exist in the environment in large concentrations and cannot gain a foothold in healthy individuals. Nevertheless, they can assume dominance in seriously ill patients in the hospital, where they spread quickly and become resistant to commonly used antibiotics. Each hospital and ICU is likely to have a single dominant organism, although the particular species may change as antibiotics are introduced and the formerly resistant bacteria are replaced by new resistant ones.

Host Factors

Several studies have demonstrated that, regardless of the organism(s) involved, the likelihood of developing nosocomial infection relates primarily to the health of the human host. Patients at higher risk are those who are immunocompromised because of malignant disease, its treatment, chronic respiratory failure, or extremes of age.

Hospital Factors

The vulnerability of susceptible patients to respiratory tract colonization and infection may be exacerbated in the hospital by the following practices:

a. Transmitting of pathogenic organisms to patients through person-to-person contact, particularly via the hands.
b. Exposing patients to contaminated equipment, including that used for respiratory care.
c. Grouping patients in ICUs, which increases their exposure to each other's bacterial flora and to the flora present in their shared environment.
d. Using artificial airways that nullify the gag reflex and prevent adequate coughing.

e. Employing improper suctioning techniques that may damage the tracheal epithelium.
f. Suppressing alveolar macrophage function by oxygen (O_2), corticosteroids, and other medications.
g. Positioning and feeding patients in such a way that aspiration is encouraged.
h. Administering sedatives, narcotics, and other drugs that depress ventilation, the gag reflex, and cough.

Routes of Respiratory Infection

Aspiration of Oropharyngeal Flora. Although the lower airways of patients with chronic bronchitis, bronchiectasis, and cystic fibrosis may be colonized with bacteria, the tracheobronchial tree is sterile below the level of the larynx in normal individuals. Pathogenic organisms gain access to the lower airways in quantities sufficient to cause tracheobronchitis and pneumonia primarily through the aspiration of oropharyngeal contents. Oropharyngeal aspiration and perhaps minor aspiration of gastric contents occurs to some degree in normal people and is impossible to prevent in seriously ill patients, including those with endotracheal tubes as discussed in Chapter 8. Aspiration of large amounts of oropharyngeal or gastric contents, however, should be preventable.

Hematogenous Dissemination. Bacterial invasion of the lung through the pulmonary circulation may occur when the right-sided heart valves (tricuspid and pulmonic valves) are infected in endocarditis. Invasion may also occur through hematogenous dissemination from a distant site of infection, such as perirenal abscess, or from the skin when cutaneous burns are present. Intravascular catheters and peripheral arterial and venous lines also may serve as a nidus of infection.

Inhalation in Inspired Gas. Most bacteria are too large to remain suspended in air after being coughed from the lungs of infected patients. The size of the bacteria also causes them to settle out or impact in the upper airway before they can diffuse as far as the alveoli. Viruses and mycobacteria, however, may be spread by the inhaled route because they form tiny droplet nuclei and remain airborne after the water that once surrounded them has evaporated. Gram-negative aerobic rods and other bacteria may also be inhaled into the lungs if they are aerosolized in small particles.

Inhalation of microorganisms in quantities sufficient to cause pneumonia generally does not occur from contaminated mouthpieces, tubing, and other forms of respiratory therapy equipment that may harbor bacteria but do not aerosolize them. Humidifiers used to moisten supplemental O_2 and the gases of mechanical ventilators also are not associated with infections because they provide water in molecular form rather than the droplet or particle form characteristic of aerosol generators. However, epidemics of nosocomial gram-negative bacterial pneumonia have been reported with nebulizers of the spinning disc, ultrasonic, and Venturi types that generate aerosols. Because of this, nebulizers should be used sparingly, and the devices should be changed frequently.

DIAGNOSIS OF RESPIRATORY COLONIZATION OR INFECTION

Colonization per se should not be associated with clinical signs or symptoms because pathogenic organisms have not invaded body tissues and stimulated an inflammatory reaction. In contrast, tracheobronchitis often causes burning substernal pain, cough, and the production of purulent sputum. These symptoms also may be seen with pneumonia, but high fever, pleuritic chest pain, and hemoptysis are more common in the latter condition. Hypoxemia also is more likely in pneumonia, and signs of consolidation should be present on auscultation of the chest and seen on the chest roentgenogram.

The issue of colonization versus infection may also be resolved by examining Gram stains of respiratory secretions. Specimens should be expectorated, aseptically suctioned into sterile containers, or obtained by the diagnostic methods outlined in Chapter 6. Secretions contaminated by oropharyngeal contents and those taken from areas of airway colonization usually demonstrate several types of gram-positive and gram-negative aerobic and anaerobic organisms, none of which is predominant in number, and few white blood cells. Specimens from infected areas usually have only one or at most two kinds of bacteria and should show an abundance of white blood cells if patients are capable of mounting an inflammatory response.

Bacterial and other microbial culture and sensitivity testing should generally be performed only on infected secretions from the lower airways, and many hospital laboratories refuse to study specimens that do not have a clearly labeled source or that contain mainly saliva. However, serial culturing of oropharyngeal secretions may be helpful in determining which flora are becoming dominant in burn victims and other immunologically suppressed patients. These results may be used to direct initial therapy when the volume of respiratory secretions increases, suggesting severe tracheobronchitis, or when a new infiltrate is noted on chest roentgenogram.

TREATMENT OF RESPIRATORY INFECTION

Some clinicians treat any respiratory infection in hospitalized patients, reasoning that even if only tracheobronchitis is present, pneumonia cannot be far behind. Most, however, prefer not to give antibiotics for mild-to-moderate tracheobronchitis lest this should lead to overgrowth with resistant organisms; they therefore treat only when tracheobronchitis is severe or, more often, when pneumonia is documented by chest roentgenogram. Antibiotic therapy should be based on culture and sensitivity results, including those discussed above regarding colonization, whenever possible. Otherwise, seriously ill patients with pneumonia noted more than 24 hours after hospital admission should receive broad coverage for presumed gram-negative aerobic organisms, including *Pseudomonas,* and for gram-positive *Staphylococcus aureus.* A comprehensive outline of the treatment of infectious pneumonia in the ICU and other settings is provided in Table 20–1.

PREVENTION OF RESPIRATORY COLONIZATION AND INFECTION

Patient Placement

A variety of forms of isolation previously were used to separate infected patients and their secretions from noninfected patients and hospital personnel, and vice versa. Today, isolation techniques have been largely replaced by the adoption of unusual body substance precautions, which are the topic of Chapter 21. For example, "reverse isolation" of neutropenic or otherwise immunocompromised patients is no longer practiced, and such patients are cared for by using precautions that are no different from routine, good patient care techniques, such as the appropriate hand washing before and after patient contact and use of gloves.

Despite these changes, private rooms may be recommended for immunocompromised patients. Furthermore, until satisfactory treatment is accomplished, patients with airborne diseases still should be managed with an approach traditionally called respiratory isolation. Such patients include those with documented or suspected active tuberculosis, varicella (chickenpox), pharyngeal diphtheria, rubella (measles), rubeola (German measles), pneumonic plague, anthrax, and pertussis (whooping cough). Respiratory precautions in such patients usually include assignment to a private room with the door closed and a red "stop sign" affixed. People entering the room should wear masks, as should the patient when he or she leaves for another area of the hospital.

Hand Washing

Studies suggest that hospital personnel wash their hands less than 50 per cent of the time after they contact patients and that physicians are the worst offenders. This is unfortunate, because hand washing is the single most important—and certainly the simplest—technique to curb the spread of nosocomial infections.

Table 20–1. INFECTIOUS PNEUMONIAS

KIND OF PATIENT	LIKELY OFFENDING MICROORGANISMS	INITIAL ANTIMICROBIAL THERAPY (Pending Sensitivities)	AVERAGE DOSE	ROUTE	INTERVAL
Normal young host with community-acquired pneumonia	Mycoplasma *Mycoplasma pneumoniae*	Erythromycin or	0.5 gm	PO	q.i.d.
		Tetracycline	0.5 gm	PO	q.i.d.
	Gram-positive aerobic bacteria *Streptococcus pneumoniae*	Penicillin G or	600,000 units	PO, IM, IV	b.i.d.
		Erythromycin	0.5 gm	PO	b.i.d.
	Viruses *Influenza A* *Adenovirus*	No therapy or			
	Respiratory syncytial virus	Amantadine	0.2 gm	PO	q.i.d.
		Ribavirin	1.1 gm	aerosol	q.d.
	Fungi (in endemic areas) *Coccidioides immitis* *Histoplasma capsulatum*	Usually untreated unless dissemination occurs or pulmonary infection becomes chronic. Then use amphotericin B as below.			
Elderly host, heavy smoker, or alcoholic individual with community-acquired pneumonia	Gram-positive aerobic bacteria *Streptococcus pneumoniae*	Penicillin G or	600,000 units	IM, IV	b.i.d
		Erythromycin	0.5 gm	IV	q.i.d
	Staphylococcus aureus	Nafcillin or	1–2 gm	IV	q. 4 h
		Vancomycin	1 gm	IV	q. 12 h
	Gram-negative aerobic bacteria *Hemophilus influenzae*	Cefuroxime	1 gm	IV	t.i.d.
	Klebsiella pneumoniae	Cefazolin and	0.2 gm	IV	q. 8 h
		Gentamicin or tobramycin	1.5 mg/kg	IV	q. 8 h
	Legionella pneumophila	Erythromycin	0.5–1 gm	IV	q.i.d.

Table continued on following page

Table 20–1. INFECTIOUS PNEUMONIAS *Continued*

KIND OF PATIENT	LIKELY OFFENDING MICROORGANISMS	INITIAL ANTIMICROBIAL THERAPY (Pending Sensitivities)	AVERAGE DOSE	ROUTE	INTERVAL
	Anaerobic bacteria (following aspiration)				
	Bacteroides fragilis	Penicillin G	1,200,000 units	IV	q.i.d.
		or			
		Clindamycin	0.3 gm	IV, PO	q.i.d.
	Mycobacteria				
	Mycobacterium tuberculosis	Isoniazid	300 mg	PO	q.d.
		and			
		Rifampin	600 mg	PO	q.d.
	Viruses and fungi (as in young hosts)	As above			
Normal young or elderly host with hospital-acquired pneumonia	Gram-positive aerobic bacteria				
	Staphylococcus aureus	Nafcillin	1–2 gm	IV	q. 4 h
		or			
		Vancomycin	1 gm	IV	q.i.d.
	Streptococcus fecalis (non-endocarditis)	Ampicillin	1 gm	IV	q.i.d.
	Gram-negative aerobic bacteria				
	Escherichia coli	Ampicillin alone	1 gm	IV	q.i.d.
		or			
		Gentamicin or tobramycin	1.5 mg/kg	IV	q.i.d.
		and			
		Carbenicillin or ticarcillin	3–6 gm	IV	q. 4 h

Pseudomonas aeruginosa	Carbenicillin or ticarcillin and	3–6 gm	IV	q. 4 h
	Gentamicin or tobramycin	1.5 mg/kg	IV	q.i.d
Proteus mirabilis	Ampicillin	1 gm	IV	q.i.d.
	or			
Klebsiella pneumoniae	Ticarcillin	3–6 gm	IV	q. 4 h
	Cefazolin and	1–2 gm	IV	q. 8 h
	Gentamicin or tobramycin	1.5 mg/kg	IV	q.i.d.
Enterobacter species	Ceftriaxone and	1 gm	IV	q.i.d.
	Gentamicin or tobramycin	1.5 mg/kg	IV	q.i.d.
Immunocompromised host with community- or hospital-acquired pneumonia	As above; prefer combination			
Viruses				
Cytomegalovirus	No therapy	to be released		
Varicella-zoster	Acyclovir			
Herpes simplex	Acyclovir			
Fungi				
Candida albicans	Amphotericin B	0.025–0.1 gm	IV	q.d.
Aspergillus fumigatus	Amphotericin B	0.025–0.1 gm	IV	q.d.
Cryptococcus neoformans	Amphotericin B	0.025–0.1 gm	IV	q.d.
Protozoa				
Pneumocystis carinii	Trimethoprim-sulfamethoxazole	5–25 mg/kg	IV, PO	q.i.d.
	or			
	Pentamidine isethionate	4 mg/kg	IV	q.d.

Most organisms acquired from brief contact with patients can be removed from the hands by washing for 30 seconds with ordinary soap and water, assuming that ample friction is applied. Scrubbing the skin with special soaps, iodines, or alcohol should be done prior to surgical procedures and the insertion of intravascular lines. However, more frequent scrubbing abrades the skin; special soaps dry it and may cause a dermatitis that invites infection.

Suctioning Techniques

Aseptic suctioning is mandatory in all mechanically ventilated patients and in those from whom respiratory tract secretions are collected. Proper technique is outlined in Chapter 8.

Use of Respiratory Apparatus

General Principles. Because respiratory therapy equipment has been implicated in the transmission of nosocomial infection and is costly to use, it should be used only when medically indicated. This is especially true of nebulizers employed either for humidifying respiratory gases or for delivering aerosolized medications. Disposable equipment, including patient mouthpieces and breathing circuits, may help lower the incidence of infection and should be discarded daily. If equipment is recycled, it should be changed and decontaminated as determined by institutional guidelines. (Recent evidence suggests that changing every 48 to 72 hours is effective.) Gas humidifiers and reservoirs on mechanical ventilators require special care as potential sources of contamination. Whenever possible, these devices and their water supply should constitute a closed system. Reservoirs should never be filled without first being emptied of stale contents. Sterile water should be used unless the manufacturer specifies otherwise. One water container should be employed with each patient. Containers should be dated and timed when opened and should not be kept longer than 24 hours. Refrigeration can be used with the knowledge that it does not protect against bacterial contamination but does slow bacterial growth. Medication chambers on intermittent positive pressure breathing machines and mechanical ventilators should be emptied and rinsed and dried before each treatment.

Specific Decontamination Techniques

Pasteurization. Pasteurization is effective against all microorganisms except spore-forming fungi, which are not an issue in the majority of patients. It involves immersing respiratory apparatus in a hot water bath at 70° to 90° C for 30 minutes. All equipment must be cleansed with soap and water and rinsed before immersion. The equipment should be dried under laminar conditions after pasteurization, and care must be taken to avoid contamination during its reassembly. The advantages of this approach are its low cost, its availability, and the lack of a toxic residue after pasteurization. Potential disadvantages include the fact that some plastic products may not be disinfected because of lack of water contact in tiny areas.

Cold Sterilization. Sterilization with aqueous glutaraldehyde solution is bactericidal, tuberculocidal, virucidal, and fungicidal, providing that equipment is soaked in the solution for an appropriate length of time. Only ten minutes are required for most bacterial and fungal cells, whereas ten hours are recommended to destroy more resistant spores, mycobacteria, and viruses. Immersible respiratory apparatus can be cleansed by this method, which requires a one-step process when used with an automatic decontamination system that cleans, disinfects, and dries equipment automatically. However, cold sterilization is relatively costly, and the residue often irritates the skin and mucous membranes.

Gas Sterilization. Sterilization with ethylene oxide completely kills all organisms if performed at the proper concentration and at a temperature of 50° C over four hours. This process is satisfactory for plastics, electrical equipment, and delicate instruments that cannot withstand high heat or moisture. However, gas sterilization is potentially dangerous owing to the liberation of chemical fumes, especially from gamma-irradiated items; sterilizers usually must be used in a central supply area and cannot be housed in the respiratory therapy department. Furthermore, items must be aerated for 8 to 24 hours after sterilization to prevent the formation of ethylene glycol, thus preventing their immediate reuse. This mode of decontamination is particularly useful for machines and surgical materials and for respiratory therapy equipment exposed to highly infectious organisms. However, recent and expected restrictions on the use of chlorofluorocarbons are making this an increasingly expensive and unattractive method of sterilization.

Steam Sterilization. Autoclaving involves exposing respiratory therapy equipment to steam at a pressure of 15 pounds per square inch at 121° C for 15 minutes or more. This is effective against all microorganisms. However, autoclaving cannot be used on materials that are distorted or melted at high temperatures and is not acceptable for machines or electrical devices. Continued use with anesthesia rubber also results in a decrease in conductivity.

Gamma Irradiation. This is performed with radiation emitted from radioactive isotopes and is toxic to all pathogenic materials. Although this procedure is used in the initial packaging of antiseptic materials, its hospital application is limited because of equipment costs. Gamma-irradiated items should not be reprocessed by ethylene oxide.

Local Disinfectants. Products such as alcohol, phenol, quaternary ammonium compounds, hexachlorophene, iodine, and acetic acid have a limited range of antibacterial activity and often are not effective against gram-negative organisms. They do improve the efficiency of hand washing with soap and water if used sparingly. Acetic acid is active against gram-negative organisms, including *Pseudomonas*, but its application is limited to reducing the growth of these organisms in nebulizers.

Use of Bacterial Filters

Bacterial filters should be positioned on the inspiratory limb of all mechanical ventilators. Bar scavenging systems also are recommended on the exhalation ports of ventilators and other devices used with patients with tuberculosis.

Prophylactic Antibiotics Administered by Respiratory Apparatus and Other Routes

Polymyxin, gentamicin, and other drugs have been administered intratracheally or via nebulizers to prevent gram-negative aerobic pneumonia in some ICUs. Although this practice led to a decline in the incidence of colonization and infection with *Pseudomonas* in several studies, it caused the emergence of other organisms and did not improve morbidity or mortality. Because of this, prophylactic antibiotics given by respiratory apparatus should be avoided unless they are being studied as part of an experimental protocol. The usefulness of inhaled or intratracheally administered antibiotics in treating documented infections is unclear, although they appear to benefit some patients. Although selective decontamination of the digestive tract has been advocated to reduce the microorganisms that cause nosocomial pneumonia, this approach cannot be generally recommended.

Education and Surveillance

Hospital infection-control personnel should assist in the education of their colleagues and in surveillance. Hand cultures may be performed on a monthly basis on ICU personnel to monitor the emergence of resistant organisms.

Improving Host Defenses

White blood cell transfusion, hyperalimentation, and other medical procedures have been undertaken in an effort to improve host defense mechanisms but have had limited effectiveness. The same is true for immunization of high-risk patients with the lipopolysaccharide antigens of common *Pseudomonas* species. Treatment of the underlying disease process remains the most important and practical way to aid the host.

Minimizing Hospital Factors

Studies have indicated that early identification of high-risk patients, close attention to hand washing and other preventive measures, and vigorous education and surveillance on the part of infection-control personnel can reduce the incidence of hospital-acquired infections, especially those involving the respiratory system. Given the pathogenicity of microorganisms in the hospital environment and the difficulty of improving host defenses, it is incumbent upon nurses, respiratory therapists, physicians, and all other staff members to minimize the contribution of hospital factors to the generation of nosocomial infections by the methods cited in this chapter.

RECOMMENDED READING

1. Albert RK, and Condie F: Handwashing patterns in medical intensive care units. *N Engl J Med*, 304:1456–1466, 1981.
2. Britt MR, et al.: Severity of underlying disease as a predictor of nosocomial infection. Utility in the control of nosocomial infection. *JAMA*, 239:1047–1051, 1978.
3. Cahill CK, and Heath J: Sterile water used for humidification in low-flow oxygen therapy: Is it necessary? *Am J Infect Control*, 18:13–17, 1990.
4. Craven DE, et al.: Contamination of mechanical ventilators with tubing changes every 24 or 48 hours. *N Engl J Med*, 306:1505–1509, 1982.
5. Craven DE, and Steger KA: Nosocomial pneumonia in the incubated patient. New concepts of pathogenesis and prevention. *Infect Dis Clin North Am*, 3:843–866, 1989.
6. Feeley TW, et al.: Aerosol polymyxin and pneumonia in seriously ill patients. *N Engl J Med*, 293:471–475, 1975.
7. Craman PS, and Hall CB: Nosocomial viral respiratory infections. *Semin Respir Infect*, 4:253–260, 1989.
8. Johanson WG: Infectious complications of respiratory therapy. *Respir Care*, 27:445–452, 1982.
9. Kelsen SG, et al.: Airborne contamination of fine-particle nebulizers. *JAMA*, 237:2311–2314, 1977.
10. Lareau SC, et al.: The relationship between frequency of ventilator circuit changes and infectious hazard. *Am Rev Respir Dis*, 118:493–496, 1978.
11. Meijer K, et al: Infection control in patients undergoing mechanical ventilation: Traditional approach vein, a new development: Selective decontamination of the digestive tract. *Heart Lung*, 19:11–20, 1990.
12. Nardeli EA: Judging droplet nuclei, reducing the probability of nosocomial tuberculosis transmission in the AIDS era. *Am Rev Respir Dis*, 142:501–503, 1990.
13. Pierce AK, and Sanford JP: Aerobic gram-negative bacillary pneumonias. *Am Rev Respir Dis*, 110:647–658, 1974.

21

INFECTION CONTROL

UNIVERSAL BODY SUBSTANCE PRECAUTIONS

Rationale

The possibility of infection with the human immunodeficiency virus (HIV) and subsequent development of the acquired immunodeficiency syndrome (AIDS) has prompted many health care professionals to become concerned about infection control. This is particularly the case among physicians, nurses, and respiratory care practitioners who care for large numbers of known or suspected HIV-infected patients in intensive care units (ICUs), AIDS wards, bronchoscopy suites, areas where aerosolized pentamidine is administered, and other locations where exposure to blood and body secretions may occur. Concern about HIV infection in such locations is appropriate, but of equal importance is the occupational exposure to other agents that are common among HIV-infected patients, including hepatitis B virus (HBV), cytomegalovirus (CMV), and *Mycobacterium tuberculosis* (MTB).

Of course, infection with HBV, MTB, and other organisms is not unique to HIV-infected patients. Indeed, significant numbers of alcoholics and immigrants have active tuberculosis, for example, and HBV infection is common among intravenous drug abusers and renal dialysis patients. In addition, the viruses responsible for influenza, varicella (chickenpox), and rubella (measles) are now carried by these and other hospitalized patients, and new viruses similar to HIV may be identified in the future.

Awareness of the risk of exposure to this large number of pathogens has led to a revision of infection control procedures by the United States Centers for Disease Control (CDC). Whereas infection control once involved primarily the identification and isolation of patients with potentially communicable diseases, it now is based on the principle that all patients—all people, for that matter—are potentially infectious, and that the best protection against infection, in the hospital or the home, is to avoid contamination by their blood and body fluids.

Introduction of universal body substance precautions (UBSP) has not totally supplanted the identification and isolation of certain patients who are considered highly infectious because they harbor organisms that are spread by the airborne rather than the blood-borne route. Thus, respiratory isolation remains mandatory for patients who are known or suspected to be infected by the influenza, varicella, and rubella viruses, by MTB, and by other organisms as described in Chapter 20. However, such isolation is intended to augment UBSP in such patients, who also may be infected by HBV or HIV.

Mandatory Patient Testing

Some health professionals have proposed mandatory HIV testing in lieu of or in addition to UBSP. Proponents of this approach argue that knowledge of HIV infection will allow surgical personnel and others to employ special infection control precautions or to increase compliance with UBSP, thereby reducing outpatient risk. However, a recent observational study of more than 1300 surgical procedures at San Francisco General Hospital showed that awareness of HIV seropositivity did not lead to a reduction in the frequency of accidental exposure to blood. Other factors, including duration of the procedure and volume loss, were predictive of accidental exposure.

The use of HIV testing as a requisite for surgical or medical intervention has several drawbacks. For example, mandating HIV testing confers a substantial degree of emotional and economic risk to patients. In addition, altering the course of care or refusing to treat patients because of HIV infection is unethical and may carry a legal risk. Results of HIV testing may be falsely negative if patients have been infected by the virus but have not yet developed the anti-HIV antibodies that are detected in the current test. And finally, HIV testing cannot reduce the risk of infection by other blood-borne pathogens, including HBV.

Although mandatory patient testing has drawbacks and should not be viewed as an alternative to UBSP, voluntary testing is of potential advantage to patients and health care workers who may have HIV or HBV infection. Like hepatitis, AIDS is now regarded as a chronic disease that can be successfully treated, although it cannot yet be cured. Because counseling, medical therapy, and social benefits are available for HIV-positive patients, they should know their antibody status. At the same time, this knowledge should be shared with sexual contacts and loved ones.

Mandatory Testing of Health Care Personnel

Documentation of HIV infection of five patients of a dentist who had antibodies to HIV has sparked concern over the possibility that patients could be infected with HIV from seropositive health care workers. Transmission of the virus in the five patients appeared to result from inadequate sterilization of dental instruments, not from direct exposure to the dentist's blood or other body fluids. Indeed, very few patients in general are exposed to the body fluids of health professionals in a medical setting, and the likelihood of being infected during surgery, for example, is infinitesimally small. Mandatory testing of health professionals would cost millions of dollars, money better spent in legitimate AIDS prevention and therapy. Nevertheless, voluntary testing is recommended for the reasons given earlier.

RISK OF AND PRECAUTIONS AGAINST BLOOD-BORNE AGENTS

Risk of Infection from Discrete Exposure

Several dozen documented cases of occupational HIV infections have been reported in the United States since 1981. In each of these reports, occupational infection has been documented by a negative baseline HIV antibody test at the time of exposure and followed by positive antibody testing within weeks or months. Parenteral exposure to blood by needlesticks or lacerations was implicated in 12 of the first 18 documented cases. In four cases infection occurred via the penetration of nonintact skin or mucous membranes by blood, and in two others it involved exposure to viral concentrates in research laboratories.

Although case reports are useful in documenting the occupational transmission of HIV, incidence can be determined only by examining denominator data. For this reason, a number of prospective cohort studies have been performed that identify health care workers with direct exposure and observe them after the exposure to determine HIV serostatus. Combined data from 14 ongoing studies that together include more than 2000 percutaneous exposures to HIV-infected material in 2000 individuals have documented new infections in only six, for an overall HIV transmission rate of 0.31 per cent. This compares with a transmission rate of approximately 20 per cent for percutaneous exposure to HBV.

There have been no observed cases of HIV seroconversion following exposure of mucous membranes or nonintact skin to infected blood or other body fluids in these prospective studies, despite the fact that more than 1000 exposures of this type have been observed. There also have been no documented reports of occupational HIV infection following exposure of intact skin to infectious material. Furthermore, although HIV may be present in small droplets of blood, there is no evidence that supports aerosolization as a viable mode of HIV transmission. In studies of dialysis units and dental offices, CDC investigation was unable to detect the presence of HBV surface antigen in aerosols. Of course, aerosols may contain other viruses and MTB.

Although HIV has been isolated from a variety of body fluids, including saliva, tears, and aerosolized fluid, exposure to these fluids has not been shown to be responsible for HIV transmission. This presumably is due to the fact that the low titer of virus found in nonbloody fluids is considerably less than that found in blood. For example, HIV is rarely isolated from the saliva of infected individuals, and when present, the HIV concentration is low. Occupational exposure to saliva during oral or respiratory tract procedures, or via bites from uncooperative patients, is unlikely to pose a risk of HIV infection. However, saliva may harbor other organisms such as CMV.

At present, the factors that influence the risk of HIV infection following parenteral exposure are largely unknown. Reported seroconversions following needlestick injury generally involve deeply penetrating needlesticks with larger-bore hollow needles or inadvertent injections of blood, although a small number of documented seroconversions have occurred as a result of superficial needlesticks. The small number of occupational HIV infections documented in case reports involving mucocutaneous exposures were typically associated with large volumes of blood, prolonged periods of contact, and a viable portal of entry through a mucous membrane or a cutaneous lesion. Seroconversion probably is more likely following exposure to the HIV-infected blood of a symptomatic patient than an asymptomatic patient because the former generally has higher viral titers than the latter. This is not necessarily the case with exposure to blood containing HBV.

Cumulative Occupational Risk

Many investigators believe that the cumulative risk of HIV and HBV infection can be approximated by the product of the prevalence of HIV- or HBV-infected patients encountered, the frequency occupational exposure to blood, and the risk of infection carried by each exposure. Using a similar model that considered only needlestick injuries, one group of investigators calculated a 50 per cent chance that one health care worker will occupationally acquire HIV for every 105,000 HIV-infected patient care days at one New York center. Unfortunately, it is impossible to obtain accurate values for any of the variables in the above model because the prevalence of HIV infection among patients is rarely known, the frequency of exposure is not well quantified, and the risk of infection is highly variable.

Prevention of Occupational Exposures

Prevention of occupational exposure is the best method to reduce occupational risk of infection with HIV and HBV. In particular, extensive care should be taken when performing invasive procedures requiring needles or other "sharps." Inasmuch as approximately one third of all needlestick injuries occur during needle recapping, improving needle disposal behavior, including the avoidance of recapping and the disposal of uncapped needles in widemouth, impermeable containers, is a high priority.

Latex gloves are impermeable to HIV and HBV if intact and should be worn when coming in contact with blood or body fluids; two or more pairs may be useful during surgery. Use of gloves is also acceptable as barrier protection. Other forms of barrier protection, including eyeglasses or goggles, masks, and waterproof gowns, should be used during performance of procedures in which blood may be splashed or liberated in droplets. Although HIV is not likely to be transmitted by nonbloody fluids, HBV and other agents can be. It therefore is prudent to use barrier precautions when in contact with all body fluids. It is hoped that more effective barriers, safer needles, and other equipment will soon be available.

Hand washing is an essential part of UBSP. Hands generally should be washed with soap, running water, and friction. Hand washing is indicated after contact with body substances or surfaces visibly soiled with body substances and after removal of gloves if gloves on hands have been soiled, before clean or sterile invasive procedures, before eating or preparing food, and after urinating or defecating. Cuts, abrasions, or minor skin infections on hands should be covered with gloves or finger cots while working, and personnel with draining skin lesions should not work in direct patient care involving physical contact.

MANAGEMENT OF OCCUPATIONAL EXPOSURES

Even the most scrupulous adherence to UBSP will not eliminate all occupational exposures. Although such exposures rarely were reported in the past, most hospitals now are encouraging and facilitating reporting. Proper reporting is important because it allows (1) appropriate counseling and reassurance of health care workers; (2) determination of the severity of the exposure; (3) evaluation of the source patient and the possible need for prophylaxis against HBV or HIV; (4) the rare diagnosis of occupational HIV infection; and (5) documentation of the exposure so that the relationship between exposure and infection can be established to ensure entitlement to benefits.

The CDC currently recommends cleansing exposed cutaneous areas with soap and water and thorough rinsing of exposed mucosal surfaces with water. Following decontamination, the nature and severity of the exposure should be evaluated, with characterization of the instrument, the depth of penetration, the type of body fluid involved, and the possibility of fluid injection. Mucous membrane or cutaneous exposures should be evaluated in terms of the type and volume of fluid involved, the duration of contact, and the area and condition of the exposed membrane or skin.

Serological tests for HIV and HBV should be performed immediately after exposure because negative baseline results followed temporally by positive results are the most appropriate documentation of occupational infection. Following the baseline assay, tests for HBV antigen and antibodies may be performed within months after exposure. HIV antibody tests generally are performed six weeks, three months, and six months after exposure. Testing of the source patient is helpful, although not legally mandated in many areas, in determining the further management, as well as the psychological well-being, of the exposed health care worker. The presence of documented infection with HIV, HBV, or both in the source patient prompts immediate consideration of postexposure prophylaxis.

The documented success of zidovudine (AZT) in altering the course of HIV infection in symptomatic patients has prompted the use of this agent on an experimental basis for prophylaxis against HIV following accidental exposure. Although no detailed information is available concerning the efficacy of AZT in preventing infection with HIV, animal studies suggest that the drug can prevent infection and viremia following exposure to retroviruses. Nevertheless, cases in which AZT was given to patients immediately after exposure to HIV-infected blood have not documented the drug's efficacy. At present, AZT is available for postexposure prophylaxis for health care workers with massive parenteral exposure at a number of centers. Whether this or other antiretroviral agents will become more widely available is unknown.

Documented occupational exposure to HBV in health care workers who are not already HBV infected should prompt anti-HBV prophylaxis. Such prophylaxis includes parenteral administration of hyperimmune globulin to provide passive immunization and of anti-HBV vaccine to provide active immunization. There is no evidence of HIV transmission with anti-HBV vaccine prepared from the serum of human volunteers. Furthermore, a synthetic monoclonal vaccine is now available.

Perhaps the most important aspect of postexposure management is counseling. Individuals familiar with the concerns of health care professionals facing possible HIV or HBV infection can be very helpful in providing accurate information about the risk of infection, the need for postexposure prophylaxis, and other matters. Counselors also can advise health care workers how to utilize barrier methods of contraception until HIV infection is definitely excluded by negative antibody results. Finally, counselors can facilitate interchange among exposed personnel and their friends and families.

RECOMMENDED READING

1. Centers for Disease Control: Update: Acquired immunodeficiency syndrome and human immunodeficiency virus among health-care workers. *MMWR*, 37:229–239, 1988.
2. Centers for Disease Control: Update: Universal precautions for prevention of transmission of human immunodeficiency virus, hepatitis B virus, and other blood-borne pathogens in health-care settings. *MMWR*, 37:377–382, 1988.

3. Centers for Disease Control: Public health service statement on management of occupational exposure to human immunodeficiency virus, including considerations regarding zidovudine use. *MMWR*, 39:1–14, 1990.
4. Ciesielski CA, et al: When a house officer gets AIDS (letter). *N Engl J Med*, 322:1156–1157, 1990.
5. Gerberding JL, et al: Risk of exposure of surgical personnel to patient's blood during surgery at San Francisco General Hospital. *N Engl J Med,* 322:1788–1793, 1990.
6. Ho DD, et al: Quantitation of human immunodeficiency virus type 1 in the blood of infected persons. *N Engl J Med*, 321:1621–1625, 1989.
7. Jagger J, et al: Rates of needle-stick injury caused by various devices in a University hospital. *N Engl J Med,* 319:284–288, 1988.
8. Mast ST, and Gerberding JL: The risk of occupationally acquired HIV infection in health care workers. Pulmonary and critical care update. *Am Coll Chest Physicians*, 6(21):1–8, 1991.
9. Wormser GP, et al: Frequency of nosocomial transmission of HIV infection among health care workers. *N Engl J Med*, 319:307–308, 1988.

INDEX

Note: Page numbers in *italics* refer to illustrations; page numbers followed by *t* refer to tables.